AF333535

Recent Results in Cancer Research

154

Managing Editors

P. M. Schlag, Berlin · H.-J. Senn, St. Gallen

Associate Editors

V. Diehl, Cologne · D.M. Parkin, Lyon
M.F. Rajewsky, Essen · R. Rubens, London
M. Wannenmacher, Heidelberg

Founding Editor

P. Rentchnik, Geneva

Springer

*Berlin
Heidelberg
New York
Barcelona
Budapest
Hong Kong
London
Milan
Paris
Singapore
Tokyo*

M. Schwab   H. Rabes   K. Munk
P. H. Hofschneider   (Eds.)

Genes and Environment in Cancer

With 58 Figures and 60 Tables

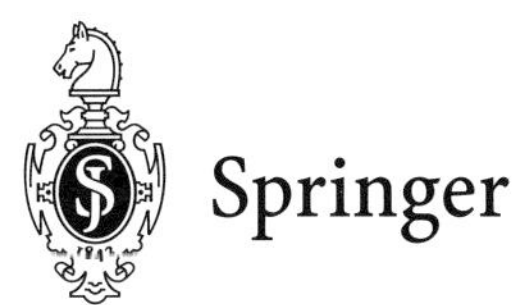

Springer

Prof. Dr. rer. nat. Manfred Schwab
Deutsches Krebsforschungszentrum
Abteilung Zytogenetik
Im Neuenheimer Feld 280
D-69120 Heidelberg
e-mail: m.schwab@dkfz-heidelberg.de

Prof. Dr. med. Hartmut M. Rabes
Pathologisches Institut der Universität München
Thalkirchner Straße 36
D-80377 München
e-mail: HM.Rabes@lrz.uni-muenchen.de

Prof. Dr. med. Klaus Munk
Deutsches Krebsforschungszentrum
Im Neuenheimer Feld 280
D-69120 Heidelberg

Prof. Dr. med. Hans Peter Hofschneider
Max-Planck-Institut für Biochemie
Am Klopferspitz 18a
D-82152 Martinsried
e-mail: coutts@biochem.mpg.de

ISBN 3-540-64430-X Springer-Verlag Berlin Heidelberg New York
ISSN 0080-0015

Library of Congress Cataloging-in-Publication Data
Genes and environment in cancer / M. Schwab ... [et al.] (eds.). p. cm. – (Recent results in cancer research; 154). Based on an international expert meeting held from Nov. 16 to 19, 1997 in Bonn, Germany. Includes bibliographical references and index. ISBN 3-540-64430-X (hardcover: alk. paper). 1. Carcinogenesis–Congresses. 2. Cancer–Genetic aspects–Congresses. 3. Cancer–Environmental aspects–Congresses. I. Schwab, M. (Manfred), 1945– . II. Series. [DNLM: 1. Neoplasms–genetics congresses. 2. Neoplasms-epidemiology congresses. 3. Environmental Exposure–adverse effects congresses. 4. Risk Assessment congresses. [W1 RE106P v. 154 1998QZ 200 G327 1998] RC261.R35 vol. 154 [RC268.48] 616.99′4 s–dc21 [616.99′4071] DNLM/DLC for Library of Congress

Production: PRO EDIT GmbH, D-69126 Heidelberg
Typesetting: K+V Fotosatz GmbH, D-64743 Beerfelden

SPIN 10676489   19/3133-5 4 3 2 1 0 – Printed on acid-free paper

Preface

The XIth International Expert Meeting of the Dr. Mildred Scheel Foundation for Cancer Research was held in Bonn, Germany, on 16–17 November 1997. Thirty-two invited speakers from 10 countries, together with 80 additional participants, discussed the topic "Genes and Environment in Cancer", a field of research that has developed rapidly in recent years.

The homeostatic balance of an organism is the result of a delicate network of interactions between genes and environment. This balance may be suspended if genes are structurally or functionally aberrant, either due to an endogenous genetic condition or to external genotropic influences.

The historical hypothesis "Cancer is a genetic disease" has convincingly been supported by a wealth of recent information. On the one hand, a hereditary genetic condition may predispose to cancer development, as evident from pedigree studies and molecular genetic analyses. Various genes have been found to be related to an individual hereditary cancer predisposition, for example, hereditary *TP53* or *RB1* defects in several types of familial cancer, loss of mismatch repair genes in hereditary nonpolyposis colon cancer (HNPCC), *BRCA-1* or *-2* germline mutations in a subgroup of breast carcinomas, or a well-defined mutation spectrum in tumors of multiple endocrine neoplasia syndromes. On the other hand, identical, similar and many other genetic aberrations may arise spontaneously or can be induced by endogenous factors formed during pathological and even physiological processes and also as a result of interaction with external environmental factors. When Percival Pott described scrotal cancer of chimney-sweeps in England 200 years ago, he opened up the search for an ever-increasing number of cancer risk factors in our environment. The list of putative or confirmed human carcinogenic factors is long and far from complete. Among them, most chemical carcinogens have to be metabolically converted into short-living, highly reactive electrophiles which form DNA adducts. Recently observed polymorphisms of both activating and detoxifying enzymes contribute to individual cancer predisposition after carcinogen exposure.

Determination of promutagenic DNA adducts in surrogate cells may help to evaluate the personal cancer risk. However, the persistence and biological effects of promutagenic DNA adducts or structural changes that are induced by chemical carcinogens or physical carcinogenic factors, ionizing radiation and UV in particular, may be influenced by DNA repair. The individual's genetically predetermined or adaptive DNA repair capacity is critical to the probability of cancer development. In patients suffering from hereditary or acquired DNA repair disorders, the risk of cancer is increased. The final result of interaction with a carcinogenic factor appears to also be dependent on the particular conditions of the genomic target. Genome instability or chromosomal fragile sites are important determinants at the genomic level.

In recent years, molecular epidemiology has become a most effective tool in bridging the gap between a typical genetic lesion (be it a mutation hotspot or a specific form of mutation), a putatively involved class of physical or chemical carcinogen and the actual cancer incidence. Although early enthusiasm for the hypothesis "Carcinogens leave fingerprints," a very attractive term indeed, has quieted down, the information obtained by combining molecular and population genetics, biochemistry and classical epidemiology is of utmost importance for elucidating relationships between risk factors and actual human cancer incidence. Molecular epidemiology may provide insights into mechanisms of initiation and progression of human cancer and may have a considerable impact on cancer prevention.

Despite sophisticated analyses of genetic aberrations and the effects of carcinogenic factors, it should not be overlooked that the mysteries of the latency period between the initiating event at the start of the carcinogenic process and the clinical manifestation of a malignant tumor have not yet been unravelled. Research on the role of genetic and environmental factors that modify the susceptibility to spontaneous and hereditary carcinogenesis is a very important issue.

Last, but not least, environmental exposure to viruses may serve as a paradigm of the contribution of transmissible carcinogenic factors to the development of human cancer. The pathway from epidemiological facts to the elucidation of molecular mechanisms and, further, to practical tumor prevention by appropriate vaccination illustrates a promising and successful line of cancer research for which hepatitis B virus is prototypic.

The idea of the XIth International Expert Meeting was to bring together recognized scientists who are familiar with the multifaceted interplay between genes and environment in cancer. Recent achievements and promising trends in different disciplines of cancer research are presented in this volume. Apart from the pure heuristic value, we hope that advances in the assessment of cancer risk and the involved hereditary, genetic and environmental parameters, as reported here, will improve the chances for developing new strategies for cancer detection and prevention.

H. M. Rabes, Chairman, Scientific Committee, Dr. Mildred Scheel Foundation for Cancer Research

Contents

IV. Induced Chromosome Damage and Cancer

V. Genetic Susceptibility and Environmental Exposure: 'The RET Paradigm'

VI. Population Genetics of Cancer Susceptibility

VII. Virus and Cancer: The HBV/HCV Paradigm

List of Contributors [*]

Aaltonen, L. A. [306]
Alexandrov, K. [86]
Arand, M. [47]
Asai, N. [229]
Bartsch, H. [86]
Bertoletti, A. [330]
Bertoni, R. [330]
Bonassi, S. [177]
Bongarzone, I. [237]
Boni, C. [330]
Bootsma, D. [147]
Bos, J. L. [271]
Buttin, G. [216]
Capen, C. C. [265]
Cavalli, A. [330]
Cho, J.-Y. [265]
Coignet, L. J. A. [156]
Colombo, M. [337]
Coquelle, A. [216]
Croce, C. M. [200]
de Boer, J. [147]
De Gregorio, L. [292]
de Wit, J. [147]
Debatisse, M. [216]
DeMarini, D. M. [97]
D'Errico, M. [97]
Dogliotti, E. [97]
Doll, R. [2]
Donker, I. [147]

Dragani, T. A. [292]
Druck, T. [200]
Engelbergs, J. [127]
Falvella, F. S. [292]
Ferrari, C. [330]
Fiaccardori, F. [330]
Furminger, T. L. [265]
Gariboldi, M. [292]
Glover, T. W. [185]
Hagmar, L. [177]
Hainaut, P. [97]
Hansteen, I.-L. [177]
Harris, C. C. [22]
Hengstler, J. G. [47]
Hernandez, T. [97]
Herrero, M. E. [47]
Hildt, E. [315]
Hillemann, M. [345]
Hoeijmakers, J. H. J. [147]
Hofschneider, P. H. [315]
Huebner, K. [200]
Hussain, S. P. [22]
Ito, S. [229]
Iwashita, T. [229]
Jhiang, S. M. [265]
Klugbauer, S. [248]
Knudsen, L. [177]
Kovatich, A. [200]
Lamonaca, V. [330]

---

[*] The address of the principal author is given on the first page
of each contribution.
[1] Page on which contribution begins.

Lando, C. [177]
Lucek, P. [285]
Manenti, G. [292]
Mazzaferri, E. L. [265]
McCredie, M. [298]
McCue, P. A. [200]
Mikoczy, Z. [177]
Missale, G. [330]
Montagud, A. H. [177]
Murakami, H. [229]
Norppa, H. [177]
Oesch, F. [47]
Ott, J. [285]
Penna, A. [330]
Perera, F. P. [39]
Pierotti, M. A. [237, 292]
Rabes, H. M. [248]
Rajewsky, M. F. [127]
Reuterwall, C. [177]
Risch, A. [86]
Rojas, M. [86]

Sagartz, J. E. [265]
Schweer, T. [127]
Scognamiglio, P. [330]
Siprashvili, Z. [200]
Strömberg, U. [177]
Takahashi, M. [229]
Thomale, J. [127]
Tinnerberg, H. [177]
Toledo, F. [216]
Tong, Q. [265]
Urbani, S. [330]
Valli, A. [330]
van der Horst, G. T. J. [147]
van Weering, D. H. J. [271]
Vermeulen, W. [147]
Vigneri, P. [237]
Weeda, G. [147]
Winkler, S. B. [147]
Yuille, M. A. R. [156]
Zanesi, N. [292]

I. Key Notes

Epidemiological Evidence of the Effects of Behaviour and the Environment on the Risk of Human Cancer

R. Doll

ICRF Clinical Trial Service Unit and Epidemiological Studies Unit, Harkness Building, Radcliffe Infirmary, Oxford OX2 6HE, UK

Abstract

The incidence of cancer in middle and old age can, in principle, be reduced by 80%–90% and the risks worldwide could be halved, although the methods required are not always socially acceptable. The proportions of fatal cancers attributable to different causes are examined under 17 headings: smoking, alcohol, pharmaceutical products, infection (parasites, bacteria, viruses) electromagnetic radiation (ionizing, ultraviolet, lower frequency) occupation, industrial products, pollution (air, water, food), physical inactivity, reproductive hormones, and diet.

Smoking is the most important factor. It contributes to the production of seven types of cancer in addition to the eight that were recognized by the International Agency for Research on Cancer in 1986 and is estimated to have been responsible for 38% of cancers in men and 6% in women in Germany in 1985. Firm estimates can also be made of the proportions of fatal cancers attributable to alcohol and ionizing radiation, and reasonable guesses can be made at the maximum effect of some of the other categories.

Many of the factors act synergistically with one another, so that the risk of developing specific cancers can be modified in different ways. When all the avoidable causes are known, the sum of the proportions avoidable in different ways may add up to several hundred per cent.

Introduction

Knowledge of the environmental and behavioural causes of cancer grew rapidly in the first few decades of the second half of this century. By 1980 we were able to assert that, in principle, it should be possible to reduce the incidence of the disease in middle and early old age by 80%–90%. It was not known precisely how such a large reduction could be brought about, but it was known how the risk could be approximately halved, though the methods required were not always socially acceptable. Since then the rate of accumulating knowledge of the means of avoiding cancer has slowed, while knowl-

Recent Results in Cancer Research, Vol. 154
© Springer-Verlag Berlin · Heidelberg 1998

edge of the mechanisms by which cancer is produced at the cellular level has increased dramatically. This increase has facilitated the discovery of viral causes of cancer, but it remains to be seen how far it will help in identifying the nature of other avoidable causes that are as yet unknown. Here, I describe the causes that are now known and draw attention to the areas where the gaps that should be capable of being filled are most glaring. I have, of necessity, had to use British data for some of my examples, as these were the only ones available to me, but I have used German data whenever I could.

Avoidable Causes

Smoking

The most important known avoidable cause continues to be smoking. This, it is now known, contributes to the production of cancer of many different types. Eight forms of cancer were recognized to be largely attributable to smoking by the International Agency for Research on Cancer (IARC) in 1986. These are listed in Table 1. For these eight cancers prolonged consumption of about 20 cigarettes per day increases the risk between 2 and 20 times. With further research since the IARC's report it has become clear that several other types of cancer are also somewhat more common in cigarette smokers than in non-smokers. These are listed in Table 2. For some, the mortality in smokers is only slightly greater than in non-smokers, but the consistency of the findings in different countries, the evidence for a dose-response relationship, the lower mortality in ex-smokers than in continuing smokers, the presence of many different carcinogens in tobacco smoke, and the lack of evidence of confounding provide grounds for believing that most of the observed relationships are causal. For one, cancer of the liver, the association in developed countries has generally been attributed to confounding with the consumption of alcohol and cirrhosis of the liver, but evidence from parts of China, where little alcohol is consumed, confirm the finding by Trichopoulos et al. (1980) that smoking plays an independent part in its causation (Liu et

Table 1. Cancers largely attributable to smoking

Cancers of:
  Mouth
  Pharynx[a]
  Oesophagus
  Larynx
  Lung
  Pancreas
  Kidney, pelvis
  Bladder

[a] Excluding nasopharynx. From: International Agency for Research on Cancer (1986).

Table 2. Other cancers associated with smoking[a]

Nature of association	Type of cancer
Causal	Lip, nose, stomach, body of kidney, myeloid leukaemia
Causal and confounding	Liver
Confounding and possibly causal	Large bowel, cervix uteri

[a] Principally or entirely cigarette smoking except for lip cancer, principally pipe smoking.

Table 3. Risk of childhood cancer associated with paternal smoking

Father's smoking (cigarettes a day)	Risk relative to father not smoking		
	Sorahan et al. (1995)	Sorahan et al. (1997)	13 other studies[a]
1–9	1.20	1.03	
10–19	1.24	1.31*	
20-29	1.26*		–
30-39	1.35*	1.42*	
40 or more	1.47*		
1 or more	–	–	1.20*
Number of children with cancer	1641	1549	2731

* $p < 0.05$.
[a] Sorahan et al. (1997 and personal communication).

al. 1997). For two (cancers of the large bowel and cervix uteri) the associations may be wholly due to confounding with, respectively, diet and some particular sexually transmitted infection(s); but smoking may still play a part in the former indirectly by causing dietary modification, and, in the latter, by causing excretion of tobacco specific mutagens in the cervical mucus.

Recently childhood cancers have been added to the list, as a small proportion appear to be produced by parental smoking; *not* by causing exposure to environmental smoke after birth or to smoke products in maternal blood in utero, but as a result of genetic mutations caused by *paternal* smoking before the child's conception. This, to me, surprising finding is strongly suggested by the massive data from the Oxford Childhood Cancer Study reported in two papers by Sorahan et al. (1995, 1997) and by the sum of the findings in 13 smaller studies, as is shown in Table 3. It is made plausible by the finding of oxidative damage to the sperm of smokers (Fraga et al. 1996).

Altogether Peto et al. (1994; Peto, personal communication) have estimated that smoking has been responsible for about 38% of all deaths from cancer in men in Germany since 1985 and that the proportion in women has gone up from 3% in 1985 to 6%–still a long way to go to catch up with the

Table 4. Per cent change in mortality 1970–1974 to 1990–1991: Cancers closely associated with smoking

Type of cancer	Per cent change			
	Males aged, years		Females aged, years	
	35–49	50–69	35–49	50–69
Lung	−49	−34	−21	+50
Mouth	+82	+80	+33	+37
Pharynx	+46	+12	−59	−37
Oesophagus	+36	+58	−31	+26
Larynx	−5	+7	−41	+9
Pancreas	−23	−15	−15	+3
Bladder	−47	−19	−33	−4

proportions of 52% in men in the UK in 1975 (now down to 40%) and the current 20% in women.

In general, smoking interacts synergistically with other agents and, although the cessation of smoking, or better still the avoidance of smoking altogether, is the most effective way of reducing the risk, there are other ways in which the risk of smoking associated cancers might be influenced – for example, by increasing the consumption of green and yellow vegetables in the case of cancer of the lung. For some types of cancer these other agents may have substantial effects, as is illustrated by the change in mortality from cancers closely related to smoking in England and Wales since the early 1970s that are shown in Table 4. The sex-specific trends in the mortality from lung cancer, which closely reflect the trends in incidence, because the fatality continues to be so high, parallel the trends in the prevalence of cigarette smoking adjusted for tar yield, after appropriate allowance has been made for latent period and cohort effects (Doll et al. 1997), but the same is not true for several of the other cancers that are caused in large part by smoking. Clearly there have been other factors, some of which will have interacted with smoking, while others may have acted independently. One that will have interacted to affect the risk of cancer of the upper digestive tract in men and cancer of the mouth in young women will have been the increased consumption of alcohol and another may be an increased prevalence of infection with carcinogenic varieties of the human papilloma virus. There must, however, have been other factors that have caused the reduction in mortality from cancers of the pharynx in women and from cancer of the bladder in older women, the last being perhaps the elimination of carcinogenic dyes.

Table 5. Mortality from breast cancer in american women by consumption of alcohol

Consumption (g/day)[a]	Annual death rate per 100 000	Relative risk (95% CI)	
None	30.3	1.0	
Less than 12	33.3	1.1	(0.9, 1.3)
12–23	37.6	1.2	(1.0, 1.6)
24–47	45.8	1.5	(1.2, 1.9)
48 or more	29.1	1.0	(0.7, 1.4)

After Thun et al. (1997).
CI, confidence interval.
[a] The unit drink is defined as containing 12 g ethanol, 50% more than the unit drink is assumed to contain in the UK.

Alcohol

Alcohol is another well established, but far less important, cause, responsible for perhaps 5% of all fatal cancers. Its contribution has been recognized by the International Agency for Research on Cancer (1988) which has accepted that alcohol, largely, but not wholly, in conjunction with smoking, increases the risk of cancers of the mouth, pharynx (other than the nasopharynx), larynx, and oesophagus and increases the risk of cancer of the liver if drunk in sufficient amounts to cause cirrhosis. But, as with smoking, further evidence since the Agency's review suggests that other types of cancer may have to be added to the list. One is cancer of the breast which many cohort studies show is related to alcohol, the mortality being increased by about 10% for each unit of consumption per day (Longnecker 1994). Observations on some 250 000 women with known drinking habits followed for 9 years in the American Cancer Society's most recent study are shown in Table 5. Maternal consumption during pregnancy may also increase the risk of myeloid leukaemia with characteristic abnormalities of the MLL gene at chromosome 11 q 23 in infants under 18 months of age (Shu et al. 1996). Whether it does have this effect should become clear next year with the report of two large studies of infant leukaemia that are now under way.

Pharmaceutical Products

As for other drugs, the more they are studied the more they seem to be beneficial rather than the reverse. If we leave aside those used to treat cancer, some of which cause a small risk of second cancers in patients otherwise apparently cured, and the immunosuppressive drugs used principally with organ transplants that cause a small risk of non-Hodgkin's lymphomas and skin cancers, the only important ones that may cause cancer are the combined steroid contraceptives and the oestrogens used as hormone replace-

Table 6. Risk of breast cancer in users of oral contraceptives

Use of oral combined steroid contraceptives	Risk relative to that in non-users (95% confidence interval)		$2p$
Continuing	1.24	(1.15–1.33)	<0.00001
Stopped 1–4 years	1.16	(1.08–1.23)	<0.00001
5–9 years	1.07	(1.02–1.13)	0.009
10 or more years	1.01	(0.96–1.05)	–

From Collaborative Group on Hormonal Factors in Breast Cancer (1996).

ment therapy for menopausal and postmenopausal women The steroid contraceptives we now know, from the results of a collaborative reanalysis of their data by epidemiologists who have studied the relationship of the drugs to breast cancer (Collaborative Group on Hormonal Factors in Breast Cancer 1996), do cause a small increase in the incidence of the disease of about 20%, but only during their use and up to 10 years after it is stopped, as is shown in Table 6. The excess was, however, limited to tumours that were localized to the breast and tumours that had spread were, if anything, *less* likely to occur in users than in non-users, so that breast cancer mortality cannot have been increased much, if at all. Any increased risk is certainly small, and in absolute terms less than the *reduction* of about 50% in the incidence of ovarian cancer from long term use, to which may possibly be added a small reduction in the risk of endometrial cancer.

Hormone replacement therapy also causes a small risk of breast cancer during and for up to 5 years after its use has been stopped, the increase in relative risk being about 2.3% for each year of use (Collaborative Group on Hormonal Factors in Breast Cancer 1997). Again, however, the increase appears to be limited to localised tumours and it is unclear whether mortality is affected and whether a similar effect is obtained with the combined oestrogen/progesterone pill as with oestrogen alone. Oestrogen therapy also causes an increase in the risk of endometrial cancer which may, however, be more than compensated for by a *decrease* in the risk of large bowel cancer. Three large cohort studies have reported reductions in the incidence of colorectal cancer of 18%, 20% and 48% in current users (Bostick et al. 1994; Chute et al. 1991; Calle et al. 1995). The largest also reported some reduction in ex-users (27%)and an increasing reduction with increasing duration of use (Calle et al. 1995)

Medicinal treatment aimed at reducing the risk of cancer is a new concept, but several drugs promise to be useful for the purpose. One is tamoxifen, which mimics oestrogen in some respects but also acts as an anti-oestrogen by blocking some oestrogen receptors. It reduces the risk of developing a new cancer in the second breast when given for the treatment of cancer in the first and controlled trials are under way to see whether it can reduce the risk of a first breast cancer in women at high risk of developing the disease, despite the fact that it can certainly increase the risk of endometrial cancer.

Aspirin, surprisingly, is another; for there is now evidence from six studies that it may approximately halve the risk of colorectal neoplasms and contradictory evidence from only one study (Logan et al. 1993). That it might have such an effect is supported by the experimental evidence that Sulindac (a similar non-steroidal anti-inflammatory drug) can reduce the number of both sporadic polyps (Matsuhashi et al. 1997) and polyps in patients with familial adenomatous polyposis (Giardello et al. 1993) possibly by blocking the production of prostaglandins which, among other things, can inhibit progression from the G to the S phase of the cell cycle in vitro.

Other pharmaceutical products may serve as dietary supplements, to which I will refer later, or to cure infections, an increasing number of which are being found to contribute to the production of many different cancers. These include infections with parasites and bacteria as well as with viruses.

Infection

Parasites

Infection with parasites does not affect us directly in Western Europe, as the parasites responsible for many cancers of the bladder, large bowel, liver and bile ducts in parts of Africa and Asia are not found here. Where they do occur they could be eliminated by a combination of hygienic and therapeutic measures, if sufficient public collaboration could be secured.

Bacteria

The most important bacterial infection appears to be infection of the gastric mucosa with *Helicobacter pylori*. Infection commonly occurs in youth, when colonisation of the gastric mucosa may cause antral gastritis. This can lead to duodenal ulceration, atrophic gastritis, intestinal metaplasia, and eventually gastric carcinoma, the last of which is moderately associated with *Helicobacter* infection in both case-control and cohort studies. The increased risk is not large, about twofold (Danesh 1998). Whether it will be possible to reduce the risk by antibiotic therapy, which can eliminate the infection and heal duodenal ulcers, remains to be shown. It would almost certainly eliminate some gastric lymphomas as they regress, and may even disappear, when *Helicobacter* infection is treated after the tumour is diagnosed (Bayerdörffer et al. 1995).

Other forms of bacterial infection do not appear to contribute much to carcinogenesis, except perhaps in the bladder, where chronic infection may be accompanied by the formation of carcinogenic nitrosamines. Precisely what role bacteria play in the large bowel is still a matter for debate.

Viruses

Viral infection is not as important as Nixon was advised when he ordered the National Cancer Institute's research programme in the United States to be focused on the discovery of "the cancer virus"; but it may yet prove to be important in the production of many cancers, which may become avoidable by appropriate immunization.

The hepatitis B virus is partly responsible for most cases of hepatocarcinoma in Africa and Asia, where the disease is so common that liver cancer ranks eight in the list of common cancers worldwide. Immunization in childhood prevents lifelong chronic infection and there is reason to hope that the mass immunization of children now being carried out in some tropical and semi-tropical countries will lead to a large reduction in the incidence of the disease. Some hepatocarcinomas, however, are attributable to hepatitis C virus, which is an RNA virus, and infection with this cannot be prevented in the same way, although it can sometimes be cured by interferon.

In Europe, the principal carcinogenic viruses thus far identified are certain specific types of the human papilloma virus. These, International Agency for Research on Cancer, 1995, are responsible for the great majority of cancers of the cervix and probably also for most cancers of the vulva, vagina, and penis and for some cancers of the anus, and they may be responsible for some cancers of the mouth, larynx, and skin. Genital cancers due to infection can be avoided if both sexes have only a very small number of sexual partners and, less effectively, if the male partner uses condoms; but at present the best hope for a major reduction in their incidence is by screening for and treating premalignant lesions. In the future, immunization against the carcinogenic types of the human papilloma virus may be possible. Immunization with gene segments of specific papilloma types has been shown to be effective in animals and the use of a similar type of vaccine has begun to be tested in humans in the UK.

Four other viruses that contribute to the production of other cancers are listed in Table 7. The roles of the Epstein-Barr (EB) virus, now known as herpes virus type 4, and the human T cell leukaemia virus are firmly established and there is strong evidence to relate the Kaposi-associated herpes virus (herpes virus type 8) to all types of Kaposi's sarcoma, the classical East European type, the tropical type, and the type associated with AIDS. The association of simian virus 40-like viruses with four mostly rare types of cancer is, however, still tentative.

As with nearly all other causes, the viruses are not associated with every case of any of the cancers that they cause and they often require other factors to be present as well, such as intensive infection with malaria parasites to produce Burkitt's lymphomas, amphibole asbestos to produce pleural mesotheliomas, and aflatoxin to produce a high incidence of liver cancer. With so many newly discovered virus-associated cancers it would be surprising if there were not still more to be discovered.

Table 7. Viral causes of cancer

Virus	Cancer
Hepatitis B	Cancer of liver
Hepatitis C	Cancer of liver
Human papilloma (types 16, 18 and others)	Cancers of cervix, vulva, vagina, penis, anus
Human herpes type 4 (Epstein-Barr virus)	Burkitt's lymphoma, immunoblastic lymphoma, nasal T cell lymphoma, Hodgkin's desease, nasopharyngeal cancer
Human herpes type 8 (Kaposi associated herpes virus)	Kaposi's sarcoma, body cavity lymphoma
Human T cell leukaemia type 1	Adult T cell leukaemia/lymphoma
Simian virus 40-like	Ependymoma, choroid plexus tumours, mesothelioma, bone tumours

Electromagnetic radiation

A group of causes whose effects can be better quantified than those of infection are the various categories of electromagnetic radiation.

Ionizing Radiation

Ionizing radiation is estimated to cause some 4%–5% of all cancers, mostly due to the natural radiation to which everyone is exposed from radon in air, cosmic rays from outer space, external radiation from the radionuclides in rocks, soils, and building materials, and internal radiation from radioactive traces of potassium, lead, and polonium in food. Of this natural radiation only some of that from radon, which worldwide provides about half the total dose, can be avoided. In Germany, as in many other countries, the dose varies more than 100-fold from one part of the country to another. Where the dose is high, it can be reduced by ventilation or, in the future, by building regulations that would ensure that relatively little radon enters homes. Precisely how much lung cancer in the general population is caused by radon is still uncertain, as the effect has had to be extrapolated from observations on heavily exposed miners. For the former West Germany, Steindorf et al. (1995) estimated that it might account for about 7%, mostly in conjunction with smoking, and this would fit in with the early results of the few direct observations that have yet been reported. Action to reduce the risk is, however, a reasonable precaution for the relatively few people who are very heavily exposed. Some further reduction in exposure to medical uses of radiation, which, in the UK, now accounts for 97% of the exposure from man-made sources and 14% of the total exposure, is doubtless possible; but the total benefit to be gained is likely to be small, as much of the medical exposure is of people who are already near the end of their lives.

Ultraviolet Light

More benefit could be expected from a reduction in exposure of the skin to strong sunlight; for sunlight, and presumably the ultraviolet component, is responsible for nearly all melanomas and basal cell carcinomas of the skin and, now that occupational exposure to coal tar and pitch has been effectively eliminated, for nearly all squamous carcinomas of the skin as well. Of the three, squamous carcinoma is the most closely related to cumulative exposure, while melanoma is specially related to intermittent exposure and the frequency of sunburn, particularly in youth (Elwood and Jopson 1997). The incidence of melanoma has been increasing steadily in all white skinned populations for many years. In England and Wales the mortality more than doubled in men aged 50–69 years between 1970–1974 and 1991–1992 and increased by 53% in women. This can be attributed to the increased exposure from changes in clothing, exposure of the skin, and travel to hot countries. The obvious way to avoid these cancers is to avoid prolonged and intensive exposure to sunlight, but such advice is socially unattractive in many countries, where a tan is regarded as an indication of health, and there has been a tendency to emphasise the alternative use of sun-screen ointments. Now, however, there is accumulating evidence that such ointments, particularly if they contain psoralen, may actually *increase* the risk of the most serious type of skin cancer: namely, melanoma. Several studies have pointed in the same direction, the results of the latest of which are summarized in Table 8. It may be that all that this is telling us is that sun-screens increase risk in so far as they allow people to be exposed for longer without getting sunburn; but that would not explain the specific risk associated with the use of psoralen. At present we can suggest only the avoidance of unnecessary exposure, particularly when the sun is high in the sky. Whether any other type of cancer can be caused by ultraviolet light is uncertain, but there is some evidence to suggest that increased exposure may be responsible for some of the increase in non-Hodgkin's lymphoma (Adami et al. 1995), which is too large and began too soon to be explained as a diagnostic artefact or as attributable to the increased risks associated with AIDS and with the use of immunosuppressive drugs.

Table 8. Risk of skin melanoma by skin type and sunscreen use

Sunscreen use	Odds ratio[a] for skin phototype	
	I–II	III–IV
Never (142, 197)*	1.0	1.8
Ever, standard type only (230, 210)	1.8	2.2
Ever, psoralen sunscreen (43, 26)	2.1	9.8

After Autier et al. (1995).
* Numbers of cases and controls in parentheses.
[a] All odds ratios greater than 1.0 ($p < 0.05$).

Table 9. Relative risk of acute lymphatic leukaemia in children exposed to different magnetic fields from 60 Hz electricity at home in the USA.

Magnetic field (μT)	Number of cases/ matched controls	Odds ratio	
<0.065	206/215	1.00	
0.065–0.099	92/98	0.96	
0.100–0.199	107/106	1.13	
0.200–0.299	29/26	1.31	1.53*
0.300–0.399	14/11	1.46	
0.400–0.499	10/2	6.41	
≥0.500	5/5	1.01	

After Linet et al. (1997).
* 95% CI 0.91–2.56.

Low and Extremely Low Frequency Radiation

Whether the radiation from other parts of the electromagnetic spectrum, or the separate electric and magnetic fields, can cause any risk of cancer is uncertain. Experimentally there was no reason to think that they could, unless perhaps the radiation was heavy enough to produce local heating, until Repacholi et al. produced an excess of lymphomas in mice that had been genetically modified to be highly susceptible to the development of the disease (Repacholi et al. 1997). But whether such a finding is relevant is open to doubt. Despite the heightened public concern, there is *no* epidemiological evidence of harm from cellular telephones, the claim for the production of brain cancer being based on single cases. There is, however, some evidence of risk for extremely low frequency magnetic fields. Occupational studies, in which exposures have been measured, have suggested – but certainly not proved – that exposures above 0.2 μT might increase the risk of adult leukaemia and brain cancer, and good quality epidemiological evidence from Fenno-Scandinavia suggests that residence near high power electricity cables producing similar fields may approximately double the risk of childhood leukaemia. This is supported by findings in Germany, based, however, on very small numbers (Michaelis et al. 1997), and something similar was observed in the largest and best US study, the results of which are summarized in Table 9. It was, however, reported by the authors as essentially negative (Linet et al. 1997). The national study of children's cancer that is now being carried out in the UK will, I hope, settle the issue by the end of next year.

Occupation, Industrial Products, and Pollution

Three potential sources of hazard cause much public concern: namely, occupation, industrial products, and pollution. In total, however, they are unlikely to be responsible for more than 3% or 4% of all fatal cancers, most of which were caused by uncontrolled exposure in the distant past. With one possible exception, I see little opportunity for benefit from further control.

Occupation

Occupational hazards have been substantial, causing, in the extreme case, all the most heavily exposed men to develop cancer, as occurred with some groups of manufacturers of 2-naphthylamine and benzidene, while coal tar fumes and asbestos have been so widespread that tens of thousands of skin and lung cancers have been produced. All such hazards have, however, now been eliminated or controlled for so long that few attributable cases continue to occur. Mesotheliomas due to exposure to amosite and crocidolite asbestos are an exception. The trend in the incidence of the disease continues upwards and, if Peto et al.'s prediction is correct, mesotheliomas attributable to asbestos may alone constitute 2% of all cancer deaths in 25 years time (Peto et al. 1995), instead of the 0.3% that they constitute now.

Industrial Products

Industrial products have never been a significant cause of cancer for the general public, apart perhaps from the dyes that used to be contaminated with aromatic amines and the asbestos materials that were used by the do-it-yourself home builder.

Pollution

Pollution, which was a significant hazard in the days when coal was burnt in every house, though never as great a cancer hazard as was commonly thought, is now so reduced that the risks that can be quantified – those of polycyclic aromatic hydrocarbons, trace metals, and benzene from the use of fossil fuels in industry and transport, dioxins from the combustion of waste, pesticide residues in food, and discharges from the nuclear industry – all appear to be so minute in the UK, the combustion of fossil fuels causing less than 0.1% of fatal cancers and nuclear waste less than 0.01% (National Academies Advisory Group 1995), that the social cost of trying to reduce them further may well outweigh any medical benefit. One possible exception is the pollution of drinking water with halomethanes caused by the action of chlorine on organic waste. From an overview of ten studies in the US, Morris et al. (1992) estimated that 8% of rectal cancers and 15% of bladder cancers might be attributable to chlorinated by-products in drinking water. The evidence is not compelling, but does point to the need for further study.

Pollution is often suggested as a cause of an increase in the incidence of any cancer that cannot be firmly ascribed to any other cause and pollution with pesticides has been suggested as a possible explanation for the increased incidence of non-Hodgkin's lymphoma, not attributable to the causes to which I have already referred, and for the increase of testis cancer in young men, which has continued in all developed countries for several decades – at least since 1940 in Denmark and for even longer in the UK. There is, however, no good evidence to suggest that pollution is a cause of either.

Physical Inactivity

There remains one factor that has only recently been appreciated (physical inactivity) and two important groups of causes that have been recognized for many years (namely, reproductive hormones and diet) which I have left to the end, because there is little new to say about them and little clear evidence to relate specific agents quantitatively to specific risks.

The first, physical inactivity, or rather a sedentary lifestyle without vigorous activity in leisure hours or at work, has been related to the risk of cancers of the colon and the breast. Intensive activity, such as jogging for an hour 5 days a week, may halve the risk of both diseases and smaller benefits may be obtained with moderate activity, such as brisk walking for 3h a week. Physical activity is, however, difficult to quantity and the nature of the dose-response relationships is uncertain, as is the duration required and its temporal relationship to the incidence of the disease. A recent cohort study of 25 000 Norwegian women suggested that any reduction in the incidence of breast cancer was largely limited to the premenopausal period (Thune et al. 1997) as is shown in Table 10; but the number of cases was small and the confidence limits consequently wide.

Table 10. Relative risk of breast cancer by level of physical activity

Level of physical activity	Premenopausal		Postmenopausal	
	Relative risk[a]	Number of cases	Relative risk[a]	Number of cases
At work				
Sedentary	1.0	22	1.0	39
Walking	0.8	62	0.9	148
Lifting/heavy manual	0.5	14	0.8	60
P for trend	0.02		0.24	
During leisure hours				
Sedentary	1.0	20	1.0	45
Moderate	0.8	68	1.0	177
Regular exercise	0.5	10	0.7	26
P for trend	0.03		0.15	

After Thune et al. (1997).
[a] Adjusted for age at entry, body mass index, height, county of residence, and number of children.

Reproductive Hormones

That reproduction affects the risk of breast cancer has been known for 250 years, since Ramazzini (1743) drew attention to the high risk of the disease in nuns. Now we know that pregnancy increases the risk temporarily, but that multiparity, early first birth, late age at menarche, and early menopause all reduce it in the long run and do so incrementally. None has a large effect alone, but in combination they could account for a reduction in risk of some 90% under the conditions of life of women in hunter-gatherer societies. Precisely what the mechanisms are is unknown, but oestrogen must play a large part and a high blood oestradiol has now been shown to predict a high risk of developing the disease (Thomas et al. 1997). Multiparity, late age at menarche, and early menopause similarly reduce the risk of endometrial cancer, by reducing exposure to unopposed oestrogen, and the same factors plus prolonged lactation reduce the risk of ovarian cancer by reducing the number of ovulations and consequently the repeated trauma to the surface epithelium of the ovary.

Hormonal factors also seem likely to play a part in the development of cancers of the testis and prostate, but apart from early maturity causing an increase of the former and vasectomy possibly causing an increase of the latter no direct relationships have yet been established.

Diet

Last, but certainly not least in importance, is diet. Its effect on the incidence of cancer has been the subject of intensive research for many years, but the extent to which such major components as fat, meat, and fibre contribute to the effect is still uncertain. A high content of fat, and particularly of saturated fat, was long thought to be a probable cause of breast cancer; but the evidence from cohort studies, which are less likely to be influenced by recall bias than case-control studies, suggest that it is not (Hunter et al. 1996). One type of fat, olive oil, may indeed be protective (Cohen and Wynder 1990; Willett 1997). Meat has often been associated with an increased risk of colorectal cancer, but again the evidence is conflicting. No evident reduction in risk has been found in a pooled analysis of five cohort studies of vegetarians (Key, personal communication), and the International Agency for Research on Cancer (1993) could not find any human evidence of a harmful effect of cooking meat, despite the production of many products that were carcinogenic in the laboratory.

Five relationships have, however, been established sufficiently clearly to justify intervention. Two have no relation to life in the developed world: namely, that of liver cancer with aflatoxin, a metabolic product of fungal contamination of oily foods under hot and humid conditions which interacts with hepatitis B infection, and that of nasopharyngeal cancer with a peculiar type of salted fish typically consumed in south China which interacts with

Table 11. Relationship between food consumption and risk of cancer: cohort and case-control studies

Food	Number of studies	Relationship in studies: percent of total		
		Inverse	Null	Positive
Vegetables, any	68	81	6	13
Vegetables, raw	39	85	10	5
Vegetables, green	79	77	6	17
Vegetables, cruciferous	54	70	15	15
Vegetables, allium	34	79	9	12
Legumes	36	39	17	44
Carrots	64	78	11	11
Tomatoes	50	70	10	20
Fruit	46	63	26	11
Citrus fruit	40	65	20	15

After Steinmetz and Potter (1996).

infection with the EB virus. A third has less relevance in most developed countries now, but used to be important worldwide: namely, the relationship of gastric cancer with the consumption of salted and salt preserved foods. The two that continue to be highly relevant in Europe are over-consumption leading to obesity and a relative deficiency of vegetables and fruit.

Dietary restriction is a powerful means of reducing cancer incidence in laboratory experiments. In humans, in the wild, restriction in youth leads to diminished growth, delayed sexual maturity in both sexes, and a diminished risk of cancers of the testis and the breast. It is not a practicable means of reducing risk, but the avoidance of obesity is, and will reduce the risk of cancers of the endometrium and gallbladder and of cancer of the breast after the menopause.

Precisely what is meant by a relative deficiency of vegetables and fruit is unclear, but it has been interpreted by the National Cancer Institute in the US and the British Department of Health to be anything less than five servings a day. Investigators have mostly estimated odds ratios for different types of cancer in people in the highest category of consumption compared with people in the lowest and have found reductions in risk of the order of 50%. The results reported for different types of vegetable or fruit are summarized from a review by Steinmetz and Potter (1996) in Table 11. Inverse relationships have been observed most consistently with cancers of the lung, stomach, and oesophagus, less consistently with cancers of the mouth, pharynx, colon, breast, pancreas, and bladder and not at all with cancer of the prostate.

On this evidence, trials of some of the potentially anti-carcinogenic compounds found in vegetables and fruit would seem to be justified. Priority was given to β-carotene and this has already been shown not to be beneficial, at least not when given in middle age, and most current interest centres on vitamin E.

Other components of food that may be specifically beneficial include calcium and vitamin D, which, in large amounts, may reduce the risk of colorectal cancer. The most recent results of the cohort study of nurses being carried out in the United States suggests that vitamin D is likely to be the more important factor in relation to colorectal cancer, though it may of course act by facilitating the absorption of calcium (Martinez et al. 1996).

Others are the oestrogenic isoflavones from soy food, which it was thought might be important because of the low incidence of breast and prostate cancer in China and Japan, where large amounts of soy foods are consumed. Mechanisms are easy to postulate, since soy has many potentially relevant physiological effects. The epidemiological evidence is weak; but was strengthened recently when Ingram et al. reported that a high urinary excretion of phyto-oestrogens (both isoflavones from soy and lignans from dietary fibre) was inversely related to the risk of breast cancer (Ingram et al. 1997).

Relative Importance of Different Avoidable Causes

It follows from this review that any attempt to allocate proportions of all cancers that might be avoidable by the control of different environmental and behavioural factors is still largely guesswork. We are still ignorant of the precise importance of different dietary components, different reproductive hormones, the principal causes of some of the most common cancers, and the reasons for the increasing incidence of two, as yet, relatively uncommon cancers, which I have referred to only *en passant*: namely, that of non-Hodgkin's lymphoma and cancer of the testis. Firm estimates can, however, be made of the proportions attributable to smoking, alcohol, and ionizing radiation, and reasonable guesses can be made of the maximum effect of some of the other categories of cause. These are shown in Table 12 along with tentative estimates of the effect of other categories.

The maximum proportions shown, it will be noted, add up to more than 100%. This is only to be expected, as several changes are required in a cell

Table 12. Proportion of fatal cancers attributable to different avoidable factors (UK)

Percent	Factor	Percent	Factor
29–31	Smoking	2–4	Occupation
4–6	Alcohol	<1	Industrial products
<1	Pharmaceutical products	1–5	Pollution
10–20	Infection		Air
	Parasites		Water
	Bacteria		Food
	Viruses	1–2	Physical inactivity
5–7	Electromagnetic radiation	10–20	Reproductive hormones
	Ionizing		
	UV light	20–50	Diet
	Lower frequency		

before it can initiate a cancer clone and many factors interact with one another to multiply each other's effects. Any one cancer may, consequently, often be avoided in several different ways. Indeed, when all avoidable causes of all cancers are known the proportions avoidable in different ways may well add up to 300% or even more.

Envoi

Taken by itself, the evidence I have reviewed points clearly to some actions that we can take as individuals to reduce the risk of cancer. Cancer is not, however, the only risk to life and preventive action has to take into account its impact on the total risk of disease, which can sometimes be much greater than its impact on the risk of cancer and may be in the opposite direction, as could be the case with both alcohol and hormone replacement therapy.

The evidence also serves to highlight the gaps in knowledge which, I hope, may be filled in by epidemiologists and molecular biologists working together.

References

Adami J, Frisch M, Yuen J, Climelius B, Belbye M (1995) Evidence of an association between non-Hodgkin's lymphoma and skin cancer. Br Med J 310:1491–1495

Autier P, Doré J-F, Schiffler SE, Cesarini J-P, Bullaerts A, Hoelmel KF, Geffeller O, Liabeuf A, Lejeune F, Lienard D, Joarlette M, Chemaly P, Kleeberg UR, for the EORTC Melanoma Cooperative Group (1995) Melanoma and use of sun-screens: an EORTC case-control study in Germany, Belgium and France. Int J Cancer 61:749–755

Bayerdörffer E, Neubauer A, Rudolph B, Thiede C, Lehn N, Eidt S, Stolte M, for Malt Lymphoma Study Group (1995) Regression of primary gastric lymphoma of mucosa-associated lymphoid tissue type after cure of Helicobacter pylori infection. Lancet 345:1591–1593

Bostick RM, Potter JD, Kushi LH et al (1994) Sugar, meat and fat intake, and non-dietary factors for colon cancer incidence in Iowa women (United States). Cancer Causes Control 5:38–52

Calle EE, Miracle-McMahill HL, Thun MJ, Heath CW (1995) Estrogen replacement therapy and risk of fatal colon cancer in a prospective cohort of postmenopausal women. J Natl Cancer Inst 87:517–523

Chute CG, Willett WC, Colditz GA et al (1991) A prospective study of reproductive history and exogenous estrogens on the risk of colorectal cancer. Epidemiology 2:201–207

Cohen LA, Wynder EL (1990) Do dietary monounsaturated fatty acids play a protective role in carcinogenesis and cardiovascular disease? Med Hypotheses 31:83–89

Collaborative Group on Hormonal Factors in Breast Cancer (1996) Breast cancer and hormonal contraceptives. Collaborative reanalysis of individual data on 53 297 women with breast cancer and 100,239 women without breast cancer from 54 epidemiological studies. Lancet 347:1713–1727

Collaborative Group on Hormonal Factors in Breast Cancer (1997) Breast cancer and hormone replacement therapy: collaborative reanalysis of data from 51 epidemiological studies of 52,705 women with breast cancer and 108,411 women without breast cancer. Lancet 350:1047–1059

Danesh JN (1998) Is Helicobacter pylori infection a cause of stomach cancer? In: Beral V, Weiss R, Newton R (eds) Cold Spring Harbor Laboratory Press, New York (in press)

Doll R, Darby S, Whitley E (1997) Trends in mortality from smoking-related diseases. In: Charlton J, Murphy M (eds) Cancer surveys: infections in cancer. The health of adult Britain, 1841–1994, vol 1. pp 128–155. The Stationary Office, London

Elwood JM, Jopson J (1997) Melanoma and sun exposure: an overview of published studies. Int J Cancer 73:198–203

Fraga CG, Motchnik PA, Wyrobek AJ, Rempel DM, Ames BN (1996) Smoking and low anti-oxidant levels increase oxidative damage to sperm DNA. Mutat Res 351:199–203

Giardello FM, Hamilton SR, Krush AJ, Piantadosi S, Hylind LM, Celano P, Booker SV, Robinson CR, Offerhaus GJ (1993) Treatment of colonic and rectal adenomas with sulindac in familial adenomatous polyposis. N Engl J Med 328:1313–1316

Hunter DJ, Spiegelmand, Adam H-O, Beeson L, Van den Brandt P, Folsom AB, Fraser GE, Goldbohm RA, Graham S, Howe Gr, Kushi LH, Marshall JR, McDermott A, Miller AB, Speizer FE, Wolk A, Yuan SS, Willett W (1996) Cohort studies of fat intake and risk of breast cancer – a pooled analysis. N Engl J Med, 334:356–360

Ingram D, Sanders K, Kolybabh M, Lopez D (1997) Case-control study of phyto-oestrogens and breast cancer. Lancet 350:990–994

International Agency for Research on Cancer (1986) Tobacco smoking. IARC Monogr Eval Carcinog Risks Chem Hum 38, IARC, Lyon

International Agency for Research on Cancer (1988) Alcohol drinking. IARC Monogr Eval Carcinog Risks Hum 44, IARC, Lyon

International Agency for Research on Cancer (1993) Some naturally occurring substances: food items and constituents, heterocyclic aromatic amines and mycotoxins. IARC Monogr Eval Carcinog Risks Human 56, IARC, Lyon

International Agency for Research on Cancer (1995) Human papilloma viruses IARC Monogr Eval Carcinog Risks Hum 64, IARC, Lyon

Linet MS, Hatch EE, Kleinerman RA, Robison LL, Kaune WT, Friedman DR, Severson RK, Haines CM, Hartsock BS, Niwa S, Wacholder S, Tarone RE (1997) Residential exposure to magnetic fields and acute lymphoblastic leukaemia in children. N Engl J Med 337:1–7

Liu B-Q, Peto R, Chen Z-M, Boreham J, Wu Y-P, Campbell TC, Chen J-S, Li J-Y (1997) Tobacco hazards in China: case-control study of 300 000 deaths and proportional mortality study of 1 000 000 deaths. Br Med J (in press)

Logan RFA, Little J, Hawtin PG, Hardcastle JD (1993) Effect of aspirin and non-steroidal anti-inflammatory drugs on colo-rectal adenomas: case-control study of subjects participating in the Nottingham faecal occult blood screening programme. Br med J 307:285–289

Longnecker MP (1994) Alcoholic beverage consumption in relation to risk of breast cancer: meta-analysis and review. Cancer Causes Control 5:73–82

Martinez ME, Giovanucci EL, Colditz GA, Stampfer MJ, Hunter DJ, Speizer FE, Wing A, Willett WC (1996) Calcium, vitamin D, and the occurrence of colorectal cancer among women. J Natl Cancer Inst 88:1375–1382

Matsuhashi N, Nakajima A, Fukushima Y, Yazaki Y, Oka T (1997) Effects of sulindac on sporadic colorectal adenomatous polyps. Gut 40:344–349

Michaelis J, Schüz J, Meinert R, Menger M, Grigat J-P, Kaatsch P, Kaletsch U, Miesner A, Stamm A, Brinkman K, Kärner H (1997) Childhood leukaemia and electromagnetic fields: results of a population-based case-control study in Germany. Cancer Causes Control 8:167–174

Morris RD, Audet A, Angelillo IF, Chalmers TC, Mosteller F (1992) Chlorination, chlorination by-products, and cancer: a metaanalysis. Am J Public Health 82:955–963

National Academies Advisory Group (1995) Energy and the environment in the 21st century. Royal Society, London

Peto J, Hodgson JT, Matthews FE, Jones JR (1995) Continuing increase in mesothelioma increase in Britain. Lancet 345:535–539

Peto R, Lopez AD, Boreham J, Thun M, Heath C (1994) Mortality from smoking in developed countries. Oxford University Press, Oxford

Ramazzini B (1743) De morbis artificum Diatriba. Corona, Venice

Repacholi MH, Basten A, Gebski V, Noonan D, Finnie J, Harris AW (1997) Lymphomas in Eµ-Pim1 Transgenic mice exposed to pulsed 900 MHz electromagnetic fields. Radiat Res 147:631–640

Shu X-O, Ross JA, Pendergrass TW, Reaman GH, Lampkin B, Robison LL (1996) Parental alcohol consumption, cigarette smoking, and risk of infant leukaemia: a children's cancer group study. J Natl Cancer Inst 88:24–31

Sorahan T, Lancashire R, Prior P, Peck I, Stewart AM (1995) Childhood cancer and parental use of alcohol and tobacco. Ann Epidemiol 5:354–359

Sorahan T, Lancashire RJ, Hulten MA, Peck I, Stewart AM (1997) Childhood cancer and parental use of tobacco: deaths from 1953 to 1955. Br J Cancer 75:134–138

Steindorf K, Lubin J, Wichman HE, Becher H (1995) Lung cancer deaths attributable to indoor radon. Int J Epidemiol 24:485–492

Steinmetz K, Potter JD (1996) Vegetables, fruit, and cancer prevention: a review. J Am Diet Assoc 96:1027–1039

Thomas HV, Key TJ, Allen DS, Moore JW, Dowsett M, Fentiman IS, Wang DY (1997) A prospective study of endogenous serum hormone concentrations and breast cancer risk in post-menopausal women. Br J Cancer 76:401–405

Thun MJ, Peto R, Lopez AD, Monaco JH, Henley SJ, Heath CW, Doll R (1997) Alcohol consumption and mortality in middle-aged and elderly US adults. N Engl J Med 337:1705–1741

Thune I, Brenin T, Lund E, Gaard M (1997) Physical activity and the risk of breast cancer. N Engl J Med 336:1269–1275

Trichopoulos D, MacMahon B, Sparrow L, Merikas G (1980) Smoking and hepatitis B-negative primary hepatocellular carcinoma. J Natl Cancer Inst 65:111–114

Willett WC (1997) Diet and risk of breast cancer. In: Fortner JG, Sharp PA (eds) Accomplishments in cancer research. Lippincott-Raven, New York, pp 125–133

Molecular Epidemiology of Human Cancer

S. P. Hussain and C. C. Harris

Laboratory of Human Carcinogenesis, National Cancer Institute, NIH, Bldg. 37, Rm. 2C01, 37 Convent Dr. MSC 4255, Bethesda, MD 20892-4255, USA

Abstract

A challenging goal of molecular epidemiology is to identify an individual's risk of cancer. Molecular epidemiology integrates molecular biology, in vitro and in vivo laboratory models, biochemistry and epidemiology to infer individual cancer risk. Molecular dosimetry of carcinogen exposure is an important facet of molecular epidemiology and cancer risk assessment. Carcinogen macromolecular adduct levels, cytogenetic alterations and somatic cell mutations can be measured to determine the biologically effective doses of carcinogens. Molecular epidemiology also explores host cancer susceptibilities, such as carcinogen metabolism, DNA repair, and epigenetic and genetic alterations in tumor suppressor genes. *p53* is a prototype tumor suppressor gene and is well suited for analysis of mutational spectrum in human cancer. The analyses of germ line and somatic mutation spectra of the *p53* tumor suppressor gene provide important clues for cancer risk assessment in molecular epidemiology. For example, characteristic *p53* mutation spectra have been associated with: dietary aflatoxin B_1 exposure and hepatocellular carcinoma; sunlight exposure and skin carcinoma; and cigarette smoking and lung cancer. The mutation spectrum also reveals those *p53* mutants that provide cells with a selective clonal expansion advantage during the multistep process of carcinogenesis. The *p53* gene encodes a multifunctional protein involved in the cellular response to stress including DNA damage and hypoxia. Certain *p53* mutants lose tumor suppressor activity and gain oncogenic activity, which is one explanation for the commonality of *p53* mutations in human cancer. Molecular epidemiological results can be evaluated for causation by inference of the Bradford-Hill criteria, i.e., strength of association (consistency, specificity and temporality) and biological plausibility, which utilizes the "weight of the evidence principle."

Recent Results in Cancer Research, Vol. 154
© Springer-Verlag Berlin · Heidelberg 1998

Molecular Epidemiology

Molecular epidemiology is a field that integrates molecular biology, in vitro and in vivo laboratory models, biochemistry and epidemiology to infer individual cancer risk (Harris 1991; Shields and Harris 1991; Perera and Santella 1993). Identification of individuals at high cancer risk in the general population is an important step towards cancer prevention. Achieving this goal is challenging both current molecular technologies and epidemiological designs, and exposing bioethical dilemmas.

The two facets of molecular epidemiology of human cancer risk are assessment of carcinogen exposure and inherited or acquired host cancer susceptibility factors (reviewed in Harris 1991; Perera 1996). The interaction between these two facets determines an individual's cancer risk. This paradigm can also improve cancer risk assessment (Fig. 1). When combined with carcinogen bioassay in laboratory animals, laboratory studies of molecular carcinogenesis and classical epidemiology, molecular epidemiology can contribute to the four traditional aspects of cancer risk assessment: hazard identification, dose response assessment, exposure assessment and risk characterization. Improved cancer risk assessment has broad public health and economic implications (National Research Council 1994).

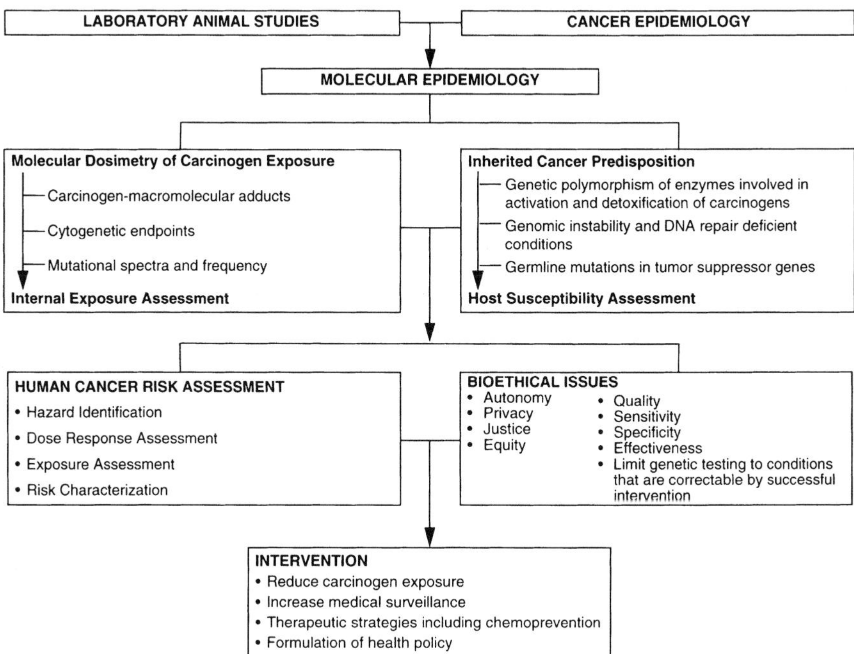

Fig. 1. Human cancer risk assessment and bioethical issues associated with molecular epidemiology and human cancer

Another important aspect that needs to be addressed is the bioethical issues that may arise following the identification of high risk individuals (Li et al. 1992). One can argue that the knowledge of one's risk can be beneficial. However more encompassing bioethical issues arise such as an individual's responsibility to family members and psychosocial concerns regarding the genetic testing of children (Li et al. 1992). Therefore the uncertainty of the current individual risk assessments and the limited availability of genetic counseling services dictate caution and, many argue, the restriction of genetic testing to those conditions amenable to preventative or therapeutic intervention.

Inherited gene mutations that increase the risk of cancer can be divided into two general categories. Predetermining genes increase the risk of cancer with little modulation by environmental factors. For example, inheritance of a defective gene involved in nucleotide excision repair (xeroderma pigmentosum) increases the risk of skin cancer only in individuals exposed to ultraviolet light, so that protection from sunlight is an obvious preventive strategy. Whereas in individuals inheriting a defective predetermining gene, e.g., Li-Fraumeni syndrome with a germline mutation in the *p53* tumor suppressor gene, modification of the environment may be a less effective strategy.

Cancer Susceptibility Genes

Germline mutations in genes, e.g., *p53*, *RB* and *APC*, that also are frequently somatically mutated in sporadic cancers, have been identified. The altered genes encode proteins that perform diverse cellular processes, including transcription, cell cycle control, xenobiotic metabolism and DNA repair. The increased cancer risk of an individual carrying one of these germline mutations can be extraordinarily high, i.e., more than 1000-fold in xeroderma pigmentosum (complementation group A–G) (Fig. 2). More common inherited

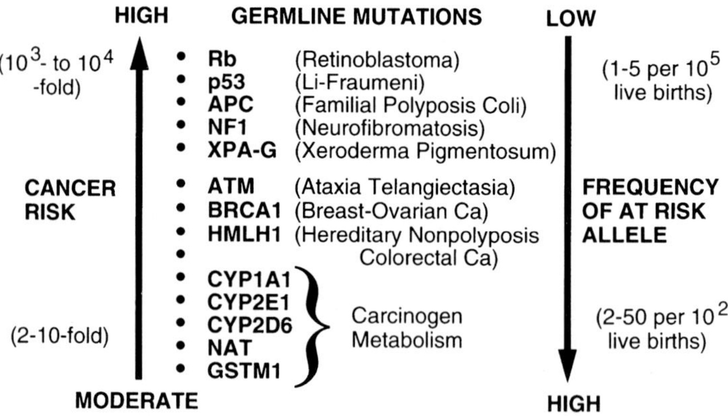

Fig. 2. Example of cancer susceptibility genes and cancer risk

cancer susceptibility conditions, e.g., deficiencies in the N-acetyltransferase (NAT) genes or glutathione S-transferase genes may contribute a more substantial attributable risk in a carcinogen-exposed population.

p53 Structure and Function

DNA Damage and Apoptotic Response Pathways

The p53 protein is clearly a component of one of the pathways activated in response to DNA damage (Fig. 3) (Maltzman and Czyzyk 1984; Kastan et al. 1991, 1992; Guillouf et al. 1995; Powell et al. 1995; Nelson and Kastan 1994). Cell cycle arrest at the G1 and G2 checkpoints prior to DNA replication and mitosis, respectively, aid the DNA repair processes and prevents mutations and aneuploidy, whereas apoptosis can be considered a failsafe mechanism to

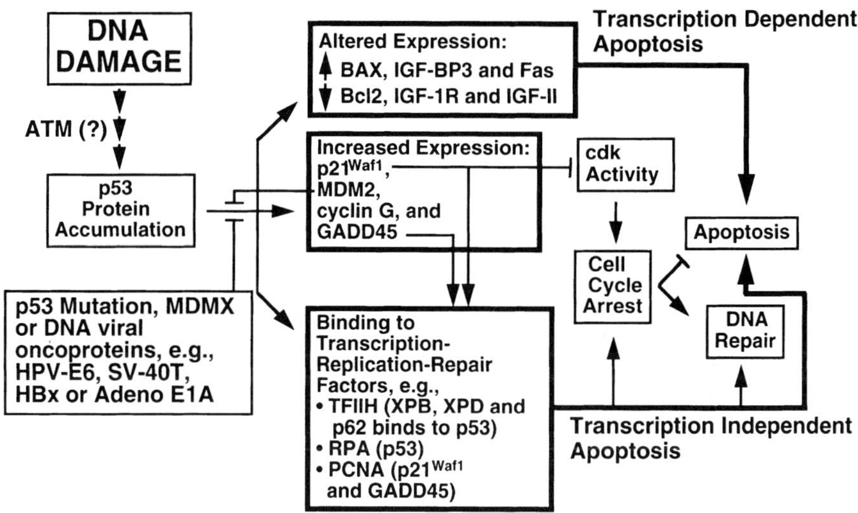

Fig. 3. Cell cycle arrest, DNA repair, and apoptosis induced by DNA damage. *p53* is a component of a DNA damage, [e.g., which may involve the ataxia telangiectasia gene product (ATM)], response pathway. This simplifed model does not consider qualitative or quantitative differences due to either cell type or microenvironment. *p53* accumulation leads to the regulation of cellular genes involved in apoptosis, e.g., *BAX, IGF-1R, IGF-BP3, Fas,* and Bcl2; cell cycle arrest, e.g., p21^{Waf1}, an inhibitor of cyclin-dependent kinases, cdk; and DNA synthesis and repair, e.g., p21^{Waf1} and *GADD45* (growth arrest and DNA damage factor) binding to PCNA (proliferating cell nuclear antigen). MDM2 protein can bind to p53 protein and inhibit its functions in a negative feedback loop. p53 can also bind directly to proteins involved in DNA synthesis (e.g., *RPA,* replicating protein antigen) and transcription, nucleotide excision, and apoptosis (e.g., *XPD,* xeroderma pigmentosum group D DNA helicase; *XPB,* xeroderma pigmentosum group B DNA helicase; and p62 of the *TFIIH,* transcription factor complex IIH). Therefore, p53 may mediate apoptosis by two interactive pathways. One dependent on p53 function as a transcription *trans*-activator and *trans*-repressor and a second pathway independent of its transcriptional activities and dependent on p53 protein-protein interactions. *MDMX,* X homologue of murine double minute gene; MDM2, murine double minute protein; HPV-E6, human papillomavirus protein E-6; *SV-40T,* simian virus-40 large T antigen; HBx, hepatitis B viral X protein; Adeno E1A, adenovirus protein E1A

rid the organism of cells either with severely damaged DNA or cells with a low apoptotic threshold. Double stranded DNA breaks are especially efficient in causing p53 protein accumulation possibly by reducing its degradation through the ubiquitin-dependent proteolytic pathway (Scheffner et al. 1990; Maltzman and Czyzyk 1984; Kastan et al. 1991, 1992; Nelson and Kastan 1994; Lu and Lane 1993; Di Leonardo et al. 1994; Huang et al. 1996). The molecular pathway between DNA damage and p53 protein accumulation is not understood. p53 protein may be involved as one of the sensors of DNA damage. The COOH-terminal of p53 can bind nonspecifically to ends of DNA molecules and catalyze DNA renaturation and strand transfer (Jayaraman and Prives 1995; Brain and Jenkins 1994; Oberosler et al. 1993; Foord et al. 1991; Reed et al. 1995). This region of the protein can also bind to extra-helical regions of DNA damage involved in forming insertion/deletion mismatches (Lee et al. 1995). It will be interesting to determine if p53 recognizes other types of DNA damage including carcinogen-DNA adducts.

Wild-type p53 protein can transcriptionally transactivate genes involved in cell cycle arrest (e.g, $p21^{waf1}$, a potent inhibitor of most cyclin-dependent kinases: Harper et al. 1993; El-Deiry et al. 1993; Xiong et al. 1993) and interact either with the DNA repair and synthetic machinery, e.g., proliferating cellular nuclear antigen (PCNA), GADD45 and $p21^{waf1}$ (Smith et al. 1994; Li et al. 1994) or proteins modulating apoptosis (e.g., Bax and Fas: Selvakumaran et al. 1994; Miyashita and Reed 1995). Certain other genes containing TATA boxes in their promoter regions, e.g., *bcl-2* (Miyashita et al. 1994), can be *trans*-repressed perhaps by p53 binding to the TATA binding protein (TBP) and inhibiting its function as a basal transcription factor (Seto et al. 1992; Liu et al. 1993; Truant et al. 1993; Chen et al. 1993). p53 can also inhibit DNA synthesis by a transcription- independent mechanism binding to putative origins of DNA replication and either prevent initiation or early replication fork unwinding (Miller et al. 1995; Cox et al. 1995). p53 forms protein-protein complexes with cellular proteins involved in DNA synthesis (e.g., RPA, replicating protein antigen: Dutta et al. 1993), DNA repair (e.g., RPA, XPB, XPD, p62, topoisomerase I and CSB: Dutta et al. 1993; Wang et al. 1994, 1995b; Xiao et al. 1994; Leveillard et al. 1996; Gobert et al. 1996), and apoptosis (e.g., XPB and XPD: Wang et al. 1996). Cellular context determines whether p53 can induce apoptosis, independent or dependent of its transcription transactivation function and in the absence of RNA and protein synthesis (Wang et al. 1996; Caelles et al. 1994; Haupt et al. 1995; Wagner et al. 1994; Del Sal et al. 1995; Sakamuro et al. 1995). Interestingly, cycloheximide, an inhibitor of protein synthesis, can induce apoptosis (Harris et al. 1968; Martin 1993; Bazar and Deeg 1992) and a temperature-sensitive mutant of a basal transcription factor, $GG1/TAF_{II}250$, when inactivated at a nonpermissive temperature, induces apoptosis (Sekiguchi et al. 1995). Cells from patients with Cockayne's B syndrome, which are deficient in transcribed strand specific repair, have increased sensitivity to ultraviolet (UV) light-induced apoptosis (Ljungman and Zhang 1996). Since the induction of apoptosis was positively correlated with p53 accumulation and inhibition of transcription,

Ljungman and Zhang (1996) have speculated that blockage of RNA polymerase by UV damage in the transcribing DNA strand initiates the apoptosis response to UV. All of these results are consistent with the hypothesis that the apoptotic protein machinery is constitutively present in a latent state and does not require the synthesis of additional proteins. Nevertheless, p53 regulation of genes, whose products (e.g., Bax, Bcl2 and p21$^{\text{Waf1}}$) may be involved in apoptosis, could modulate a cell's sensitivity to inducers of apoptosis. p53 initiated G1/S cell cycle arrest is primarily mediated by up-regulation of p21$^{\text{Waf1}}$ (Harper et al. 1993; El-Deiry et al. 1993; Xiong et al. 1993), but p21$^{\text{Waf1}}$ is not an inducer of apoptosis in that ionizing radiation induces a p53-dependent apoptosis in p21$^{-/-}$ cells from p21$^{\text{Waf1}}$ gene knockout mice (Brugarolas et al. 1995; Deng et al. 1995). Therefore, p53 may function by transcription transactivator-dependent and -independent mechanisms in interactive, yet distinct pathways of cell cycle arrest and apoptosis.

Molecular Archaeology of Tumor Suppressor Genes

Several endogenous and exogenous mutagens have been described to induce a characteristic pattern of DNA alteration. Mutational spectrum analysis is required to study the type, location and frequency of DNA changes. Alterations of cancer-related genes found in tumors not only represents the interaction of a carcinogen with DNA and cellular DNA repair processes, but also reflect the selection of those mutations that provide premalignant and malignant cells with a clonal growth advantage. Study of the frequency, timing and mutational spectra of p53 and other cancer related genes provide insight into the etiology and molecular pathogenesis of cancer and generate hypotheses for future investigations. These include questions regarding carcinogen-DNA interactions, function of the affected gene products, mechanism of carcinogenesis in specific organs or tissues and features of general cell biology, such as DNA replication and repair.

Nonsense mutations, deletions and insertions are the most frequent types of mutations in tumor suppressor genes that produce either an absentee or truncated protein product. These mutations are clearly loss-of-function mutations. In contrast, the p53 tumor suppressor gene shows an unusual spectrum of mutations when compared with other suppressor genes, e.g., *APC*, *BRCA-1* or *ATM* (Fig. 4). Missense mutations in which the encoded protein contains amino acid substitutions are commonly found in the p53 tumor suppressor gene. The missense class of mutations can cause both a loss of tumor suppressor function and a gain of oncogenic function by changing the repertoire of genes whose expression are controlled by this transcription factor (Lane and Benchimol 1990; Dittmer et al. 1993; Hsiao et al. 1994). The p53 gene was initially classified as an oncogene, until it was discovered in the late 1980s that the cDNAs cloned from murine and human tumor cells contained missense mutations; it was correctly classified when a true wild-type p53 gene construct suppressed the growth of tumor cells (Eliyahu et al.

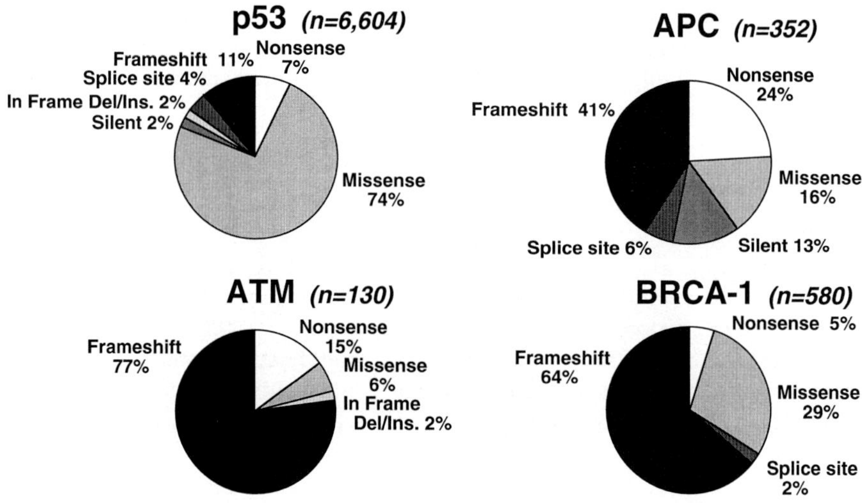

Fig. 4. Class of mutations found in tumor suppressor genes

1989; Finlay et al. 1989; Baker et al. 1990; Diller et al. 1990; Mercer et al. 1990; Chen et al. 1991; Cariello et al. 1994). This functional duality may be one explanation for the high frequency of p53 mutations in human cancer.

The p53 gene is well suited to mutational spectrum analysis for several reasons. First, since p53 mutations are common in many human cancers, a sizeable data base of more than 7000 entries has accrued, the analysis of which can yield statistically valid conclusions (Hainaut et al. 1997). The modest size of the p53 gene (11 exons, 393 amino acids) permits study of the entire coding region, and it is highly conserved in vertebrates, allowing extrapolation of data from animal models (Soussi et al. 1990). Point mutations that alter p53 function are distributed over a large region of the molecule, especially in the hydrophobic midportion (Hollstein et al. 1991; Levine et al. 1991; Greenblatt et al. 1994), where many base substitutions alter p53 conformation and sequence-specific *trans*-activation activity; thus correlation between distinct mutants and functional changes are possible (Fig. 5). Frameshift and nonsense mutations that truncate the protein can be located outside of these regions, so evaluation of the entire DNA sequence yields relevant data. This situation differs from the *ras* oncogenes whose transforming mutations occur primarily in three codons, a few sequence-specific motifs and a critical functional domain (Park and Vande Woude 1989). The diversity of p53 mutational events permits more extensive inferences regarding mechanisms of DNA damage.

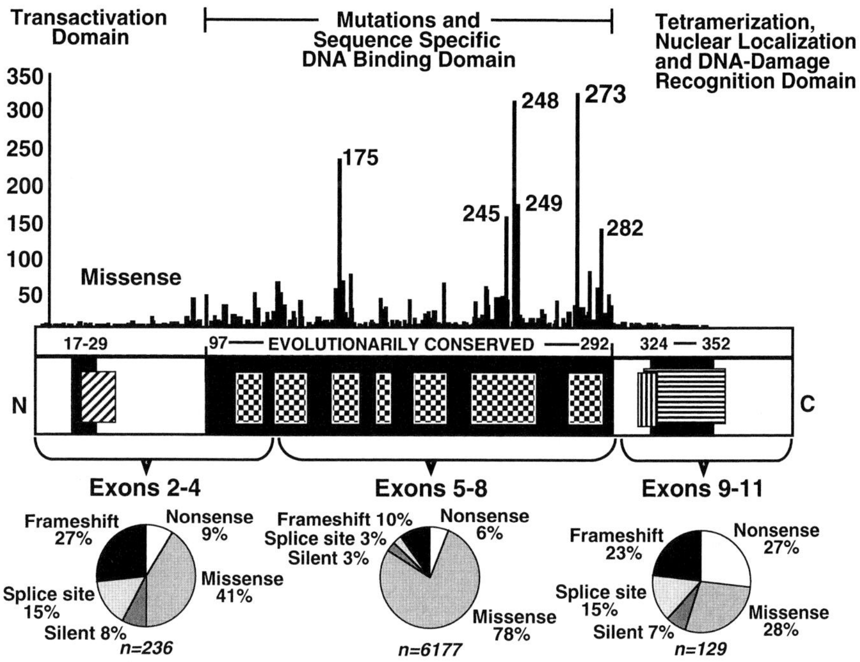

Fig. 5. The p53 molecule. The human p53 protein consists of 393 amino acids with functional domains, evolutionary conserved domains, and regions designated as mutational hotspots (reviewed in Greenblatt et al. 1994). Missense or nonsense mutation: functional domains include the transactivation region (*diagonally striped block*), sequence-specific DNA binding region (amino acids 100–293), nuclear localization sequence (amino acids 316–325, *vertical-striped block*), and oligomerization region (amino acids 319–360, *horizontal-striped block*). Evolutionary conserved domains (amino acids 17–29, 97–292, and 324–352; black areas) were determined using the MACAW program. Seven mutational hotspot and evolutionarily conserved regions within the large conserved domain are also identified (amino acids 130–142, 151–164, 171–181, 193–200, 213–233, 234–258, and 270–286, *checkered blocks*). *Vertical lines* above the schematic are missense mutations. The majority of missense mutations are in the conserved hydrophobic midregion of the protein that is required for the sequence-specific binding to DNA, the nonmissense (nonsense, frameshift, splicing, and silent mutations) are distributed throughout the protein, determined primarily by sequence context. Deletions and insertions are more common in the NH_2-terminal and COOH-terminal of the p53 gene

Molecular Linkage Between Carcinogen Exposure and Cancer

A number of specific p53 mutational hotspots have been identified in different human cancers (Fig. 6). Molecular linkage between carcinogen exposure and cancer can be well exemplified by the p53 mutational spectrum of hepatocellular carcinoma, skin cancer and lung cancer. In liver tumors from persons living in geographic areas in which aflatoxin B_1 and hepatitis B virus (HBV) are cancer risk factors, most p53 mutations are at the third nucleotide pair of codon 249 (Hsu et al. 1991; Bressac et al. 1991; Scorsone et al. 1992; Li et al. 1993). A dose-dependent relationship between dietary aflatoxin B_1 intake and codon 249^{ser} p53 mutations is observed in hepatocellular carcino-

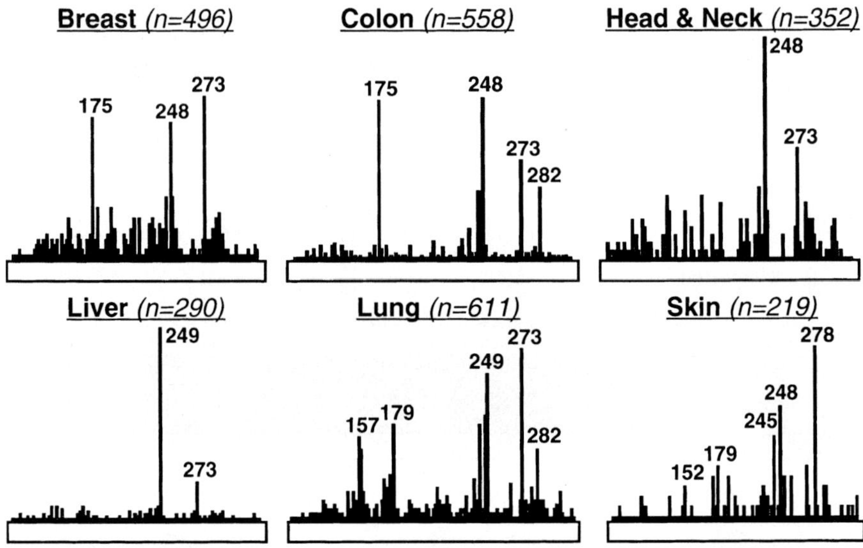

Fig. 6. p53 mutational hotspots in human cancers

ma from Asia, Africa and North America (reviewed in Harris, 1996). The mutation load of 249^{ser} mutant cells in nontumorous liver also is positively correlated with dietary aflatoxin B_1 exposure (Aguilar et al. 1994). Exposure of aflatoxin B_1 to human liver cells in vitro produces 249^{ser} (AGG to AGT) p53 mutants (Aguilar et al. 1993; Mace et al. 1997). These results indicate that expression of the 249^{ser} mutant p53 protein provides a specific growth and/or survival advantage to liver cells and are consistent with the hypothesis that p53 mutations can occur early in liver carcinogenesis.

Sunlight exposure is a well known risk factor for skin cancer. CC to TT double mutations are frequently found in squamous and basal cell skin carcinoma (Brash et al. 1991), while it is rarely reported in other forms of cancers (Greenblatt et al. 1994). In vitro studies have shown the induction of the characteristic CC to TT mutations by ultraviolet exposure (Hsia et al. 1989; Bredberg et al. 1986; Brash 1988; Kress et al. 1992; Tornaletti et al. 1993). Sunlight exposed normal and precancerous skin contains CC to TT double mutations (Nakazawa et al. 1994; Ziegler et al. 1994). These results indicate that CC to TT mutations which can be induced by sunlight exposure, may play a role in the occurrence of skin cancer.

Cigarette smoking is a major risk factor for the incidence of lung cancer. Benzo(a)pyrene, a chemical carcinogen in tobacco smoke, causes p53 hotspot mutations at codons 157, 248 and 273 in lung cancer. A dose-response increase in p53 G to T transversion mutations with cigarette smoking has been reported in lung cancer (Takeshima et al. 1993). Interestingly, codon 157 (GTC to TTC) mutations are uncommon in other types of cancer and have not been found in lung cancer from never smokers (Greenblatt et al. 1994).

Table 1. Assessment of causation by the Bradford-Hill criteria. Hypothesis: Dietary aflatoxin B$_1$ (AFB$_1$) exposure can produce 249^{ser} (AGG to AGT) *p53* mutations during human liver carcinogenesis

Strength of association	Biological plausibility

Consistency
  Positive correlation between estimated dietary AFB$_1$ exposure and frequency of 249^{ser} *p53* mutations in three different ethnic populations on three continents (Hsu et al. 1991; Bressac et al. 1991; Soini et al. 1996).
Specificity
  249^{ser} *p53* mutant cells are observed in non-tumorous liver in high HCC incidence geographic areas (Aguilar et al. 1994).
	AFB$_1$ is enzymatically activated by human hepatocytes (Autrup et al. 1984; Pfeifer et al. 1993) and the 8,9-AFB$_1$ oxide binds to the third base (G) in codon 249 (Puisieux et al. 1991). AFB$_1$ exposure to human liver cells(Aguilar et al. 1993; Mace et al. 1997) in vitro produces codon 249^{ser} *p53* mutations.
	249^{ser} *p53* expression inhibits apoptosis (Wang et al. 1995a), *p53* mediated transcription (Forrester et al. 1995) and enhances liver cell growth in vitro (Ponchel et al. 1994).

Table 2. Assessment of causation by the Bradford-Hill criteria. Hypothesis: Chemical carcinogens, e.g., benzo[a]pyrene (BP), in tobacco smoke cause *p53* hotspot mutations at codons 157, 248 and 273 in human lung carcinogenesis

Strength of association	Biological plausibility

Consistency
  Cigarette smoking is associated with a dose-response increase in *p53* mutations (G to T transversions) in human lung cancer (Takeshima et al. 1993).
Specificity
  Codon 157 (GTC toTTC) mutations are uncommon in other types of cancer and have not been found in lung cancer from never smokers (Greenblatt et al. 1994).
Temporality
  p53 mutations can be found in bronchial dysplasia (Vahakangas et al. 1992).
	BP is metabolically activated and forms BP diol epoxide-DNA adducts in human bronchus in vitro (75-fold interindividual variation) (Harris et al. 1974; Jeffrey et al. 1977).
	BP diol epoxide binds to Gs in codons 157, 248 and 273, which are *p53* mutational hotspots (Denissenko et al. 1996).
	BP exposure to human cells in vitro produces codon 248 (CGG to CTG) *p53* mutations (Cherpillod and Amstad 1995).
	Cigarette smoke condensates or BP can neoplastically transform human bronchial epithelial cells in the laboratory (Klein-Szanto et al. 1992; Iizasa et al. 1993).

Recently it was shown that BP diol epoxide, the metabolically activated form of BP, binds to guanosine residues in codons 157, 248 and 273 which are mutational hotspots in lung cancer (Denissenko et al. 1996). Cigarette smoke condensate or BP also neoplastically transforms human bronchial epithelial cells (Klein-Szanto et al. 1992).

Assessment of Causation by Bradford-Hill Criteria

Results obtained from molecular epidemiological studies can be used for the assessment of causation. Using "weight of the evidence" principle, Bradford-Hill (Hill, 1965) proposed criteria in the assessment of cancer causation including strength of association (consistency, specificity and temporality) and

Table 3. Assessment of causation by the Bradford-Hill criteria. Hypothesis: Sunlight exposure can cause a characteristic CC to TT tandem double mutation in *p53* in human skin cancer

Strength of association	Biological plausibility
Consistency Commonality of CC to TT tandem double mutation in squamous and basal cell skin carcinoma (Brash et al. 1991; Ziegler et al. 1994; Daya-Grosjean et al. 1995). Specificity Tandem dipyrimidine CC to TT mutations are uncommon in other types of cancer (Greenblatt et al. 1994). Temporality CC to TT mutations are found in normal and precancerous skin (Nakazawa et al. 1994; Ziegler et al. 1994).	Cyclobutane pyrimidine dimers and pyrimidine photoproducts are the two major adducts produced by UV- irradiation and induces C to T, at non-CpG sites, and CC to TT mutations (Tornaletti et al. 1993; Brash 1988; Cherpillod and Amstad, 1995). Skin cancer in xeroderma pigmentosum patients, with defective nucleotide excision repair, contains a high frequency of CC to TT mutations (Dumaz et al. 1993). UV exposure produces CC to TT mutations in studies using phage, bacteria and mice (Hsia et al. 1989; Bredberg et al. 1986; Brash 1988; Kress et al. 1992).

biological plausibility. For example, there is a considerable amount of evidence now consistent with the hypotheses that dietary aflatoxin B_1 exposure can produce codon 249^{ser} (AGG to AGT) p53 mutations during human liver carcinogenesis (Table 1), the chemical carcinogen, e.g., benzo(a)pyrene, in tobacco smoke cause p53 hotspot mutations in human lung carcinogenesis (Table 2), and sunlight exposure causes the characteristic CC to TT double mutations in p53 in human skin cancer (Table 3).

Acknowledgements. We thank Dorothea Dudek for her editorial and graphic assistance.

References

Aguilar F, Hussain SP, Cerutti P (1993) Aflatoxin B1 induces the transversion of G→T in codon 249 of the p53 tumor suppressor gene in human hepatocytes. Proc Natl Acad Sci USA, 90:8586–8590

Aguilar F, Harris CC, Sun T, Hollstein M, Cerutti P (1994) Geographic variation of p53 mutational profile in nonmalignant human liver. Science 264:1317–1319

Autrup H, Harris CC, Wu SM, Bao LY, Pei XF, Lu S, Sun TT, Hsia CC (1984) Activation of chemical carcinogens by cultured human fetal liver, esophagus and stomach. Chem. Biol. Interact 50:15–25

Baker SJ, Markowitz S, Fearon ER, Willson JK, Vogelstein B (1990) Suppression of human colorectal carcinoma cell growth by wild-type p53. Science 249:912–915

Bazar LS, Deeg HJ (1992) Ultraviolet B-induced DNA fragmentation (apoptosis) in activated T-lymphocytes and Jurkat cells is augmented by inhibition of RNA and protein synthesis. Exp Hematol 20:80–86

Brain R, Jenkins JR (1994) Human p53 directs DNA strand reassociation and is photolabelled by 8-azido ATP. Oncogene 9:1775–1780

Brash DE (1988) UV mutagenic photoproducts in Escherichia coli and human cells: a molecular genetics perspective on human skin cancer. Photochem Photobiol 48:59–66

Brash DE, Rudolph JA, Simon JA, Lin A, McKenna GJ, Baden HP, Halperin AJ, Ponten J (1991) A role for sunlight in skin cancer: UV-induced p53 mutations in squamous cell carcinoma. Proc Natl Acad Sci USA 88:10124–10128

Bredberg A, Kraemer KH, Seidman MM (1986) Restricted ultraviolet mutational spectrum in a shuttle vector propagated in xeroderma pigmentosum cells. Proc Natl Acad Sci USA 83: 8273–8277

Bressac B, Kew M, Wands J, Ozturk M (1991) Selective G to T mutations of p53 gene in hepato-cellular carcinoma from southern Africa. Nature 350:429–431

Brugarolas J, Chandrasekaran C, Gordon JI, Beach D, Jacks T, Hannon GJ (1995) Radiation-induced cell cycle arrest compromised by p21 deficiency. Nature 377:552–557

Caelles C, Helmberg A, Karin M (1994) p53-dependent apoptosis in the absence of transcriptional activation of p53-target genes [see comments]. Nature 370:220–223

Cariello NF, Cui L, Beroud C, Soussi T (1994) Database and software for the analysis of mutations in the human p53 gene. Cancer Res 54:4454–4460

Chen PL, Chen Y, Bookstein R, Lee WH (1991) Genetic mechanisms of tumor suppression by the human p53 gene. Science 250:1576–1580

Chen X, Farmer G, Zhu H, Prywes R, Prives C (1993) Cooperative DNA binding of p53 with TFIID (TBP): a possible mechanism for transcriptional activation [published erratum appears in Genes Dev 1993 Dec;7(12B):2652]. Genes Dev 7:1837–1849

Cherpillod P, Amstad PA (1995) Benzo[a]pyrene-induced mutagenesis of p53 hot-spot codons 248 and 249 in human hepatocytes. Mol Carcinog 13:15–20

Cox LS, Hupp T, Midgley CA, Lane DP (1995) A direct effect of activated human p53 on nuclear DNA replication. EMBO J 14:2099–2105

Daya-Grosjean L, Dumaz N, Sarasin A (1995) The specificity of p53 mutation spectra in sunlight induced human cancers. J Photochem Photobiol B 28:115–124

Del Sal G, Ruaro EM, Utrera R, Cole CN, Levine AJ, Schneider C (1995) Gas1-induced growth suppression requires a transactivation-independent p53 function. Mol Cell Biol 15:7152–7160

Deng C, Zhang P, Harper JW, Elledge SJ, Leder P (1995) Mice lacking p21CIP1/WAF1 undergo normal development, but are defective in G1 checkpoint control. Cell 82:675–684

Denissenko MF, Pao A, Tang M, Pfeifer GP (1996) Preferential formation of benzo[a]pyrene adducts at lung cancer mutational hotspots in p53. Science 274:430–432

Di Leonardo A, Linke SP, Clarkin K, Wahl GM (1994) DNA damage triggers a prolonged p53-dependent G1 arrest and long-term induction of Cip1 in normal human fibroblasts. Genes Dev 8:2540–2551

Diller L, Kassel J, Nelson CE, Gryka MA, Litwak G, Gebhardt M, Bressac B, Ozturk M, Baker SJ, Vogelstein B (1990) p53 Functions as a cell cycle control protein in osteosarcomas. Mol Cell Biol 10:5772–5781

Dittmer D, Pati S, Zambetti G, Chu S, Teresky AK, Moore M, Finlay C, Levine AJ (1993) Gain of function mutations in p53. Nature [Genet] 4:42–46

Dumaz N, Drougard C, Sarasin A, Daya-Grosjean L (1993) Specific UV-induced mutation spectrum in the p53 gene of skin tumors from DNA-repair-deficient xeroderma pigmentosum patients. Proc Natl Acad Sci USA 90:10529–10533

Dutta A, Ruppert JM, Aster JC, Winchester E (1993) Inhibition of DNA replication factor RPA by p53. Nature 365:79–82

El-Deiry WS, Tokino T, Velculescu VE, Levy DB, Parsons R, Trent JM, Lin D, Mercer WE, Kinzler KW, Vogelstein B (1993) WAF1, a potential mediator of p53 tumor suppression. Cell 75:817–825

Eliyahu D, Michalovitz D, Eliyahu S, Pinhasi-Kimhi O, Oren M (1989) Wild-type p53 can inhibit oncogene-mediated focus formation. Proc Natl Acad Sci USA 86:8763–8767

Finlay CA, Hinds PW, Levine AJ (1989) The p53 proto-oncogene can act as a suppressor of transformation. Cell 57:1083–1093

Foord OS, Bhattacharya P, Reich Z, Rotter V (1991) A DNA binding domain is contained in the C-terminus of wild type p53 protein. Nucleic Acids Res 19:5191–5198

Forrester K, Lupold SE, Ott VL, Chay CH, Band V, Wang XW, Harris CC (1995) Effects of p53 mutants on wild-type p53-mediated transactivation are cell type dependent. Oncogene 10:2103–2111

Gobert C, Bracco L, Rossi F, Olivier M, Tazi J, Lavelle F, Larsen AK, Riou JF (1996) Modulation of DNA topoisomerase I activity by p53. Biochemistry 35:5778–5786

Greenblatt MS, Bennett WP, Hollstein M, Harris CC (1994) Mutations in the p53 tumor suppressor gene: clues to cancer etiology and molecular pathogenesis. Cancer Res 54:4855–4878

Guillouf C, Rosselli F, Krishnaraju K, Moustacchi E, Hoffman B, Liebermann DA (1995) p53 Involvement in control of G2 exit of the cell cycle: role in DNA damage-induced apoptosis. Oncogene 10:2263–2270

Hainaut P, Soussi T, Shomer B, Hollstein M, Greenblatt M, Hovig E, Harris CC, Montesano R (1997) Database of p53 gene somatic mutations in human tumors and cell lines: updated compilation and future prospects. Nucleic Acids Res 25:151–157

Harper JW, Adami GR, Wei N, Keyomarsi K, Elledge SJ (1993) The p21 cdk-interacting protein Cip1 is a potent inhibitor of G1 cyclin-dependent kinases. Cell 75:805–816

Harris CC (1991) Chemical and physical carcinogenesis: advances and perspectives for the 1990's. Cancer Res 51:5023s–5044s

Harris CC (1996) The 1995 Walter Hubert Lecture – Molecular epidemiology of human cancer: insights from the mutational analysis of the p53 tumor suppressor gene. Br J Cancer 73:261–269

Harris CC, Grady H, Svoboda D (1968) Alterations in pancreatic and hepatic ultrastructure following acute cycloheximide intoxication. J Ultrastruct Res 22:240–251

Harris CC, Genta VM, Frank AL, Kaufman DG, Barrett LA, McDowell EM, Trump BF (1974) Carcinogenic polynuclear hydrocarbons bind to macromolecules in cultured human bronchi. Nature 252:68–69

Haupt Y, Rowan S, Shaulian E, Vousden KH, Oren M (1995) Induction of apoptosis in HeLa cells by trans-activation-deficient p53. Genes Dev 9:2170–2183

Hill AB (1965) The environment and disease: association or causation. Proc R Soc Med 58:295–300

Hollstein M, Sidransky D, Vogelstein B, Harris CC (1991) p53 Mutations in human cancers. Science 253:49–53

Hsia HC, Lebkowski JS, Leong PM, Calos MP, Miller JH (1989) Comparison of ultraviolet irradiation-induced mutagenesis of the lacI gene in Escherichia coli and in human 293 cells. J Mol Biol 205:103–113

Hsiao M, Low J, Dorn E, Ku D, Pattengale P, Yeargin J, Haas M (1994) Gain-of-function mutations of the p53 gene induce lymphohematopoietic metastatic potential and tissue invasiveness. Am J Pathol 145:702–714

Hsu IC, Metcalf RA, Sun T, Welsh JA, Wang NJ, Harris CC (1991) Mutational hotspot in the p53 gene in human hepatocellular carcinomas. Nature 350:427–428

Huang LC, Clarkin KC, Wahl GM (1996) Sensitivity and selectivity of the DNA damage sensor responsible for activating p53-dependent G1 arrest. Proc Natl Acad Sci USA 93:4827–4832

Iizasa T, Momiki S, Bauer B, Caamano J, Metcalf R, Lechner J, Harris CC, Klein-Szanto AJ (1993) Invasive tumors derived from xenotransplanted, immortalized human cells after in vivo exposure to chemical carcinogens. Carcinogenesis 14:1789–1794

Jayaraman L, Prives C (1995) Activation of p53 sequence-specific DNA binding by short single strands of DNA requires the p53 C-terminus. Cell 81:1021–1029

Jeffrey AM, Weinstein IB, Jennette KW, Grzeskowiak K, Nakanishi K, Harvey RG, Autrup H, Harris CC (1977) Structures of benzo(a)pyrene-nucleic acid adducts formed in human and bovine bronchial explants. Nature 269:348–350

Kastan MB, Radin AI, Kuerbitz SJ, Onyekwere O, Wolkow CA, Civin CI, Stone KD, Woo T, Ravindranath Y, Craig RW (1991) Levels of p53 protein increase with maturation in human hematopoietic cells. Cancer Res 51:4279–4286

Kastan MB, Zhan Q, El-Deiry WS, Carrier F, Jacks T, Walsh WV, Plunkett BS, Vogelstein B, Fornace Jr (1992) A mammalian cell cycle checkpoint pathway utilizing p53 and GADD45 is defective in Ataxia-Telangiectasia. Cell 71:587–597

Klein-Szanto AJ, Iizasa T, Momiki S, Garcia-Palazzo I, Caamano J, Metcalf R, Welsh J, Harris CC (1992) A tobacco-specific N-nitrosamine or cigarette smoke condensate causes neoplastic transformation of xenotransplanted human bronchial epithelial cells. Proc Natl Acad Sci USA 89:6693–6697

Kress S, Sutter C, Strickland PT, Mukhtar H, Schweizer J, Schwarz M (1992) Carcinogen-specific mutational pattern in the p53 gene in ultraviolet B radiation-induced squamous cell carcinomas of mouse skin. Cancer Res 52:6400–6403

Lane DP, Benchimol S (1990) p53: oncogene or anti-oncogene. Genes Dev 4:1–8

Lee S, Elenbase B, Levine A, Griffith J (1995) p53 and its 14kDa C-terminal domain recognize primary DNA damage in the form of insertion/deletion mismatches. Cell 81:1013–1020

Leveillard T, Andera L, Bissonnette N, Schaeffer L, Bracco L, Egly JM, Wasylyk B (1996) Functional interactions between p53 and the TFIIH complex are affected by tumour-associated mutations. EMBO J 15:1615–1624

Levine AJ, Momand J, Finlay CA (1991) The p53 tumour suppressor gene. Nature 351:453–456

Li D, Cao Y, He L, Wang NJ, Gu J (1993) Aberrations of p53 gene in human hepatocellular carcinoma from China. Carcinogenesis 14:169–173

Li FP, Garber JE, Friend SH, Strong LC, Patenaude AF, Juengst ET, Reilly PR, Correa YP, Fraumeni JF Jr (1992) Recommendations on predictive testing for germ line p53 mutations among cancer-prone individuals. J Natl Cancer Inst 84:1156–1160

Li R, Waga S, Hannon GJ, Beach D, Stillman B (1994) Differential effects by the p21 CDK inhibitor on PCNA-dependent DNA replication and repair. Nature 371:534–537

Liu X, Miller CW, Koeffler PH, Berk AJ (1993) The p53 activation domain binds the TATA box-binding polypeptide in Holo-TFIID, and a neighboring p53 domain inhibits transcription. Mol Cell Biol 13:3291–3300

Ljungman M, Zhang F (1996) Blackage of RNA polymerase as a possible trigger for UV light-induced apoptosis. Oncogene

Lu X, Lane DP (1993) Differential induction of transcriptionally active p53 following UV or ionizing radiation: defects in chromosome instability syndromes? Cell 75:765–778

Mace K, Aguilar F, Wang JS, Vautravers P, Gomez-Lechon M, Gonzalea FJ, Groopman J, Harris CC, Pfeifer AMA (1997) Aflatoxin B1 induced DNA adduct formation and p53 mutations in CYP450-expressing human liver cell lines. Carcinogenesis 18:1291–1297

Maltzman W, Czyzyk L (1984) UV irradiation stimulates levels of p53 cellular tumor antigen in nontransformed mouse cells. Mol Cell Biol 4:1689–1694

Martin SJ (1993) Protein or RNA synthesis inhibition induces apoptosis of mature human CD4+ T cell blasts. Immunol Lett 35:125–134

Mercer WE, Shields MT, Amin M, Sauve GJ, Appella E, Romano JW, Ullrich SJ (1990) Negative growth regulation in a glioblastoma tumor cell line that conditionally expresses human wild-type p53. Proc Natl Acad Sci USA 87:6166–6170

Miller SD, Farmer G, Prives C (1995) p53 inhibits DNA replication in vitro and in a DNA-binding-dependent manner. Mol Cell Biol 15:6554–6560

Miyashita T, Reed JC (1995) Tumor suppressor p53 is a direct transcriptional activator of the human bax gene. Cell 80:293–299

Miyashita T, Krajewski S, Krajewska M, Wang HG, Lin HK, Liebermann DA, Hoffman B, Reed JC (1994) Tumor suppressor p53 is a regulator of bcl-2 and bax gene expression in vitro and in vivo. Oncogene 9:1799–1805

Nakazawa H, English D, Randell PL, Nakazawa K, Martel N, Armstrong BK, Yamasaki H (1994) UV and skin cancer: specific p53 gene mutation in normal skin as a biologically relevant exposure measurement. Proc Natl Acad Sci USA 91:360–364

National Research Council (1994) Science and judgement in risk assessment: assessment of toxicology. National Academy Press, Washington, DC, pp 56–67

Nelson WG, Kastan MB (1994) DNA strand breaks: the DNA template alterations that trigger p53-dependent DNA damage response pathways. Mol Cell Biol 14:1815–1823

Oberosler P, Hloch P, Ramsperger U, Stahl H (1993) p53-catalyzed annealing of complementary single-stranded nucleic acids. EMBO J 12:2389–2396

Park M, Van de Woude GF (1989) Cancer. In: DeVita VT Jr, Hellman S et al (eds) Principles of molecular cell biology of cancer: oncogenes, 3rd edn. Lippincott, New York, pp 45–66 (Principles and practice of oncology)

Perera FP (1996) Molecular epidemiology: insights into cancer susceptibility, risk assessment, and prevention. J Natl Cancer Inst 88:496–509

Perera FP, Santella R (1993) Molecular epidemiology. In: Schulte P, Perera FP (eds) Principles and practices: carcinogenesis. Academic, New York, pp 277–300

Pfeifer AMA, Cole KE, Smoot DT, Weston A, Groopman JD, Shields PG, Vignaud J-M, Juillerat M, Lipsky MM, Trump BF, Lechner JF, Harris CC (1993) SV40 T-antigen immortalized normal human liver epithelial cells express hepatocyte characteristics and metabolize chemical carcinogens. Proc Natl Acad Sci USA 90:5123–5127

Ponchel F, Puisieux A, Tabone E, Michot JP, Froschl G, Morel AP, Frebourg T, Fontaniere B, Oberhammer F, Ozturk M (1994) Hepatocarcinoma-specific mutant p53-249ser induces mitotic activity but has no effect on transforming growth factor beta 1-mediated apoptosis. Cancer Res 54:2064–2068

Powell SN, DeFrank JS, Connell P, Eogan M, Preffer F, Dombkowski D, Tang W, Friend S (1995) Differential sensitivity of p53(–) and p53(+) cells to caffeine-induced radiosensitization and override of G2 delay. Cancer Res 55:1643–1648

Puisieux A, Lim S, Groopman J, Ozturk M (1991) Selective targeting of p53 gene mutational hotspots in human cancers by etiologically defined carcinogens. Cancer Res 51:6185–6189

Reed M, Woelker B, Wang P, Wang Y, Anderson ME, Tegtmeyer P (1995) The C-terminal domain of p53 recognizes DNA damaged by ionizing radiation. Proc Natl Acad Sci USA 92:9455–9459

Sakamuro D, Eviner V, Elliott KJ, Showe L, White E, Prendergast GC (1995) c-Myc induces apoptosis in epithelial cells by both p53-dependent and p53-independent mechanisms. Oncogene 11:2411–2418

Scheffner M, Werness BA, Huibregtse JM, Levine AJ, Howley PM (1990) The E6 oncoprotein encoded by human papillomavirus types 16 and 18 promotes the degradation of p53. Cell 63:1129–1136

Scorsone KA, Zhou YZ, Butel JS, Slagle BL (1992) p53 Mutations cluster at codon 249 in hepatitis B virus-positive hepatocellular carcinomas from China. Cancer Res 52:1635–1638

Sekiguchi T, Nakashima T, Hayashida T, Kuraoka A, Hashimoto S, Tsuchida N, Shibata Y, Hunter T, Nishimoto T (1995) Apoptosis is induced in BHK cells by the tsBN462/13 mutation in the CCG1/TAFII250 subunit of the TFIID basal transcription factor. Exp Cell Res 218:490–498

Selvakumaran M, Lin HK, Miyashita T, Wang HG, Krajewski S, Reed JC, Hoffman B, Liebermann D (1994) Immediate early up-regulation of bax expression by p53 but not TGF beta 1: a paradigm for distinct apoptotic pathways. Oncogene 9:1791–1798

Seto E, Usheva A, Zambetti GP, Momand J, Horikoshi N, Weinmann R, Levine AJ, Shenk T (1992) Wild-type p53 binds to the TATA-binding protein and represses transcription. Proc Natl Acad Sci USA 89:12028–12032

Shields PG, Harris CC (1991) Molecular epidemiology and the genetics of environmental cancer. JAMA 266:681–687

Smith ML, Chen IT, Zhan Q, Bae I, Chen CY, Gilmer TM, Kastan MB, O'Connor PM, Fornace AJ Jr (1994) Interaction of the p53-regulated protein Gadd45 with proliferating cell nuclear antigen. Science 266:1376–1380

Soini Y, Chia SC, Bennett WP, Groopman JD, Wang JS, DeBenedetti VM, Cawley H, Welsh JA, Hansen C, Bergasa NV, Jones EA, DiBisceglie AM, Trivers GE, Sandoval CA, Calderon IE, Munoz Espinosa LE, Harris CC (1996) An aflatoxin-associated mutational hotspot at codon 249 in the p53 tumor suppressor gene occurs in hepatocellular carcinomas from Mexico. Carcinogenesis 17:1007–1012

Soussi T, Caron de Fromentel C, May P (1990) Structural aspects of the p53 protein in relation to gene evolution. Oncogene 5:945–952

Takeshima Y, Seyama T, Bennett WP, Akiyama M, Tokuoka S, Inai K, Mabuchi K, Land CE, Harris CC (1993) p53 Mutations in lung cancers from non-smoking atomic-bomb survivors. Lancet 342:1520–1521

Tornaletti S, Rozek D, Pfeifer GP (1993) The distribution of UV photoproducts along the human p53 gene and its relation to mutations in skin cancer [published erratum appears in Oncogene 1993 Dec; 8(12):3469]. Oncogene 8:2051–2057

Truant R, Xiao H, Ingles CJ, Greenblatt J (1993) Direct interaction between the transcriptional activation domain of human p53 and the TATA box-binding protein. J Biol Chem 268:2284–2287

Vahakangas KH, Samet JM, Metcalf RA, Welsh JA, Bennett WP, Lane DP, Harris CC (1992) Mutations of p53 and ras genes in radon-associated lung cancer from uranium miners. Lancet 339:576–580

Wagner AJ, Kokontis JM, Hay N (1994) Myc-mediated apoptosis requires wild-type p53 in a manner independent of cell cycle arrest and the ability of p53 to induce p21waf1/cip1. Genes Dev 8:2817–2830

Wang XW, Forrester K, Yeh H, Feitelson MA, Gu JR, Harris CC (1994) Hepatitis B virus X protein inhibits p53 sequence-specific DNA binding, transcriptional activity, and association with transcription factor ERCC3. Proc Natl Acad Sci USA 91:2230–2234

Wang XW, Gibson MK, Vermeulen W, Yeh H, Forrester K, Sturzbecher HW, Hoeijmakers JHJ, Harris CC (1995a) Abrogation of p53-induced apoptosis by the hepatitis B virus X gene. Cancer Res 55:6012–6016

Wang XW, Yeh H, Schaeffer L, Roy R, Moncollin V, Egly JM, Wang Z, Friedberg EC, Evans MK, Taffe BG, Bohr VA, Hoeijmakers JH, Forrester K, Harris CC (1995b) p53 Modulation of TFIIH-associated nucleotide excision repair activity. Nature [Genet] 10:188–195

Wang XW, Vermeulen W, Coursen JD, Gibson M, Lupold SE, Forrester K, Xu G, Elmore L, Yeh H, Hoeijmakers JHJ, Harris CC (1996) The XPB and XPD helicases are components of the p53-mediated apoptosis pathway. Genes Dev 10:1219–1232

Xiao H, Pearson A, Coulombe B, Truant R, Zhang S, Regier JL, Triezenberg SJ, Reinberg D, Flores O, Ingles CJ, Greenblatt J (1994) Binding of basal transcription factor TFIIH to the acidic activation domains of VP16 and p53. Mol Cell Biol 14:7013–7024

Xiong Y, Hannon GJ, Zhang H, Casso D, Kobayashi R, Beach D (1993) p21 is a universal inhibitor of cyclin kinases. Nature 366:701–704

Ziegler A, Jonason AS, Leffell DJ, Simon JA, Sharma HW, Kimmelman J, Remington L, Jacks T, Brash DE (1994) Sunburn and p53 in the onset of skin cancer. Nature 372:773–776

II. Risk Assessment and DNA Lesions

Molecular Epidemiology of Environmental Carcinogenesis

F. P. Perera

Columbia University School of Public Health,
Division of Environmental Health Science, 60 Haven Avenue,
B-116, New York, NY 10032, USA

Abstract

Environmental factors such as smoking, diet, and pollutants act in concert with individual susceptibility to cause most human cancers. This article briefly reviews molecular evidence that two types of susceptibility factors – common predisposing genetic traits and young age at exposure – convey heightened risk from certain exposures. Examples are drawn from molecular epidemiologic studies of common environmental carcinogens such as polycyclic aromatic hydrocarbons (PAH) and aromatic amines. Understanding of both genetic and acquired susceptibility in the population will be instrumental in developing health and regulatory policies that adequately protect of the more susceptible groups from risks of environmental carcinogens.

Introduction

The greatest potential of molecular epidemiology in cancer prevention lies in its ability to shed light on the complex interaction between the environment and individual susceptibility. That is, to elucidate relationships between exposures to tobacco smoke, dietary constituents, workplace and ambient pollutants, on the one hand, and individual susceptibility traits on the other. Known or suspected susceptibility factors include not only genetic polymorphisms affecting the metabolic activation and detoxification of carcinogens but a number of "acquired" factors (Table 1). An estimated 80% of cancer is thought to be related to these interactions and thus to be theoretically preventable through the identification and control of the environmental factors involved.

Molecular epidemiology can be a useful tool in this regard by enhancing our understanding of mechanisms in human carcinogenesis, identifying groups and ultimately individuals at greatest risk, and designing and tracking interventions to ensure their efficacy. It must be stressed that achievement of this potential necessitates the thorough validation of biomarkers and their use in conjunction with sound epidemiologic principles.

Recent Results in Cancer Research, Vol. 154
© Springer-Verlag Berlin · Heidelberg 1998

Table 1. Known or potential biologic susceptibility factors in cancer

Type	Factor	Type of cancer	Putative mechanism
Genetic factors			
Rare inherited syndromes	Li-Fraumeni	Breast, other	
	Rb	Retinoblastoma	
	Wilms tumor	Bladder	Loss or inactivation of tumor
	BRCA1	Breast	Suppressor gene
	FAP	Colon	
	HNPCC	Colon	
	XP	Skin	Defective DNA repair
	AT	Breast, other	
Common inherited genetic variants[a]	CYP1A1	Lung, other	Altered metabolism (substrate: PAH)
	CYP2D6	Lung	Altered metabolism (substrate: NNK)
	GST	Lung, bladder	Decreased detoxification (substrates: PAH, EtO, styrene, AFB_1)
	NAT2	Bladder, breast	Decreased detoxification (substrate: 4-ABP)
	O^6-Alkyldeoxyguanosine	Lung, other	Inefficient DNA repair
	h-ras- 1 VTR	Lung, breast other	Unknown
Ethnicity	Genetic and environmental	Various	Differing prevalence of genotypes and environmental patterns of exposure
Age	Physiologic	Breast, lung, other	Decreased detoxification, DNA repair, and immune function with early or old age
Gender	Hormonal	Breast, other	Deregulation of growth and differentiation through receptor binding
	Metabolic	Lung, other	Differing metabolic/detoxification patterns
Preexisting impairment	Immunologic, chronic disease, nutritional	Liver, lung, breast cervical, other	Decreased immune function, altered metabolism, detoxification, reduced repair, deregulation of growth and differentiation

[a] Associations reported in some, but not all, studies; risks are strongly dependent on exposure.
FAP, familial adenomatous polyposis; HNPCC, hereditary nonpolyposis colon cancer; VTR, variable tandem repeat; EtO, ethylene oxide. (Perera 1997; Perera and Weinstein 1982).

Considerable molecular epidemiologic research, including our own, has focussed on widespread chemical carcinogens, since exposures to them are often readily preventable once identified as harmful. There is substantial human exposure to hundreds of carcinogens, albeit generally at low concentrations – in tobacco smoke, diet, workplace, indoor and outdoor air and drinking water. As in the case of polycyclic aromatic hydrocarbons (PAH), benzene and pesticides, exposure frequently comes from multiple sources via multiple routes.

In terms of population attributable risk, common predisposing genotypes that affect metabolic handling of such carcinogens are more significant than rare high risk syndromes such as Li-Fraumeni, Rb and BRCA1 which have frequencies of less than 10^{-3}. Other susceptibility factors – perhaps equally important as the genetic ones – are age or stage of development at exposure, preexisting nutritional and health status, gender and ethnicity. I will discuss two of these susceptibility factors, common predisposing genetic polymorphisms and age at exposure, reviewing recent molecular epidemiologic evidence that these factors are capable of modulating the risk of diverse carcinogens.

But first, a word about the history and conceptual framework of molecular epidemiology. Molecular epidemiology has its roots in prior work in clinical chemistry and pathology, seroepidemiology, genetic epidemiology, multistage carcinogenesis and molecular biology. In contrast to traditional epidemiology, in which associations are observed between exposure/risk factors and disease, molecular epidemiology seeks to directly measure the intervening "black box" interactions. In 1982, Perera and Weinstein used the term molecular epidemiology to describe a comprehensive theoretical approach using biologic markers to document dose, preclinical effects and susceptibility to carcinogens directly in human populations (Perera and Weinstein, 1982). The purpose: to obtain early warning of potential risk and an understanding of the range and distribution of both exposure and susceptibility in the population. This information could then be used to inform interventions, both regulatory and behavioral.

Genetics Susceptibility

Although they pose low individual risk, more common genetic traits, such as those that influence the metabolic activation or detoxification of carcinogenic chemicals, can be important determinants of population risk. For example, the phase I cytochrome P450 enzymes catalyze the oxidative metabolism of diverse endogenous and exogenous chemicals from steroids to pollutants; during the oxidative process electrophilic and carcinogenic intermediates can be created. Many P450 genes are polymorphic, including *CYP1A1*, whose product metabolizes PAH such as benzo[a]pyrene (BP). About 10% of the Caucasian population has a highly inducible form of the enzyme that is associated with an increased risk of lung cancer in smokers. Although not all studies have been positive, in Japanese and certain Caucasian populations, increased lung cancer risk is correlated with one or both *CYP1A1* polymorphisms, the so-called Msp I polymorphism and the closely linked exon 7 (isoleucine to valine) polymorphism (Kawajiri et al. 1996; Nakachi et al. 1991; Xu et al. 1996). The greatest incremental lung cancer risk from the "susceptible" *CYP1A1* genotype, was seen in light smokers (seven times the risk of light smokers without the genotype) whereas heavy smokers with this genotype had less than twice the risk as smokers without the genotype (Kawajiri et al. 1996; Nakachi et al. 1991). The proposed mechanisms for this phenomenon are higher *CYP1A1* inducibility or enhanced catalytic activity of the valine-type *CYP1A1* enzyme. Consistent with these mechanisms, smoking volunteers in the US with the exon 7 mutation were found to have more PAH-DNA adducts in white blood cells than smokers without the variant (Mooney et al. 1997). PAH-DNA adducts are also elevated in cord blood and placenta of newborns with the *CYP1A1* MSP1 polymorphism, which suggests that the genetic polymorphism may increase risk from transplacental PAH exposure (Whyatt et al. 1998 and in press). In lung tissue of adults, adduct concentration correlates with *CYP1A1* expression or enzyme activity (Bartsch and Hietanen 1996). Finally, lung tumors of Japanese smokers were found to be significantly more likely to have *P53* mutations if they had the susceptible *CYP1A1* genotype (Kawajiri et al. 1996; Nakachi et al. 1991). As described below, variation in other cytochrome P450 genes, (such as *CYP1A2*, whose product metabolizes aromatic and heterocyclic amines,) can also modulate cancer risk (Vineis et al. 1994).

In contrast to the phase I activating enzymes, phase II enzymes, including epoxide hydrolase, *GST*, NAT, and sulfotransferase, generally detoxify carcinogenic metabolites to produce excretable hydrophilic products. For example, *GSTM1* detoxifies reactive intermediates of the carcinogens such as PAH, ethylene oxide and styrene. In about 50% of Caucasians, the *GSTM1* locus is entirely deleted. Many studies have associated *GSTM1* deletion with an increased risk of bladder and lung cancer (McWilliams et al. 1995; Bell et al. 1993). The importance of gene-environment interactions is illustrated by the finding that individuals with the null genotype had little risk of bladder cancer in the absence of exposure to tobacco smoke. In lung biopsies, the frequencies of PAH-DNA adducts and *p53* mutations were higher in persons with the *GSTM1* null genotype (Kato et al. 1995; Ryberg et al. 1994a, b). Finally, susceptibility to aflatoxin B_1 (AFB)- B_1 induced hepatocellular carcinoma has been associated with the deletion of *GSTM1* in combination with the epoxide hydrolase genotype that is correlated with low activity of the detoxification enzyme (McGlynn et al. 1995).

NAT2 deactivates carcinogenic aromatic amines through N-acetylation; 50%–60% of Caucasians and 30%–40% of African-Americans are "slow" acetylators (Yu et al. 1994, 1995). Some, but not all, studies indicate that persons with the NAT_2 slow acetylator genotype have a higher risk of bladder cancer if they are exposed to environmental carcinogens such as 2-napthylamine and 4-aminobiphenyl (4-ABP) (Vineis et al. 1994; Landi et al. 1996). With low exposure to tobacco smoke, slow acetylators had approximately twice as many 4-ABP hemoglobin adducts as did rapid acetylators; however, with higher exposure, NAT2 had no effect on adduct concentration. Among post-menopausal women, smoking increased breast cancer risk only among those with the NAT2 slow acetylator genotype (Ambrosone et al. 1996).

Not only can multiple genes modulate the effects of environmental carcinogens, but interactions between genes can result in a greater-than-additive effect on risk. Smokers with the combined rapid CYP1A2 oxidizer slow N-acetylation phenotype had more 4-ABP-hemoglobin than other smokers, but only when the smokers' dose was low (Vineis et al. 1994; Landi et al. 1996). Research with Japanese populations has revealed that individuals with the combination of the *CYP1A1* (Val/Val) and GSTM1 null genotypes, relative to persons with neither genotype, have an eightfold increase in frequency of *p53* mutations (Kawajiri et al. 1996; Nakachi et al. 1991) and an estimated sixfold greater risk of lung cancer (Kawajiri et al. 1996; Nakachi et al. 1991; Hayashi et al. 1992). Studies of the role of *CYP1A1* and *GST* in lung cancer risk in Caucasians have yielded inconsistent results, possibly because of ethnic differences in gene prevalence or linkage.

Much of this research suggests that common genetic polymorphisms in P450s and *NAT2* have a greater impact on procarcinogenic adducts and cancer risk when exposure to carcinogens is low. Although this pattern was not seen with *GSTM1* and bladder cancer, it is plausible that at higher exposure, the effects of certain genetic traits are overwhelmed by the environmental insults.

Age-Related Susceptibility

There are important age-related differences in susceptibility to environmental toxicants (Perera and Weinstein 1982; Perera 1996; Goldman 1995; Bearer 1995; National Academy of Sciences 1993, 1994). Experimental and epidemiologic data indicate that, because of differential exposure or physiological immaturity, infants and children have greater risk than adults from a number of environmental toxicants, including PAH, nitrosamines, pesticides, tobacco smoke, air pollution and radiation. The underlying mechanisms may include increased absorption and retention of toxicants, reduced detoxification and repair, the higher rate of cell proliferation during the early stages of development, and the fact that cancers initiated in the womb and in the early years have the opportunity to develop over many decades.

Relative to body weight, infants and children take in appreciably more food, water, and air – and any carcinogens contained in them – than do adults. The very young may also have uniquely high exposures from nursing and other behaviors. For example, relative to adults with background exposure, nursing infants have an estimated 10- to 20-fold greater average daily intake of dioxin, a carcinogen that accumulates in breast milk (Mott et al. 1994). Molecular epidemiologic studies also indicate that the young have a higher internal dose of toxicants and greater genetic damage than adults who are similarly exposed to tobacco smoke and PAH. In cord blood of newborns at delivery, concentrations of cotinine were significantly higher (by 70%) than in the mothers' blood, also sampled at delivery (Whyatt et al. 1996). The newborns had 30% more PAH-DNA adducts than their mothers. (Although that difference was not statistically significant, this finding was noteworthy because the internal dose of PAH to the fetus is estimated to be about one-tenth of that to the mother). Similarly, in young children, urinary levels of 1-hydroxypyrene glucuronide, an indicator of PAH exposure, were higher than those in their mothers (Kang et al. 1995).

Adolescence and young adulthood are also viewed as sensitive life stages because of greater proliferative activity in epithelial cells of certain tissues. Women who were in their teens at the time of the atomic bombings had the greatest risk of radiation-induced breast cancer (Tokunaga et al., 1987). Similarly, initiation of smoking at an early age confers a higher risk of lung, bladder, and possibly breast cancer. The risk for women who began smoking before age 25 is almost four times that for women who began after age 25 (Hegmann et al. 1993). Breast cancer risk associated with the *NAT2* slow acetylator genotype was higher in women who began smoking before the age of 16 (Ambrosone et al. 1996). Similarly, long-term use of oral contraceptives by young women and exposure to human papilloma virus at an early age have been associated with enhanced risk of breast and cervical cancer, respectively (see Perera 1996 for review).

Susceptibility in the elderly has received less attention in research. However, immune function and DNA repair efficiency both decrease with age, which reduces protection against environmental carcinogens.

Conclusion

I have highlighted two examples of susceptibility factors that modulate individual responses to environmental carcinogens. As reviewed elsewhere (Perera 1997), molecular data illustrate the complexity of environment-susceptibility interactions – not one gene, but multiple genes may be involved, and the effects of these genes can be modified by ethnicity, age, gender, nutritional status, and extent of carcinogen exposure (Perera 1997). Despite its complexity, this body of knowledge holds much potential in terms of cancer prevention. First, it has immediate application to the identification of environmental risk factors. In epidemiology, it has been difficult to detect relative risks of 1.5 or even 2.0. Causal relationships and underlying mechanisms may emerge more clearly when etiologic research is focused on subgroups with heightened sensitivity (Millikan et al. 1995). Second, the greatest strides in preventing cancer at the population level will come from interventions that protect the susceptible subgroups. Thus, knowledge of differential risk resulting from predisposing metabolic genetic traits, ethnicity, young age, gender, or health and nutritional impairment can be useful in developing regulations, public education, health surveillance, behavior modification programs, and chemoprevention strategies that will have the maximum impact.

References

Ambrosone CB, Freudenheim JL, Graham S, Marshal JR, Vena JE, Brasure JR, Michalek AM, Laughlin R, Nemoto T, Gillenwater KA et al (1996) Cigarette smoking, n-acetyltransferase 2 genetic polymorphisms, and breast cancer risk. JAMA 276:1494–1501

Bartsch J, Hietanen E (1996) The role of individual susceptiblity in cancer burden related to environmental exposure. Environ Health Perspect 104 (Suppl) 3:569–577

Bearer CF (1995) Environmental health hazards: how children are different from adults. Future Child 5:11–26

Bell DA, Taylor JA, Paulson DE, Robertson CN, Mohler JL, Lucier GW (1993) Genetic risk and carcinogen exposure: a common inherited defect of the carcinogen-metabolism gene glutathione S-transferase M1 (GSTM1) that increases susceptibility to bladder cancer. J Natl Cancer Inst 85:1159–1164

Goldman LR (1995) Children-unique and vulnerable. Environmental risks facing children and recommendations for response. Environ Health Perspect 103 (Suppl) 6:13–18

Hayashi S, Watanabe J, Kawajiri K (1992) High susceptibility to lung cancer analyzed in terms of combined genotype of P450IA1 and Mu-class Glutathione S-transferase genes. Jpn J Cancer Res 83:866–870

Hegmann KT, Fraser AM, Keaney RP, Moser SE, Nilasena DS (1993) The effect of age at smoking initiation on lung cancer risk. Epidemiology 4:444–448

Kang DH, Correa-Villasenor A, Breysse PN, Strickland PT (1995) Correlation of urinary 1-hydroxypyrene glucuronide concentration between children and their mothers. Proc Am Assoc Cancer Res 36:107

Kato S, Bowman ED, Harrington AM, Blomeke B, Shields PG (1995) Human lung carcinogen-DNA adduct levels mediated by genetic polymorphisms in vivo. J Natl Cancer Inst 87:902–907

Kawajiri K, Eguchi H, Nakachi K, Sekiya T, Yamamoto M (1996) Association of CYP1A1 germ line polymorphisms with mutations of the p53 gene in lung cancer. Cancer Res 56:72–76

Landi MT, Zocchetti C, Bernucci I, Kadlubar FF, Tannenbaum S, Skipper P, Bartsch H, Malaveille C, Shields P, Caporaso NE et al (1996) Cytochrome P4501A2: enzyme induction and genetic control in determining 4-aminobiphenyl-hemoglobin adduct levels. Cancer Epidemiol Biomarkers Prev 5:693–698

McGlynn KA, Rosvold EA, Lustbader ED, Hu Y, Clapper ML, Zhou T, Wild CP, Xia X-L, Baffoe-Bonnie A, Ofori-Adjei D et al (1995) Susceptibility to hepatocellular carcinoma is associated with genetic variation in the enzymatic detoxification of aflatoxin B_1. Proc Natl Acad Sci USA 92:2384–2397

McWilliams JE, Sanderson BJS, Harris EL, Richert-Boe KE, Henner WD (1995) Glutathione S-transferase M1 (GSTM1) deficiency and lung cancer risk. Cancer Epidemiol Biomarkers Prev 4:589–594

Millikan R, DeVoto E, Newman B, Savitz D (1995) Studying environmental influences and breast cancer risk: suggestions for an integrated population-based approach. Breast Cancer Res Treat 35:79–89

Mooney LA, Bell DA, Santella RM, Van Bennekum AM, Ottman R, Paik M, Blaner WS, Lucier GW, Covey L, Young TL et al (1997) Contribution of genetic and nutritional factors to DNA damage in heavy smokers. Carcinogenesis 18:503–509

Mott L, Vance F, Curtis J (1994) Handle with care: children and environmental carcinogens. Natural Resources Defense Council, New York

Nakachi K, Imai K, Hayashi S, Watanabe J, Kawajiri K (1991) Genetic susceptibility to squamous cell carinoma of the lung in relation to cigarette smoking dose. Cancer Res 51:5177–5180

National Academy of Sciences (1993) Pesticides in the diets of infants and children. National Academy Press, Washington, DC

National Academy of Sciences (1994) Science and judgement of risk assessment. National Academy Press, Washington, DC

Perera FP (1996) Molecular epidemiology: insights into cancer susceptibility, risk assessment, and prevention. J Natl Cancer Inst 88:496–509

Perera FP (1997) Environment and cancer: who are susceptible? Science 278:1068–1073

Perera FP, Weinstein IB (1982) Molecular epidemiology and carcinogen-DNA adduct detection: new approaches to studies of human cancer causation. J Chronic Dis 35:581–600

Ryberg D, Hewer A, Phillips DH, Haugen A (1194a) Different susceptibility to smoking-induced DNA damage among male and female lung cancer patients. Cancer Res 54:5801–5803

Ryberg D, Kure E, Lystad S, Skaug V, Stangeland L, Mercy K, Borresen AL, Haugen A (1994b) p53 mutations in lung tumors: relationship to putative susceptibility markers for cancer. Cancer Res 54:1551–1555

Tokunaga M, Land CE, Yamamoto T, Asano M, Tokvoka S, Ezaki H et al (1987) Incidence of female breast cancer among atomic bomb survivors. Hiroshima and Nagasaki 1950–1980. Radiat Res 112:243–272

Vineis P, Bartsch H, Caporaso N, Harrington AM, Kadlubar FF, Landl MT, Malaveille C, Shields PG, Skipper P, Talaska G et al (1994) Genetically based N-acetyltransferase metabolic polymorphism and low-level environmental exposure to carcinogens. Nature 369:154–156

Whyatt RM, Santella RM, Jedrychowski W, Garte SJ, Bell DA, Ottman R, Gladek-Yarborough A, Cosma G, Young T-L, Cooper TB, Randall MC, Manchester DK, Perera FP (1998) Relationship between ambient air pollution and procarcinogenic DNA damage in Polish mothers and newborns. Env Health Persp 106(Suppl 3):821–826

Whyatt RM, Bell DA, Jedrychowski W, Santella RM, Garte SJ, Gladek-Yarborough A, Cosma G, Manchester DK, Randall MC, Young T-L, Cooper TB, Ottman R, Perera FP: Polycyclic aromatic hydrocarbon-DNA adducts in human placenta and modulation by CYP1A1 enzyme induction and genotype. Carcinogenesis, in press

Yu MC, Skipper PL, Taghizadeh K, Tannenbaum SR, Chan KK, Henderson BE, Ross RK (1994) Acetylator phenotype, aminobiphenyl-hemoglobin adduct levels, and bladder cancer risk in white, black and Asian men in Los Angeles, California. J Natl Cancer Inst 86:712–716

Yu MC, Ross RK, Chan KK, Henderson BE, Skipper PL, Tannenbaum SR, Coetzee GA (1995) Glutathione S-transferase M1 genotype affects aminobiphenyl-hemoglobin adduct levels in White, Black and Asian smokers and nonsmokers. Cancer Epidemiol Biomarkers Prev 4:861–864

Polymorphisms of N-Acetyltransferases, Glutathione S-Transferases, Microsomal Epoxide Hydrolase and Sulfotransferases: Influence on Cancer Susceptibility

J. G. Hengstler, M. Arand, M. E. Herrero, and F. Oesch

Institute of Toxicology, Obere Zahlbacher Strasse 67, 55131 Mainz, Germany

Abstract

It has become clear that several polymorphisms of human drug-metabolizing enzymes influence an individual's susceptibility for chemical carcinogenesis. This review gives an overview on relevant polymorphisms of four families of drug-metabolizing enzymes. Rapid acetylators (with respect to N-acetyltransferase NAT2) were shown to have an increased risk of colon cancer, but a decreased risk of bladder cancer. In addition an association between a NAT1 variant allele (NAT*10, due to mutations in the polyadenylation site causing ~ two fold higher activity) and colorectal cancer among NAT2 rapid acetylators was observed, suggesting a possible interaction between NAT1 and NAT2. Glutathione S-transferases M1 and T1 (GSTM1 and GSTT1) are polymorphic due to large deletions in the structural gene. Meta-analysis of 12 case-control studies demonstrated a significant association between the homozygous deletion of GSTM1 (GSTM1-0) and lung cancer (odds ratio: 1.41; 95% CI: 1.23–1.61). Combination of GSTM1-0 with two allelic variants of cytochrome P4501A1 (CYP1A1), CYP1A1 m2/m2 and CYP1A1 Val/Val further increases the risk for lung cancer. Indirect mechanisms by which deletion of GSTM1 increases risk for lung cancer may include GSTM1-0 associated decreased expression of GST M3 and increased activity of CYP1A1 and 1A2. Combination of GST M1-0 and NAT2 slow acetylation was associated with markedly increased risk for lung cancer (odds ratio: 7.8; 95% CI: 1.4–78.7). In addition GSTM1-0 is clearly associated with bladder cancer and possibly also with colorectal, hepatocellular, gastric, esophageal (interaction with CYP1A1), head and neck as well as cutaneous cancer. In individuals with the GSTT1-0 genotype more chromosomal aberrations and sister chromatid exchanges (SCEs) were observed after exposure to 1,3-butadiene or various haloalkanes or haloalkenes. Evidence for an association between GSTT1-0 and myelodysplastic syndrome and acute lymphoblastic leukemia has been presented. A polymorphic site of GSTP1 (valine to isoleucine at codon 104) decreases activity to several carcinogenic diol epoxides and was associated with testicular, bladder and lung cancer. Microsomal expoxide hydrolase (mEH) is polymorphic due to amino acid variation at residues 113

Recent Results in Cancer Research, Vol. 154
© Springer-Verlag Berlin · Heidelberg 1998

and 139. Polymorphic variants of mEH were associated with hepatocellular cancer (His-113 allele), ovarian cancer (Tyr-113 allele) and chronic obstructive pulmonary disease (His-113 allele). Three human sulfotransferases (STs) are regulated by genetic polymorphisms (hDHEAST, hM-PST, TS PST). Since a large number of environmental mutagens are activated by STs an association with human cancer risk might be expected.

Introduction

It has become clear that interindividual differences in human susceptibility to genotoxic agents may depend on the individual's genetic makeup. Especially polymorphisms of human drug-metabolizing enzymes have been shown to influence susceptibility to genotoxic substances and to be associated with cancer risk. In addition it has become increasingly clear that polymorphisms of drug metabolizing enzymes also modulate the risk of developing specific types of cancer. Although several polymorphisms confer only a modestly increased risk of cancer, they still can be important to public health, particularly if the polymorphism and its associated cancer are common (McWilliams et al. 1995). Polymorphisms are defined as less frequent phenotypes, which occur in at least 1% of a population and are caused by gene mutations, especially point mutations, frame shift mutations, or gene deletions resulting in most cases (but not always) in enzymes with reduced or no activity. Large interethnic differences in the frequency of gene mutations responsible for polymorphisms have been observed.

This review gives an overview on polymorphisms of four important superfamilies of drug metabolizing enzymes, namely N-acetyltransferases (NAT1 and 2), glutathione S-transferases (GST M1, T1, and P1), microsomal epoxide hydrolase (mEH), and sulfotransferases (ST).

N-Acetyltransferases

The N-acetylation polymorphism was recognized already 1951 in tuberculosis patients treated with isoniazid (Evans 1968). The half-life of isoniazid in plasma was about 1 h in about 50% of the Caucasian patients compared to about 3 h in the second half of the patients. This difference could be explained by the polymorphism of NAT2 – the "classical" N-acetylation polymorphism – which inactivates isoniazid mainly in the liver (Blum et al. 1990; Hickman and Sim 1991). Rapid acetylators are either homozygous or heterozygous for the rapid acetylator allele, whereas slow acetylators are homozygous for the slow acetylator allele(s). Although a large percentage of slow acetylator phenotypes can be explained by three slow acetylator alleles (two in Caucasians, one in Asians), at least 20 rare NAT2 alleles are known (Vatsis et al. 1991; Blum et al. 1990; Martinez et al. 1995).

Later it was realized that the NAT2 polymorphism is associated with cancer risk. Rapid acetylators (NAT2) were shown to have an increased risk of colon cancer (Gonzalez and Idle 1994; Nebert 1991; Vineis and McMichael 1996). Recently, rapid acetylator phenotype (assessed by the rate of orally given sulphamethazine, a substrate specific to NAT2) was shown to be associated with colorectal cancer (odds ratio: 1.8; 95% CI: 1–3.3; number of patients: 110) (Roberts-Thomson et al. 1996). The highest risk was observed in the youngest tertile (<64 years) of patients in this study (odds ratio: 8.9; 95% CI: 2.6–30.4). The risk of colorectal cancer increased with increasing intake of meat in rapid, but not in slow, acetylators (Roberts-Thomson et al. 1996).

An association of the fast acetylator phenotype (with respect to NAT2) with increased risk of colorectal cancer may be explained by the participation of NAT2 in activation of heterocyclic aromatic amines formed during the cooking of meat and meat derived products. A principal route of metabolic activation of heterocyclic aromatic amines, e.g. 2-amino-3,8-dimethyl-imidazo[4,5-*f*]quinoxaline (MeIQx; Fig. 1) includes N-oxidation to hydroxylamines (e.g. by cytochrome P450 1A2), their subsequent activation by acetyl-transferase-catalyzed O-acetylation resulting in reactive N-acetoxy-esters, which can spontaneously lose acetate to form a nitrenium ion and covalently bind to DNA, one preferred position being the C8-position of guanine (Fig. 1). After N-hydroxylation and N,O-glucuronidation in the liver, the heterocyclic aromatic amine-derived glucuronides are secreted into the bile, due to their relatively high molecular weight. In the colon the heterocyclic hydroxylamines may then be released from the conjugates due to action of bacterial glucuronidases. Contrary to the original *not* hydroxylated heterocyclic aromatic amines the hydroxylamines represent good substrates for NAT2, which is expressed in relatively high levels in colon epithelial cells. This mechanism may explain the colon-specific carcinogenic effect of some heterocyclic amines. The role of cytochrome P450 1A2 and NAT2 in metabolic activation of heterocyclic amines has been proven by several studies. For example, expressing both cytochrome P450 1A2 and NAT2 in Chinese hamster CHL cells caused an about 100-fold increase in sensitivity to the cytotoxic and mutagenic action of MeIQx compared to the parental cell line (Yanagawa et al. 1994). However, no significant increase in sensitivity to MeIQx was observed expressing NAT2 or cytochrome P450 1A2 alone or cytochrome P450 1A2 plus NAT1. Furthermore, aberrant crypts, the earliest morphologically evident preoplastic lesion in chemical colon carcinogenesis was about three fold higher in rapid vs slow acetylator (NAT2) congenic Syrian hamsters administered 3,2'-dimethyl-4-aminobiphenyl, an aromatic amine colon carcinogen (Feng et al. 1996). Similarly, the level of DNA adducts induced by 2-amino-3-methylimidazo[4,5-*f*]quinoline (IQ) in colon tissue of C57BL/6 mice was about three fold higher in rapid vs slow acetylator (NAT2) congenic mice (Nerurkar et al. 1995).

Although evidence has been given that 2-amino-1-methyl-6-phenylimidazo[4,5-*b*]pyridine (PhIP) (which represents a predominant heterocyclic arylamine in pyrolized meat and fish) can be further activated by NAT2 (Hein et

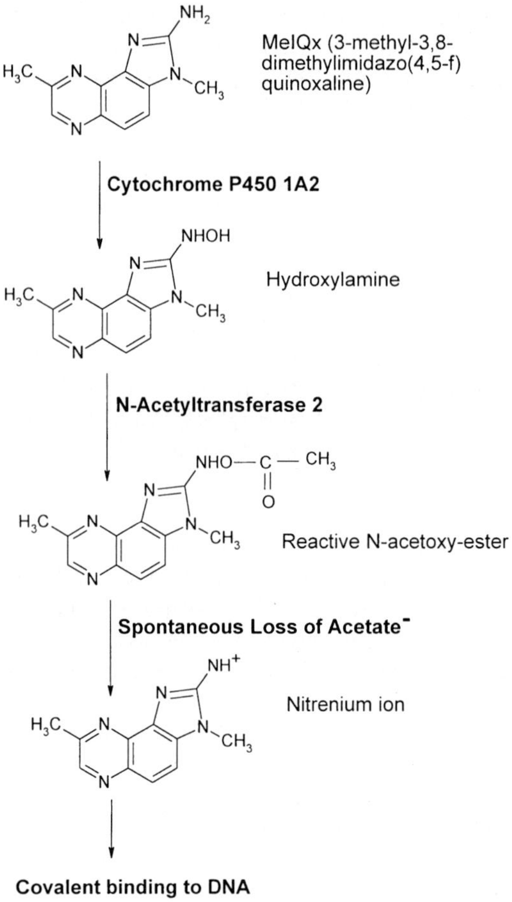

Fig. 1. Metabolic activation of MelQx (3-methyl-3,8-dimethylimidazo[4,5-*f*] quinoxaline) by cytochrome P450 1A2 and N-acetyltransferase 2

al. 1994; Turesky et al. 1991) after hydroxylation, two recent studies from independent groups suggest that PhIP may represent an exception (Wild et al. 1995; Wu et al. 1997). Chinese hamster ovary UV5P3 cells were about 50-fold more sensitive to the cytotoxic effect of PhIP than to IQ (2-amino-3-methyl-imidazo[4,5-f]quinoline), another genotoxic compound found in cooked food (Wu et al. 1997). Expression of human NAT2 in Chinese hamster ovary UV5P3 cells caused an approximately 1000-fold increase in sensitivity to the killing effect of IQ over the parental cell line. However, no increase in cytotoxicity to PhIP was observed in the NAT2-expressing cells. A similar result was obtained by expressing human NAT2 in *Salmonella typhimurium* TA 1538/1,8-DNP, a derivative of strain TA 1538 devoid of the endogeneous *Salmonella* O-acetyltransferase. In the Ames test with rat liver S-9 Mix as an activating system the mutagenic potency of several heterocyclic aromatic amines was much higher in NAT2 expressing *Salmonella typhimurium* (strain DJ 460) than in the NAT2-deficient strain (TA 1538/1,8-DNP) except for PhIP, which exhibited similar mutagenic potencies in both strains (Wild et al. 1995). These results suggest that PhIP – as an exception to the rule for heterocyclic arylamines – may be activated independent of NAT2 and, thus, genotoxic effects of PhIP will not depend on the NAT2 polymorphism.

In contrast to the colon, for bladder the rapid acetylator phenotype (NAT2) was associated with a lower incidence of cancer (Weber and Hein, 1985; Cartwright 1984; Karakaya et al. 1989; Okkels et al. 1997; Ross et al. 1996). However, exposure to bladder carcinogens, such as aromatic amines or cigarette smoking, were required to observe an association between the slow acetylator phenotype and an increased risk for bladder cancer. No association between NAT2 polymorphism and bladder cancer was observed without exposure of individuals to aromatic amines.

In a relatively large hospital based case-control study (374 patients; 373 controls), slow acetylation (NAT2) was a significant risk factor for bladder cancer in heavy smokers (not selected for occupational exposure to aromatic amines) (odds ratio: 2.7; 95% CI: 1–7.4) (Brockmöller et al. 1996a). In contrast to earlier findings, a recent study with 196 urothelial cancer patients did not show a significantly increased frequency of slow acetylators (NAT2) among bladder cancer patients compared to the normal population (Golka et al. 1996). However, in subgroups of these urothelial cancer patients with former occupational exposure to aromatic amines, a trend towards a higher representation of slow acetylators was observed. This finding suggests that the percentage of slow acetylators (NAT2) in the population of urothelial cancer patients decreased during the last few years, possibly because the production of benzidine ceased in the early 1970s (Golka et al. 1996).

The protection against bladder cancer by fast acetylation may be explained by the role of NAT and cytochrome P450 in metabolic activation of aromatic amines, some of which are well-known bladder carcinogens (Fig. 2, 4-aminobiphenyl). Toxification of aromatic amines includes N-hydroxylation by cytochrome P450 1A2 followed by the formation of a reactive O,N-ester (acetoxy-group) by N-acetyltransferase and spontaneous decomposition to an aryl-nitrenium ion, which can covalently bind to DNA. Cytochrome P450 1A2 hydroxylates 4-aminobiphenyl relatively fast, whereas the arylamide, produced by N-acetylation of 4-aminobiphenyl, is a relatively poor substrate for cytochrome P450 1A2 (Fig. 2). Thus, high activities of NAT, which may compete with cytochrome P450 1A2 for aromatic amines, will reduce the formation of aryl-nitrenium ions and consequently reduce the formation of DNA adducts. The example of NAT2 shows that polymorphisms may influence susceptibility of different organs in opposite directions.

Some investigators also observed associations between the acetylator phenotype and cancer of organs other than colon and bladder. An excess of slow acetylators (NAT2) was observed among patients with hepatocellular carcinoma (Agundez et al. 1996). In postmenopausal women NAT2 modified the association of smoking with risk of breast cancer (Ambrosone et al. 1996). For slow acetylators smoking increased breast cancer risk in a dose-dependent manner (odds ratio: 4.4; 95% CI: 1.3–14.8), whereas for rapid acetyla-

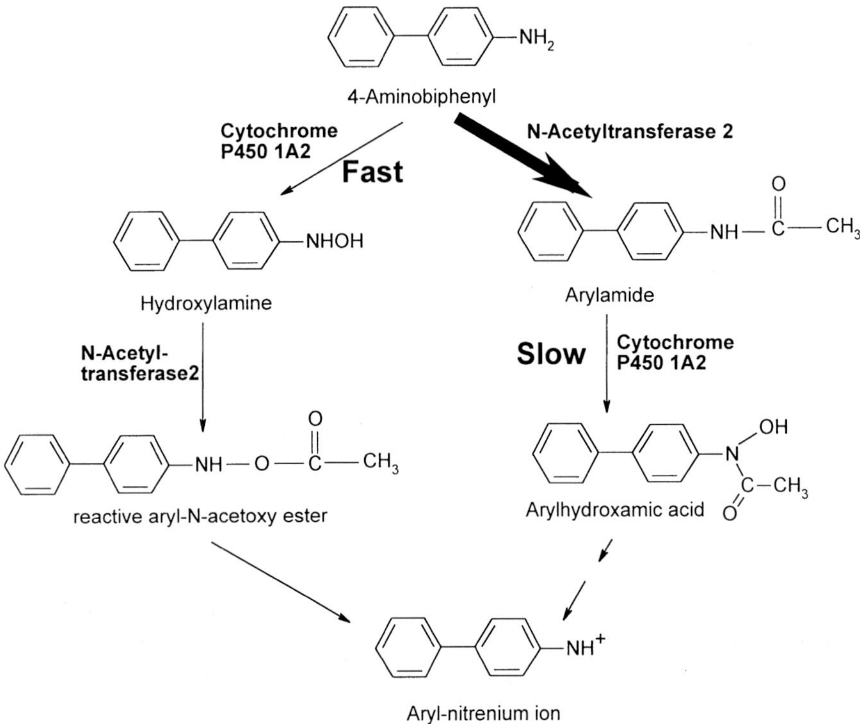

Fig. 2. Metabolic activation of 4-aminobiphenyl by cytochrome P450 1A2 and N-acetyltransferase 2. Formation of aryl-nitrenium ions is decreased by high activity of N-acetyltransferase 2, since the parent arylamine is a good substrate but the arylamide is a poor substrate for cytochrome P450 1A2

tors smoking was not associated with increased breast cancer risk. A study with 389 lung cancer patients revealed an overexpression of NAT*4/4 genotype in the lung cancer patients (odds ratio: 2.4; 95% CI: 1.05–5.32), which is associated with especially high acetylation capacity (Cascorbi et al. 1996). By contrast, the risk of asbestos-exposed individuals of developing malignant mesothelioma for individuals with a NAT2 slow-acetylator genotype was about fourfold that observed for those with a NAT2 fast-acetylator genotype as reported by another group (odds ratio: 3.8; 95% CI: 1.2–14.3; Hirvonen et al. 1996).

Activities of NAT1 and NAT2 can be differentiated by the use of diagnostic substrates, in which N-acetylation of *p*-aminosalicylic acid represents an activity specific for NAT1 and N-acetylation of sulfamethazine is specific for NAT2 (Sadrieh et al. 1996). The classical acetylation polymorphism is regulated at the NAT2 locus, although NAT1 is also expressed polymorphically in human bladder (Bell et al. 1995). Individuals who inherited a variant polyadenylation signal of the NAT1 gene (NAT*10 allele) exhibited an about two fold higher NAT1 enzyme activity in bladder and colon tissue specimens.

According to present knowledge NAT2 would be expected to be of higher toxicologic relevance than NAT1, since it has a higher affinity to several aromatic amines (Nebert et al. 1996) and heterocyclic hydroxylamines (Sinha et al. 1994; Kerdar et al. 1993; Wild et al. 1995; Yanagawa et al. 1994) than NAT1. For example, expression of human cytochrome P450 1A2 and NAT2 in Chinese hamster CHL cells caused 370- and 100-fold increases in mutagenic effects of IQ (2-amino-3-methylimidazo[4,5-f]quinoline) and MeIQx (2-amino-3,8-dimethylimidazo[4,5-f]quinoxaline) compared to the parental cell line, whereas no clear increase in sensitivity was observed after expression of human cytochrome P450 1A2 and NAT1 (Yanagawa et al. 1994). Similarly Wild et al. (1995), Hein et al. (1994) and Kerdar et al. (1993) observed a more efficient O-acetylation of heterocyclic arylamines by human NAT2 compared to NAT1 expressing both enzymes in *Salmonella typhimurium* or in COS-1 cells. The opposite situation – a more efficient O-acetylation (Minchin et al. 1992) and a more efficient activation to a mutagen (Grant et al. 1992) by NAT1 – was observed for the nonheterocyclic N-hydroxy-2-aminofluorene. Furthermore, NAT1 is expressed with relatively high activity in bladder and colon mucosa (Bell et al. 1995; Badawi et al. 1996). Bell et al. (1995) observed an association between the NAT1 variant allele (NAT1*10 genotype due to mutations in the NAT1 polyadenylation site causing about two fold higher activity) and colorectal cancer among NAT2 rapid acetylators (odds ratio: 2.8; 95% CI: 1.4–5.7). This suggests a possible interaction between NAT2 and NAT1 and is in agreement with the finding that the bladder NAT1*10 genotype and phenotype were correlated with significantly higher levels of aromatic amine-DNA adducts in human bladder as measured by ^{32}P-postlabelling (Kadlubar and Badawi 1995). However, a recent study did not observe an association between the NAT1*10 fast acetylator allele and an increased prevalence of colorectal adenomas, nor a gene-gene interaction between NAT2 and NAT1 (Probst-Hensch et al. 1996), thus, presently leaving an unclear situation with respect to the role of NAT1 for colorectal tumorigenesis.

Glutathione S-Transferase M1 and T1

The cytosolic glutathione S-transferase (GST) activity in mammalian tissues is due to the presence of multiple isoenzymes which, on the basis of their amino acid sequences, can be assigned to five classes known as, α, μ, π, σ, and θ (Hayes and Pulford 1995). These enzymes catalyze many reactions between glutathione and lipophilic compounds with electrophilic centers. When the reaction forms a covalent bond the resultant more water soluble GSH conjugate usually is no longer toxic and may be excreted. However, mutagenicity of several substances (especially haloalkanes and haloalkenes) including 1,2,3,4-diepoxybutane, epibromohydrin, 1,3-dichloroacetone and 1,2-dibromoethane, is increased by the action of GST (Thier et al. 1996; Guengerich 1996). This activation process includes formation of an episulfonium ion, which reacts with nucleophiles and may bind to DNA, preferentially to the N7 position of guanine. Within the GSTμ class there exist at least five genes encoding the isoenzymes GST M1–M5 (Hayes and Pulford 1995). The most commonly expressed gene is GST M1, which has been shown to be polymorphic and for which at least three different allelic variants exist. A null allele (GSTM1-0) contains a nearly complete deletion of the gene and produces no enzyme (review in Nebert et al. 1996; Seidegard and Ekström 1997; Rebbeck 1997). Two allelic variants have been described for GST M1, GST M1a and GST M1b. The GST M1a and GST M1b alleles differ by a C to G transversion at base position 534, causing a Lys to Asn substitution at amino acid 172. However, similar substrate specificities and enzyme activities have been observed for both variants.

For Caucasians the frequency of homozygous deletions in GST M1 is about 50%. Thus, most individuals who are phenotypically GST M1-1 are deletion heterozygotes rather than nondeletion homozygotes (approximately 42% vs 9%, respectively) (Seidegard et al. 1988). Large ethnic differences for the frequency of homozygous deletion in GST M1 have been observed. Frequencies of homozygous GST M1-0 in Pacific Islanders, Malay, Japanese, Chinese, Indians (Asia), and Africans were 64%–100%, 62%, 48%–51%, 35%–63%, 33%–36%, 22%–35%, respectively (review in Rebbeck 1997). Earlier studies used enzymatic assays with *trans*-stilbene oxide or immunological techniques for analysis of GST M1 positivity vs negativity, whereas most recent studies used PCR-based methods. The latter technique accurately distinguishes deletion homozygotes from deletion heterozygotes and nondeletion homozygotes, whereas differentiation between heterozygotes and nondeletion homozygotes is difficult, due to limitations of consistent PCR product quality. Since the variant of interest is a gene deletion, PCR based assays should include an internal positive control for PCR amplification, e.g. the albumin or the β-globin gene (Arand et al. 1996a; Hengstler et al. 1998a). Techniques which allow simultaneous amplification of the GST M1, GST T1 and albumin (positive control) genes in a single PCR reaction have been described (Arand et al. 1996a; Hengstler et al. 1998a). A list of typical substrates detoxified by GST M1 is given in Table 1.

Similarly to GST M1, GST T1 also has been shown to be polymorphic due to a large deletion in the structural gene (Pemble et al. 1994). Already in 1989 a polymorphic conjugation of methyl chloride by human erythrocytes

Table 1. Xenobiotics detoxified by human glutathione S-transferase M1. (Adapted from Hayes and Pulford 1995)

Benzo[*a*]-pyrene-4,5-oxide
(+)-*anti*-Benzo[*a*]pyrene-7,8-diol-9,10-oxide
Aflatoxin B$_1$-8,9-epoxide
Styrene oxide
trans-Stilbene oxide
Thiotepa

Table 2. Typical substrates for GST T1 and the influence of GST T1 on mutageniticity after expression in *Salmonella typhimurium* TA 1535. (From Thier et al. 1996)

Substance	Influence of GST T1 on mutagenicity[a]
1,2,3,4-Diepoxybutane	++
1,3-Dichloroacetone	++
Epibromohydrin	+
1,2-Dibromoethane	+
1,2-Epoxy-3-(4′-nitrophenoxy)propane	−

[a] Strong (++) and intermediate (+) increase in mutagenicity; decrease in mutagenicity (−).

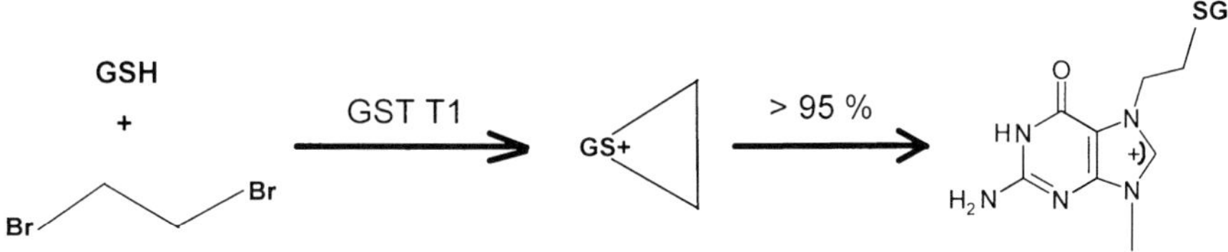

Fig. 3. Activation of dibromoethane by glutathione S-transferase T1 (GST T1) via formation of an episulfonium ion (from Guengerich, 1996)

was observed (Peter et al. 1989). The majority of human blood samples showed a significant metabolic elimination of methyl chloride (conjugators), whereas a smaller fraction did not (nonconjugators). Later, conjugator status could be explained by the polymorphism of GST T1 (Pemble et al. 1994; Kempkes et al. 1996a; Fost et al. 1995; Schröder et al. 1996). Although large ethnic differences have been observed, the homozygous null genotype of GST T1 is in general less frequent than GST M1. Frequencies of homozygous GST T1-0 in Chinese, Koreans, Africans, Caucasians, and Indians were 64%, 60%, 24%–38%, 11%–16%, and 16%, respectively. A list of substrates for GST T1 is given in Table 2.

Recently, Thier et al. (1996) expressed human GST T1 in *Salmonella typhimurium* either in a sense or antisense orientation, the latter serving as a control. Expression of GST T1 enhanced mutagenicity of all investigated substrates, except 1,2-epoxy-3-(4′-nitrophenoxy)propane, which was detoxified (Table 2). In this respect GST T1 differs from GST M1, since GST M1 detoxifies the large majority of its substrates, e.g. many diol epoxides of polycyclic aromatic hydrocarbons or the 8,9-epoxide of aflatoxin B_1. Bioactivation of haloalkanes mediated by GST T1 has been described by Guengerich (1996). Conjugation of these haloalkanes with glutathione generates episulfonium ions, which predominantly bind to the N7-position of guanine ($\geq$95%), but also to other sites including O^6-guanine (Fig. 3). The observation that GST T1 enhances mutagenicity of several of its substrates (Thier et al. 1996) is in contrast with the protective effect of GST T1 observed in humans ex vivo using various biomarkers. For example, approximately twofold more chromosomal aberrations were observed in GST T1-0 workers exposed to 1,3-butadiene (which is metabolized to 1,2,3,4-diepoxybutane and 1,2-epoxy-3-butene) than in workers without the homozygous gene defect, whereas for controls only a slight, statistically not significant, difference was observed (Sorsa et al. 1996). In addition, GST T1-0 individuals were more sensitive to induction of sister chromatid exchanges (SCEs) in lymphocytes by 1,2,3,4-diepoxybutane (Wiencke et al. 1995). Incubation of whole blood samples with dichloromethane (methylene chloride) as well as methyl bromide led to a significant increase in SCEs in the lymphocytes of nonconjugators but not in those of conjugators (Hallier et al. 1993). In addition the GST T1-polymorphism has been shown to influence the level of endogenous SCEs in human lymphocytes ex vivo with higher SCE levels in GST T1 negative individuals (Schröder et al. 1995; Wiencke et al. 1995).

Similarly, we observed a slightly ($\sim$30%; borderline significant $p<0.05$), higher level of DNA strand lesions ex vivo (determined by alkaline elution) in mononuclear blood cells of workers exposed to ethylene oxide (which represents only a relatively weak substrate for GST T1) if the GST T1 gene was homozygously deleted (Hengstler, unpublished data). In addition, incubation of venous blood with ethylene oxide in vitro resulted in slightly higher levels of DNA strand lesions in mononuclear blood cells of GST T1 negative vs positive individuals (Fig. 4). By contrast, levels of DNA strand lesions induced by ethylene oxide were almost identical between GST T1 positive and negative individuals if isolated mononuclear blood cells were incubated with ethylene oxide in vitro (Fig. 4). This is consistent with the observation that GST T1 is highly expressed in human erythrocytes, whereas expression in human lymphocytes has not been demonstrated (Schröder et al. 1996). The discrepancy between enhanced mutagenicity by GST T1 in *Salmonella typhimurium* and the protective effect of GST T1 against DNA strand lesions (single strand breaks and alkali labile sites) in blood or in vivo might be explained by the high polarity of the conjugate formed in erythrocytes, which is unlikely to pass the erythrocyte and lymphocyte plasma membranes (Thier et al. 1996). Furthermore, the mechanisms underlying the induction of point mutations and the induction of chromosomal aberrations, DNA strand lesions or SCEs are not identical (Oesch et al. 1997). The latter DNA alterations require formation of DNA single strand breaks, which mainly arise as a consequence of covalent binding to the N-7 position of guanine. By contrast, point mutations (detected by *Salmonella typhimurium* 1535) are most effectively induced by substances with a relatively high ratio of O^6 vs N7 guanine binding (Fig. 5; Dipple, 1995; Oesch et al. 1997). It might be possible that GST T1 forms metabolites (possibly episulfonium ions) that react more according to an S_N1 reaction than do the parent substances, thus forming more O^6- (and relatively less N7-) guanine adducts, consequently resulting in more point mutations and less DNA strand breaks, chromosomal aberrations and SCEs (Fig. 5). However, both explanations are hypothetical and have not yet been confirmed experimentally.

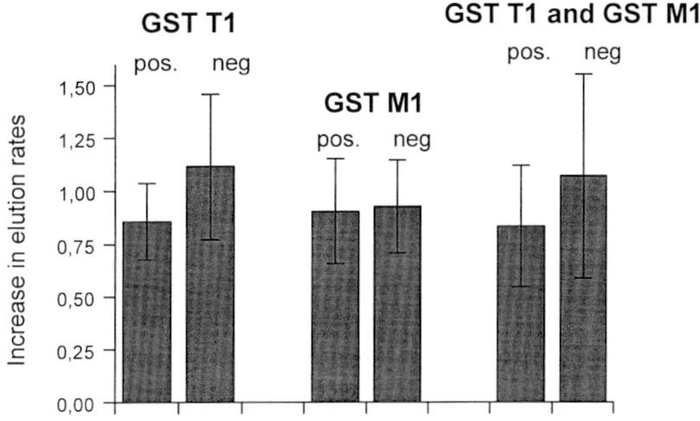

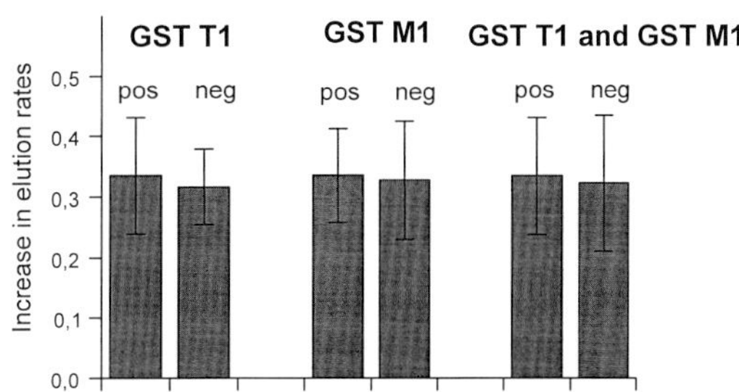

Fig. 4. Induction of DNA strand lesions (increase in elution rates) in mononuclear blood cells by ethylene oxide. Total venous blood and isolated mononuclear blood cells suspended in PBS (phosphate buffered saline) were incubated with ethylene oxide for 2 h. Individuals were genotyped by multiplex PCR as described (Arand et al 1996 a). Of the 55 healthy individuals 42 were GST T1-1, 13 GST T1-0, 22 GST M1-1, 33 GST M1-0, 9 GST M1-0 and GST T1-0, and 18 GST M1-1 and GST T1-1. Incubations were performed with 0.66 mM ethylene oxide for total venous blood and with 0.44 mM for isolated mononuclear blood cells, because the susceptibility of the isolated cells was higher. Determination of DNA strand lesions was performed by alkaline elution as described. (From Hengstler et al 1992)

A very large number of case-control studies have been performed to examine a possible influence of GST M1 and T1 polymorphisms on cancer risk. The best overview might be given if these are discussed according to tumor site.

Lung Cancer

Although it has been clear since a long time that the GST M1 polymorphism alone confers only a modestly increased risk for lung cancer (if any at all), the lung has been the tumor site which has been examined most intensively. However, this effort is justified since only a modestly increased risk of lung cancer is important to public health, as both the polymorphism and its associated cancer are common. McWilliams et al. (1995) peformed a meta-analy-

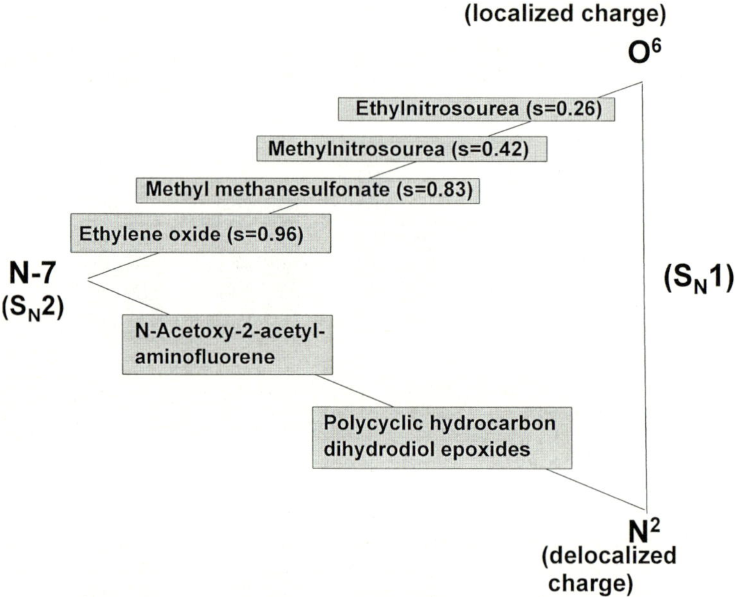

Fig. 5. Reaction of various genotoxic substances on guanine residues in DNA. (From Dipple 1995)

sis of 12 case-control studies of lung cancer risk and GST M1 status published between 1985 and 1994. In each of the studies an excess of GST M1-deficient individuals among the lung cancer cases was observed compared to the controls. However, this excess reached statistical significance in only four of the individual studies. The summary odds ratio of all 12 studies (using Mantel-Haenszel methods for stratified analysis) was 1.41 (95% CI: 1.23–1.61; $p<0.0001$), including 1593 patients and 2135 controls. According to this odds ratio GST M1 deficiency accounts for approximately 17% of lung cancer because of the high prevalence, although the increased risk is small (McWilliams et al. 1995). The increased risk is evident for all major histological subtypes of lung cancer, namely squamous cell (odds ratio: 1.49; 95% CI: 1.22–1.80), adenocarcinoma (odds ratio: 1.53; 95% CI: 1.26–1.85), and small cell carcinoma cell (odds ratio: 1.90; 95% CI: 1.27–1.85).

Summary odds ratios of three studies including only Japanese patients and controls and of six studies limited to Caucasians were calculated. The summary odds ratio for the Japanese population was 1.60 (95% CI: 1.25–2.13) compared to 1.17 (0.98–1.40) for Caucasians (McWilliams et al. 1995), suggesting ethnic differences. Interestingly, a higher odds ratio was obtained in studies, which determined GST M1 status by phenotyping (enzymatic assay with *trans*-stilbene oxide or immunological techniques; odds ratio: 1.80; 95% CI: 1.29–2.50) than in studies using genotypic methods (odds ratio: 1.34; 95% CI: 1.16–1.55; McWilliams et al. 1995). This might be plausible, since a negative genotype determined by PCR must be associated with lack of enzyme activity, but due to various possible mechanisms (e.g. deficiencies in transcription, translation, posttranslational mechanisms or even epigenetic factors) a positive genotype does not guarantee the presence of enzyme activity.

Thus, potential sources of bias, such as imbalance of racial groups or different methods for determination of GST M1 status, were excluded in McWilliam's meta-analysis. However, another source of bias, which might cause an overestimation of the summary odds ratio, was not discussed, namely unpublished negative studies. While the summary odds ratio according to McWilliams et al. (1995) was 1.41, three of the single studies (Seidegard et al. 1986, 1990; Nazar-Stewart et al. 1993) obtained ratios higher than 2.0, but not a single study reported an odds ratio equal or smaller than 1.0. In addition the two studies with the highest odds ratios (Seidegard et al. 1986; Nazar-Stewart et al. 1993) have the largest 95% confidence intervals, whereas the studies with the smallest odds ratios (four studies with odds ratios only slightly higher than 1.0: Zhong et al. 1991; Brockmöller et al. 1993; Heckbert et al. 1992; Alexandrie et al. 1994) have relatively small 95% confidence intervals. This imbalance results from small case numbers in the highly positive studies (Seidegard et al. 1986: 66 patients, 78 controls; Nazar-Stewart et al. 1993: 35 patients, 43 controls) and relatively high case numbers in the four studies with the lowest odds ratios (Zhong et al. 1991: 228 patients, 225 controls; Brockmöller et al. 1993: 117 patients, 355 controls; Heckbert et al. 1992: 113 patients, 120 controls; Alexandrie et al. 1994: 296 patients, 329 controls). This constellation suggests that negative studies, especially when case numbers were small, were not submitted for publication, or – even worse – were rejected by journals trying to improve their impact factors. Thus, it is important that all (methodologically correct) case-control studies are published, even if some might represent outsider positions, to avoid a selection of positive studies.

Several studies on GST M1 polymorphism and lung cancer risk have been published since 1995 presenting odds ratios between approximately 1.0 and 1.8, altogether suggesting a slightly increased relative risk similar to McWilliam's meta-analysis (Kelsey et al. 1997a; To-Figueras et al. 1996, 1997; Kihara et al. 1995a,b; Harrison et al. 1997; Garcia-Closas et al. 1997; London et al. 1995, Moreira et al. 1996). A study of Kelsey et al. (1997) suggested racial differences, since the GST M1 homozygously negative genotype was associated with increased lung cancer risk in Mexican-Americans (odds ratio: 1.80; 95% CI: 1.0–3.3; 60 patients, 146 controls), whereas no increase was observed for African-Americans (odds ratio: 1.0; 95% CI: 0.5–1.8; 108 patients, 132 controls). In addition an influence of gender was suggested by a Japanese study, which observed a significantly higher percentage of GST M1 null genotypes in female compared to male lung cancer patients (447 patients, 469 controls) (Kihara et al. 1995b). However, neither an influence of race nor of gender has as yet been confirmed.

Several studies have shown that the risk for lung cancer is markedly influenced by the combination of GST M1 and cytochrome P450 1A1 (CYP 1A1) genotypes. The latter refers to a phase I enzyme and is, therefore, not discussed in detail in this review. Briefly, two separate point mutations are known in CYP 1A1, one in exon 7 causing an isoleucine to valine substitution at amino acid 462 and the other in the 3' non-coding region of the gene causing an *Msp*I cleavage site. By the latter polymorphism individuals can be classified into CYP 1A1 (m1/m1) lacking the *Msp*I cleavage site, CYP 1A1 (m2/m2) homozygous for the allele with the *Msp*I cleavage site, and CYP 1A1 (m1/m2) heterozygous for the *Msp*I site. Probably both, the CYP 1A1 (m2/m2)-variant in the 3' noncoding region and the CYP 1A1 (Val/Val) variant in exon 7, are associated with higher AHH (aryl hydrocarbon hydroxylase) inducibility. Combined with the GST M1-0 genotype both variants have been shown to be associated with lung cancer. For lung cancer patients with GST M1-0 genotype and the CYP 1A1 (m2/m2) variant an odds ratio of 8.3 (95% CI: 1.44–49.7) was observed (Kihara et al. 1995a). Patients with the heterozygous CYP 1A1 (m1/m2) and GST M1-0 had an odds ratio of 5.2 (95% CI: 1.20–22.7), whereas the genotype CYP 1A1 (m1/m1) and GST M1-0 was not significantly associated with lung cancer (odds ratio: 2.3; 95% CI: 0.39–12.6). A similar interaction was observed for the CYP 1A1 polymorphism at exon 7, with the highest risk observed for the combination of CYP 1A1 (Val/Val) and GST M1-0 (Kawajiri et al. 1993). Although these findings are in agreement with several further Japanese investigations, studies with CYP 1A1 in other ethnic groups initially failed to support these observations (review: Nebert et al. 1996). However, the interaction between CYP 1A1 variants and GST M1-null genotype has meanwhile been confirmed also in non-Japanese populations (Garcia-Closas et al. 1997; Alexandrie et al. 1994), although odds ratios in general were smaller.

A finding in a Japanese population which might be of relevance was that the combination of the GST M1-1 and CYP 1A1 (m2/m2) genotypes was associated with the lowest risk of developing lung cancer. Probably individuals with this genotype are able to eliminate absorbed polycyclic aromatic hydrocarbons (e.g. from tobacco smoke) most rapidly, due to increased monooxygenation and conjugation activities (Kihara et al. 1995a).

In addition to GST M1 also GST M3, which shows catalytic activity for several electrophiles, may be important in the development of smoking-related lung cancer. Interestingly, GST M1-0 individuals showed a significantly lower expression of GST M3 protein in healthy human lung tissue (Nakajima et al. 1995), which may contribute to the limited detoxification capacity of individuals with the GST M1 gene deletion. Contrary to GST M3, which is reduced in GST M1-0 individuals, inducibility of cytochrome P450 1A1 (Vaury et al. 1995) and activity of cytochrome P450 1A2 (MacLeod et al. 1997; Bartsch et al. 1995) have been shown to be higher in individuals lacking a functional GST M1 gene. This might be explained by the fact that many inducers of cytochrome P450 1A1 and 1A2 are substrates of GST M1. Thus, the absence of GST M1 might result in longer half-lives of inducing agents, thereby exhibiting a greater inducing capacity. Since increased activity of cytochrome P450 1A may be associated with increased cancer risk (e.g. cytochrome P450 1A1 with lung cancer and cytochrome P450 1A2 with urothelial cancer) interaction between GST M1 and cytochrome P450 may be another indirect mechanism which links the GST M1 gene defect to enhanced susceptibility.

No significant association between GST T1-0 and lung cancer was observed in three independent studies, although all odds ratios were slightly higher than 1.0 (Kelsey et al. 1997a; To-Figueras et al., 1997; Deakin et al. 1996). An interaction between GST T1-0 and GST M1-0 as observed by Kelsey et al. (1997a) was not confirmed (To-Figueras et al. 1997).

Malignant Mesothelioma

In asbestos-exposed individuals a borderline significant association between GST M1-0 genotype and malignant mesothelioma has been observed (odds ratio: 1.8; 95% CI: 1.0–3.5) (Hirvonen et al. 1995), which was not confirmed in a more recent publication (Hirvonen et al. 1996). However, the NAT2 slow acetylator phenotype was associated with malignant mesothelioma (odds ratio: 3.8; 95% CI: 1.2–14.3) and the odds ratio increased markedly if the combined NAT2 slow acetylator GST M1-0 genotype was examined (odds ratio: 7.8; 95% CI: 1.4–78.7), suggesting an interaction between GST M1 and NAT2 (Hirvonen et al. 1996).

Urothelial Cancer (Bladder, Renal Pelvis, and Ureter)

At least 11 studies have been performed between 1993 and 1997 to examine a possible association between risk of urothelial cancer and GST M1-0 genotype (Table 3). Six of 11 studies obtained a statistically significant association, with odds ratios ranging between 1.5 and 7.0. However, the study with the highest odds ratio (7.0) contained only a very small number of cases ($n=22$). The data show that GST M1-0 genotype probably has a higher penetrance for urothelial cancer than for lung cancer, although the total number of lung cancer cases due to GST M1-0 genotype is higher than the total number of urothelial cancer, due to the higher incidence of lung cancer. The observed risk modification of urothelial cancer is mechanistically supported by measurements of the mutagenicity of urine, showing that smokers with the GST M1-0 genotype have several times more mutagenic urine than smokers with the functional gene (Hirvonen et al. 1994).

Cigarette smoking is known to be an important risk factor for bladder cancer. Among persons who did not smoke, the GST M1-0 genotype was only weakly associated with bladder cancer risk (odds ratio: 1.3; 95% CI: 0.6–2.7) (Bell et al. 1993). However, among smokers individuals who lacked the GST M1 structural gene had almost twice the risk of developing bladder cancer as persons with similar smoking histories who had the detoxification enzyme (GST M1-1). These data suggest a protective effect of GST M1 for smoking-induced bladder cancer.

Table 3. Association between urothelial cancer and GST M1-0 genotype: case control studies between 1993 and 1997

Authors	Nationality	Odds ratio[a]	95% CI[b]	Number of cases	Number of controls
Zhong et al.. (1993)	UK	1.1	n.p.[d]	97	225
Belle tal. (1993)	USA	1.7	1.1–2.5	213	199
Lin et al. (1994)	USA	1.4	0.9–2.1	114	1104
Brockmöller et al. (1994)	Germany	1.5	1.1–2.1	296	373
Brockmöller et al. (1996a)	Germany	1.6	1.2–2.2	374	373
Katoh et al. (1995)	Japan	2.2	1.2–3.9	85	88
Anwar et al. (1996)	Egypt	7.0	1.6–30.6	22	21
Rothman et al. (1996)[c]	USA	1.0	0.4–2.7	38	43
Okkels et al. (1996)	Denmark	1.3	0.9–1.9	234	202
Okkels et al. (1997)	Denmark	1.2	0.8–1.7	254	242
Kempkes et al. (1996b)	Germany	1.8	1.1–3.0	113	170

[a] Overall odds ratios of total cases of the respective studies
[b] 95% confidence interval.
[c] Benzidine associated cases.
[d] Not published.

The risk conferred by the GST M1-0 genotype was similar for white and black Americans (Bell et al. 1993). However, the frequency of the GST M1-0 genotype was significantly lower in blacks (35%) than in whites (49%). The incidence of bladder cancer in black men is approximately half that in the white men (Silverman et al. 1992). Thus, the lower frequency of the GST M1-0 genotype in black individuals might contribute to the lower incidence of bladder cancer among blacks.

Okkels et al. (1996, 1997) observed no significant association between the GST M1-0 genotype and bladder cancer in incident patients (odds ratio: 0.95; 95% CI: 0.58–1.58). However, a significant association between GST M1 deficiency and bladder cancer was found in patients who survived at least 2 years after diagnosis (odds ratio: 1.63; 95% CI: 1.06–2.50). These data suggest that the GST M1-0 genotype may be related to survival of bladder cancer patients and possibly plays only a minor role in carcinogenesis. Since almost all studies shown in Table 3 relied on prevalent cases (or included only small numbers of incident cases), further studies should differentiate between incident patients and survivors.

The GST T1-0 genotype has not been shown to be associated with risk of urothelial cancer if the total population including smokers and nonsmokers was examined. However, in the subgroup of nonsmoking urothelial cancer patients a significantly higher frequency of GST T1-0 genotypes was observed. Odds ratios were 2.6 (95% CI: 1.1–6; 374 patients, 373 controls) (Brockmöller et al. 1996a) and 3.8 (1.21–12.23) (Kempkes et al. 1996b), respectively.

Colorectal Cancer

Zhong et al. (1993) observed a significant association between the GST M1-0 genotype and colorectal cancer, whereas Katoh et al. (1996) observed an association only if the subgroup of distal colorectal tumors was considered. However, the overall picture of case-control studies is inconsistent with the majority of studies being negative (Chenevix-Trench et al. 1995; Katoh et al. 1996; Lin et al. 1995; Deakin et al. 1996). Nevertheless, most of the negative studies obtained odds ratios higher than 1.0. Thus, a modestly increased risk cannot be excluded. However, the number of published studies is still too small to perform a reasonable meta-analysis.

For GST T1-0 genotypes no association with colorectal cancer has been observed in three studies (Katoh et al. 1996; Chenevix-Trench et al. 1995) in contrast to a case-control study which obtained an odds ratio of 1.9 (Deakin et al. 1996). However, in one study the GST T1-0 genotype was significantly more common in colorectal cancer patients who were diagnosed before the age of 70 years than in those who were diagnosed at an older age, suggesting that the GST T1 genotype might influence the age of onset of colorectal cancer (Chenevix-Trench et al. 1995). This study has not yet been confirmed.

Esophageal Carcinoma

In a Japanese case-control study no significant association between the GST M1-0 genotype and esophageal cancer was observed (Morita et al. 1997). However, a recent study in a Japanese population obtained a significant association between the CYP 1A1 (Val/Val) variant and esophageal carcinoma in smokers (odds ratio: 6.63; 95% CI: 1.86–23.7). If patients with the GST M1-0 *and* CYP 1A1 (Val/Val) genotype were considered the odds ratio increased about twofold (12.7; 95% CI: 1.97–81.8) suggesting a significant interaction of CYP 1A1 and GST M1 (Nimura et al. 1997).

Head and Neck Cancer

The absence of GST M1 conferred an odds ratio of 2.37 (95% CI: 1.20–4.67) for tumors of the head and neck (Trizna et al. 1995). Similarly, Kihara et al. (1997) observed an association between GST M1-0 and head and neck cancer (carcinoma of the larynx excluded) in smokers (odds ratio: 1.77; 95% CI: 1.04–3.01). The absence of GST T1 conferred a slightly, but statistically not significantly increased odds ratio for head and neck cancer (odds ratio: 1.47; 95% CI: 0.71–3.02) (Trizna et al. 1995). Laryngeal carcinoma has been shown to be associated with GST T1-0 and the frequency of GST M3 B/B as well as GST M1 A/B genotype was significantly, lower in head and neck cancer patients (Jahnke et al. 1997). Coutelle et al. (1997) observed a highly significant overrepresentation of the combination GST M1-0 and ADH (aldehyde dehydrogenase) (3)1/ADH(3)1 genotype in alcoholics with laryngeal cancer (odds ratio: 12.9; 95% CI: 1.8–92).

Brain Neoplasms

GST T1-0 has been shown to be associated with both astrocytoma and meningioma, whereas GST M1-0 was not overrepresented (Elexpuru-Camiruaga et al. 1995; Hand et al. 1996). Contrary to lung cancer, no relationship between GST M1 genotype and GST M3 expression was observed in brain (Hand et al. 1996). Similarly, Wiencke et al. (1997) observed no significant association between GST M1-0 and gliomas, although women with GST M1 deletion were slightly younger on average at diagnosis than women who were GST M1 positive (44 vs 52 years). In addition GST M1-0 has been shown to be associated with pituitary adenomas (Fryer et al. 1993; Perrett et al. 1995).

Hepatocellular Cancer

A borderline significant association between GST M1-0 genotype and hepatocellular cancer has been observed (odds ratio: 1.9; 95% CI: 0.94–3.63) (McGlynn et al. 1995). In addition higher serum aflatoxin B1-albumin adduct levels were observed in GST M1-0 and/or GST T1-0 patients with hepatocellular cancer (C.J. Chen et al. 1996). Two case-control studies with relatively small case numbers did not observe an association between hepatocellular cancer and GST T1-0 and GST M1-0 genotypes (Yu et al. 1995; Hsieh et al. 1996).

Cutaneous Tumors

Basal cell carcinoma of the skin is the commonest cancer in Caucasians, although mortality is very low. A feature seen in patients who suffered from basal cell carcinoma and who were successfully treated is the risk of further separate primary tumors. The GST T1-0 genotype was associated with significantly decreased time to the next separate primary tumor (Lear et al. 1997). About two-thirds of GST T1-0 patients suffered a further tumor within 5 years in contrast to only one-third of GST T1-positive patients. GST M1 genotype alone did not influence subsequent tumor presentation time. However, GST M1-0 genotype in combination with basal cell carcinoma at a truncal tumor site (which is usually less exposed to ultraviolet radiation) demonstrated a markedly decreased time to next lesion, such that all patients (100%) suffered a further primary basal cell carcinoma within 5 years (Lear et al. 1997). Heagerty et al. (1994) observed similar frequencies of GST M1-0 genotypes in the total group of patients with cutaneous tumors (basal cell carcinoma, squamous cell carcinoma, malignant melanoma; total cases: 629) and controls ($n = 153$). However, GST M1-0 was significantly associated with patients who suffered from two or more tumors of different types (odds ratio: 2.31; 95% CI: 1.12–4.75; 45 patients, 152 controls). The heterozygote GST M1 A/B genotype was reduced in the total group of patients with cutaneous tumors (odds ratio: 0.31; 95% CI: 0.13–0.75) and in patients with basal carcinoma (odds ratio: 0.26; 95% CI: 0.10–0.72) (Heagerty et al. 1994), suggesting that GST M1 A/B might be protective.

In addition the GST M3 polymorphism (GST M3 AA) in combination with GST M1-0 genotype has been shown to confer increased risk of basal cell carcinoma (Yengi et al. 1996). Two alleles of GST M3, GST M3*A and GST M3*B, distinguished by a recognition motif for the YY1 transcription factor, have been observed. Since GST M3AA (in combination with GST M1-0) was associated with increased tumor risk, YY1 might act as an activator of the recognition motif in GST M3*B (Yengi et al. 1996).

Myelodysplastic Syndrome

Recently, a strong association between the GST T1-0 genotype with myelodysplastic syndrome has been observed (odds ratio: 4.3; 95% CI: 2.5–7.4; 96 patients, 190 controls) (H. Chen et al. 1996). However, this observation has not been confirmed in an independent study with relatively high case numbers (174 patients, 100 controls) (Preudhomme et al. 1997).

Gynecologic Tumors

No association between GST M1-0 and/or GST T1-0 with ovarian cancer (Hengstler et al. 1998b; Sarhanis et al. 1996), breast cancer (Zhong et al. 1993; Kelsey et al. 1997b; Ambrosone et al. 1995), endometrial cancer (Esteller et al. 1997) or cervical cancer (Warwick et al. 1994) has been observed. However, the GST M1-0 genotype was associated with longer survival in breast cancer (Kelsey et al. 1997b) and the proportion of patients with both GST M1-0 and GST T1-0 was significantly greater in individuals with p53 immunopositive ovarian carcinomas than in the p53 immunonegative group (Sarhanis et al. 1996). Both interesting observations have not yet been confirmed by independent groups.

Other Sites

GSTM1-0 was associated with gastric adenocarcinoma in a Japanese study (Katoh et al. 1996). The double-null genotype (GST M1-0 and GST T1-0) was significantly overrepresented in black children with acute lymphoblastic leukemia, but not in white children (Chen et al. 1997).

The GSTT1-0 genotype was significantly underrepresented in patients with renal cell cancer having been exposed to high levels of trichloroethylene over many years (odds ratio: 0.24; 95% CI: 0.07–0.86; 45 patients, 48 controls) (Brüning et al. 1997). The reference group consisted of 48 individuals with similar exposure to trichloroethylene but not suffering from cancer. Similarly, GST M1-0 was significantly underrepresented in patients with renal cell cancer (odds ratio: 0.36; 95% CI: 0.16–0.85) (Brüning et al. 1997). Thus, GST T1-0 and GST M1-0 genotypes seem to protect from renal cell cancer. This observation is interesting, since it differs from other positive case-control studies (of sites other than kidney), which all observed an association of GST M1-0 or GST T1-0 with increased cancer risk. The protective effect of GST M1-0 or GST T1-0 genotypes might be explained by the metabolic pathway of trichloroethylene, which includes formation of dichlorovinyl-S-cysteine catalyzed by glutathione S-transferases. In the proximal renal tubule dichlorovinyl-S-cysteine is further metabolized to electrophilic thioketenes, the ultimately genotoxic metabolites, by the action of β-lyase (Dekant and Vamvakas, 1993). It would be interesting to know whether the protective effect of the GST M1 and GST T1 null genotypes against renal cell cancer is limited to trichloroethylene-associated renal cancer or whether it is a general feature of renal cell carcinogenesis.

Glutathione S-Transferase P1

Glutathione S-transferase P1 (GST P1) is (together with GST A1/A2) the major GST protein in human lung tissue, whereas GST M1 is only expressed weakly (Anttila et al. 1993). GST P1 is involved in the inactivation of various cigarette smoke carcinogens, such as benzo[a]pyrene-7,8-diol-9,10-epoxide (BPDE) (and other diol epoxides of polycyclic aromatic hydrocarbons), and also other toxic cigarette smoke constituents, such as acrolein (Hayes and Pulford 1995). In addition GST P1 is known to be overexpressed in some types of tumor tissue (Hengstler et al. 1998b) and may be involved in cytostatic drug resistance (Tanner et al. 1997).

A polymorphic site of GST P1 at codon 104 has been observed (Ahmad et al. 1990; Izawa and Ali-Osman 1993; Harries et al. 1997). An A to G substitution at base pair 314 results in an amino acid difference, valine vs isoleucine, at codon 104. This residue is located close to the hydrophobic binding site of GST P1 (Garcia-Saez et al. 1994) and it has been shown that the isoleucine 104 variant exhibits a lower activity towards several carcinogenic diol epoxides compared to the valine 104 form (Hu et al. 1997a,b). For example, the V_{max} of glutathione conjugation of (+)-7β,8α-dihydroxy-9α,10α-oxy-7,8,9,10-tetrahydrobenzo[α]pyrene ((+)-anti-BPDE), which among the four BPDE isomers is the most potent carcinogen, was 3.4-fold higher for the valine 104 wild type of GST P1 compared to the isoleucine 104 variant (Hu et al. 1997a). Similarly, the V_{max} of GSH conjugation of the carcinogenic diol epoxide of chrysene, (+)-anti-1,2-dihydroxy-3,4-oxy-1,2,3,4-tetrahydrochrysene ((+)-anti-CDE) was 5.3-fold higher for the valine 104 wild type compared to the isoleucine 104-variant (Hu et al. 1997b). These results suggest that individuals with the GST P1 isoleucine 104 variant might be more susceptible to carcinogenic effects of diol epoxides of polycyclic aromatic hydrocarbons.

Recently, 297 healthy caucasians were genotyped for the GST P1 polymorphism at codon 104. Approximately 52% were homozygous for adenine at base pair 314 (valine 104 form), 39% were heterozygous and 9% were homozygous for guanine at base pair 314 (isoleucine 104 form) (Ryberg et al. 1997).

Several types of cancer have been shown to be associated with the low activity allele of GST P1 (isoleucine 104 variant). The odds ratio of testicular cancer patients ($n = 155$) homozygous for the isoleucine 104 allele vs random controls ($n = 155$) was 3.3 (1.5–7.7) (95% CI) (Harries et al. 1997). Similarly, the frequency of the homozygous isoleucine 104 allele was increased in bladder cancer patients ($n = 71$) vs controls ($n = 155$) (odds ratio: 3.6; 95% CI: 1.4–9.2) (Harries et al. 1997). Furthermore, a significant association of the GST P1 polymorphism at codon 104 with lung cancer was observed (Ryberg et al. 1997). The frequency of the homozygous isoleucine at codon 104 was significantly higher for male lung cancer patients (current or former smokers only) ($n = 138$) than for healthy controls ($n = 297$) (odds ratio: 2.41; 95% CI: 1.17–4.96). In the same population the GST M1 null genotype was associated only with a slightly, statistically not significant, increased odds ratio for lung cancer (odds ratio: 1.33; 95% CI: 0.89–1.99). In addition lung cancer patients homozygous for the isoleucine 104 variant had significantly (about twofold) more DNA-adducts in surgically obtained healthy lung tissue, as determined by ^{32}P-postlabelling, than lung cancer patients homozygous for the valine 104 form (Ryberg et al. 1997).

An increase in the proportion of individuals homozygous for the isoleucine 104 variant in lung cancer patients was observed also in another study (Harries et al. 1997). However, this did not reach statistical significance (odds ratio: 1.9; 95% CI: 0.7–4.8). Nevertheless, the preliminary data indicate that the isoleucine 104 variant of GST P1 might have a higher penetrance as a risk factor for lung cancer than the null genotype of GST M1.

In contrast to lung, bladder and testicular cancer, a marked reduction in the frequency of isoleucine, 104 homozygotes was observed in patients with prostatic cancer ($n = 36$) (Harries et al. 1997). Although this was not significant (odds ratio: 0.4; 95% CI: 0.02–3.3), there was a highly significant reduction in prostatic cancer patients homozygous for the valine 104 form ($p = 0.008$) and a significant increase in the proportion of heterozygotes ($p = 0.003$).

No significant association between the GST P1 isoleucine 104 variant and breast cancer (odds ratio: 1.3; 95% CI: 0.4–4.3) and colon cancer (odds ratio 1.3; 95% CI: 0.4–4.6) was observed (Harries et al. 1997).

These preliminary data, which have not been confirmed yet, suggest an important role for the GST P1 polymorphism in cancer susceptibility, especially in view of the almost ubiquitous expression of GST P1. Possibly this polymorphism may also be important in the success of anticancer chemotherapy with alkylating agents. It can be expected that a large number of studies on the relevance of the GST P1 polymorphism at codon 104 will be presented in the next few years, since genotyping is relatively easy by PCR and digestion of the product with *Alw*261, as described by Harries et al. (1997).

Microsomal Epoxide Hydrolase

Epoxide hydrolases comprise a group of enzymes that are functionally related in that they catalyze the addition of water to an epoxide to form the vicinal dihydrodiol, which in the cases of defined stereochemistry has the *trans*-configuration. Enzymatic hydration often results in metabolites of lower reactivity, or of metabolites which can be conjugated and excreted. Thus, in most cases the action of epoxide hydrolases is considered as detoxifying. However, numerous studies have reported its central role in formation of precursors of even more deleterious products in the metabolism of angular polycyclic aromatic hydrocarbons to diol bay region epoxides (Oesch 1988).

Four different epoxide hydrolases are known in humans. Microsomal and cytosolic epoxide hydrolases metabolize a wide range of xenobiotic alkene and arene oxides including many known carcinogens and mutagens (Herrero et al. 1997; Lacourciere and Armstrong 1994; Beetham et al. 1995; Arand et al. 1996b; Oesch et al. 1984), whereas microsomal cholesterol epoxide hydrolase (specific substrate: cholesterol 5,6-oxide) and cytosolic leukotriene A_4 hydrolase are more specific (Oesch et al. 1984; Medina et al. 1991; Seidegard and Ekström 1997).

Presently, only one of the four human epoxide hydrolases, namely microsomal epoxide hydrolase (mEH), has been shown to be polymorphic (Hassett et al. 1994; 1997; Gaedigk et al. 1994; Green et al. 1995). The discovery of a polymorphism mEH (Hassett et al. 1994) was relatively unexpected, since several studies observed large interindividual variation but a *unimodal* frequency distribution for the activity of mEH in human leukocytes (Seidegard et al. 1984; Mertes et al. 1985; Kroetz et al. 1990; Heckbert et al. 1992; for review see Daly et al. 1993). Nonetheless, already in 1990 a *trimodal* frequency distribution in the activity of mEH in human amniocytes, obtained during gestational weeks 14–16, was observed (Buehler et al. 1990). Hassett et al. (1994) identified two allelic variants of human mEH, a His vs Tyr substitution in amino acid position 113 (exon 3) and a His vs Arg substitution in position 139 (exon 4). The frequency of individuals (predominantly Caucasians; >85%) homozygous for Tyr at position 113 was 36%, whereas 8% were homozygous for His, and the remaining 56% were heterozygous (105 individuals examined). At amino acid position 139 the percentage of individuals homozygous for His was approximately 58%, 5% were homozygous for Arg and 37% were heterozygous (109 individuals examined). Expression of cDNAs containing each of the amino acids at positions 113 and 139 in COS-1 cells showed a functional relevance of the different alleles with respect to mEH protein expression and enzyme activity (Table 4). The highest activity of mEH (determined with benzo[*a*]pyrene-4,5-oxide as a substrate) was observed in S9 protein (the protein of the 9000 *g* supernatant fraction, which contains the microsomes) of COS-1 cells transfected with mEH cDNA with amino acids Tyr-113 and Arg-139 (relative activity: 100%), whereas the Tyr-113/His-139, His-113/Arg-139, and His-113/His-139 variants resulted in relative mEH activities of 80%, 70%, and 49%, respectively (Hassett et al. 1994). Since enzymatic activity correlated well with immunochemically detected levels of mEH protein and the ratio of mEH activity/mEH protein was not increased in the more active COS-1 cells (Table 4), the data suggest that amino acid variation at residues 113 and 139 does not exert a primary influence on catalytic function (Table 4). Furthermore, mEH mRNA expression was relatively uniform, despite the different alleles (Table 4). These observations might suggest an influence of amino acid residues 113 and 139 on stability of mEH protein, although – to our knowledge – this has not yet been shown directly.

To examine whether variations in mEH activity are associated with amino acid polymorphisms at positions 113 and 139, mEH activity and diploid haplotypes were determined in 40 transplant quality human liver samples (Hassett et al. 1997). mEH showed an approximately eightfold range in activity. Overall rank ordering of mean mEH activity in livers from homozygous haplotypes followed the same trend as observed in vitro (Table 4). However, the small number of cases of the homozygous haplotypes did not allow reasonable statistical evaluation. Furthermore, large interindividual differences in mEH activity were observed even for individuals with identical amino acids at positions 113 and 139, suggesting that additional factors are responsible for mEH activity. Thus, further studies with sufficient case numbers are required to examine a possible association between polymorphic 113 and 139 residues and mEH activity in various human organs.

Table 4. Expression of the polymorphic microsomal epoxide hydrolase (mEH) alleles in COS-1 cells. (From Hassett et al. 1994)

Amino acids at positions		Relative mEH activity in transfected COS-1 cells[a]	Relative immunohistochemically detected mEH protein expression in transfected COS-1 cells[b]	mEH activity/ mEH protein	relative mEH mRNA expression[2]
113	139				
Tyr	Arg	100%	100%	1.0	100%
Tyr	His	80%	65%	1.2	99%
His	Arg	70%	53%	1.3	106%
His	His	49%	36%	1.4	103%
Mock transfected		0.6%	7%	0.1	0.09%

[a] Benzo[*a*]pyrene-4,5-oxide was used as a substrate. 100% represents 938 pmol benzo[*a*]pyrene-4,5-diol formed per mg S9 protein per min.
[b] Arbitrary units.

Presently, three studies have shown a possible association between the exon 3 (Tyr-113→His) polymorphism of mEH with different types of cancer (McGlynn et al. 1995; Lancaster et al. 1996). The His-113 variant of mEH was significantly overrepresented in 52 Chinese patients with hepatocellular cancer compared to 116 healthy controls (McGlynn et al. 1995). The odds ratio associated with having at least one His-113 allele (mutant or putative low-activity allele) was 3.3 (95% CI: 0.39–28.6) in HB_sAg^- (hepatitis B surface antigen-negative) individuals. As expected, viral infection (HB_sAg^+) represented a risk factor also in individuals with the homozygous Tyr-113 allele (odds ratio: 15.0; 95% CI: 1.2–184). However, the odds ratio of HB_sAg^+ individuals carrying at least one His-113 allele was even more than five fold higher (odds ratio: 77.3; 95% CI: 8.9–666; compared to HB_sAg^- individuals with homozygous Tyr-113 allele) than the odds ratio of HB_sAg^+ individuals with the homozygous Tyr-113 allele. Mutations at codon 249 of p53 were detected in ten of the 52 hepatocellular tumor samples. All of the ten mutations occurred in tumors of individuals who had at least one His-113 allele. Since primary hepatocellular carcinoma has been shown to be caused by aflatoxin B_1 (AFB_1), which after metabolic activation binds to the N7-position of guanine and induces G to T transversions, serum AFB_1-albumin adducts were determined in 49 Ghanian males with possible exposure to AFB_1 (McGlynn et al. 1995). Individuals with detectable AFB_1-albumin adduct levels (>5 pg/ mg) were more likely to have at least one His113 allele of mEH ($p = 0.02$) than individuals without detectable AFB_1-albumin adduct levels. The observed link between the mEH polymorphism, AFB1-adducts, p53 mutations and hepatocellular cancer suggests an important role for mEH in detoxication of AFB_1exo-8,9-epoxide. AFB_1 is oxidized by human cytochrome P450 3A4 to several products. Only one of these, the 8,9-exo-epoxide, appears to be highly mutagenic (Guengerich et al. 1996). Purified human epoxide hydrolase provided no detectable enhancement of the rate of (already nonenzymatically very high) chemical hydrolysis of AFB_1-exo-8,9-epoxide (Guengerich et al. 1996; Johnson et al. 1997). Using a *Salmonella typhimurium* system (endpoint: *umu*-response) with very low concentrations of active cytochrome P450 3A4 (10 nM) and cofactors together with relatively high concentrations of purified human mEH (0.3–3 µM) only a moderate inhibition in genotoxicity of AFB_1 (20 µM), by approximately 30% could be achieved by mEH (1 µM) (Guengerich et al. 1996; Johnson et al. 1997). However, the slight effect resulting from extremely high ratios of mEH to cytochrome P450 is difficult to interpret. Furthermore, the use of AFB_1-albumin adducts to study the contribution of mEH to detoxication of AFB_1-8,9-epoxide (McGlynn et al. 1995) was criticized (Johnson et al. 1997), since the hydrolysis product of AFB_1-exo-8,9-epoxide, AFB_1-8,9-dihydrodiol, was postulated to be responsible for formation of protein adducts via formation of the electrophilic dialdehyde (Sabbioni et al. 1987). Thus, further studies with higher case numbers and more specific endpoints for biomonitoring AFB1-exo-8,9-epoxide formation are required to examine the postulated spectacular association between mEH polymorphism and AFB1-induced hepatocellular cancer.

Recently, the mEH polymorphism has been shown to be associated with ovarian cancer (Lancaster et al. 1996). The frequency of the homozygous (putative) high-activity genotype (Tyr-113 allele) was 41% in a caucasian control population (75 individuals) and 64% (75 individuals) in patients (odds ratio: 2.6; 95% CI: 1.3–5). Thus, if the reported associations between mEH polymorphisms and hepatocellular as well as ovarian cancer are reproducible, they represent another striking example of organ-specific differences in polymorphism-based modification of cancer susceptibility, since the (putative) high-activity genotype protects from hepatocellular cancer (possibly by detoxication of carcinogenic AFB1 metabolites), whereas susceptibility for ovarian cancer is increased (possibly due to formation of mutagenic precursors).

Since mEH is strongly expressed in bronchial epithelial cells, which are subject to oxidative stress from cigarette smoke, a possible association between mEH and susceptibility to lung cancer (50 patients), emphysema (94 patients) and chronic obstructive pulmonary disease (68 patients) has been examined (Smith and Harrison 1997). The homozygous exon 3 (slow) mutation (His-113 allele) was significantly associated with chronic obstructive pulmonary disease (odds ratio: 3.5; 95% CI: 1.5–8.0) and emphysema (odds ratio: 5.6; 95% CI: 2.7–11.5). Although a trend towards a higher odds ratio was observed (1.6; 95% CI: 0.6–4.8), the homozygous His-113 allele was not significantly associated with lung cancer. However, it should be considered that only a very small number of cases ($n = 50$) has been examined. The exon 4 polymorphism (histidine residue 139 to arginine) was not significantly associated with lung cancer and emphysema, whereas an increased odds ratio (1.9; 95% CI: 1.2–3.0) for carriers of the mutant (fast) exon 4 allele (His-139 to Arg; homozygous and heterozygous) was observed for patients with chronic obstructive pulmonary disease.

Further investigations (with higher numbers of cases) on possible associations between mEH polymorphisms and cancer risk are required, especially for tumors of organs with a high constitutive expression of mEH, such as kidney, pancreas, lung and liver. The scientific value of future studies will be increased if not only the Tyr-113→His, but also the His-139→Arg polymorphism is considered and if determination of genotypes are combined with measurement of mEH activity, since an association has not yet been confirmed sufficiently.

Sulfotransferases

Cytosolic sulfotransferases transfer the sulfonyl moiety from the cofactor 3′-phosphoadenosine-5′-phosphosulfate (PAPS) mainly to hydroxyl-, but also to amino-, sulfhydryl-, and N-oxide groups of endogenous or xenobiotic substrates (Glatt et al. 1996). O-sulfonation is a common step in phase II metabolism and was traditionally associated with detoxification. However, since the sulfate anion represents a good leaving group it may be cleaved off heterolytically from such sites thereby generating a relatively stable cation which, by means of its electrophilic nature, may covalently bind to DNA. Sulfotransferase-mediated genotoxicity has been demonstrated for numerous substances (e.g. hydroxylated arylamines and also benzylic alcohols derived from polycyclic aromatic hydrocarbons; for review see Glatt et al. 1996) and presently almost weekly more substances are discovered which are activated to mutagens by sulfonation (Glatt, personal communication).

Sulfotransferases are members of a gene superfamily that presently includes phenol sulfotransferases (PST), hydroxysteroid sulfotransferases (HST), and in plants flavonol sulfotransferases (Weinshilboum et al. 1997). Five cytosolic sulfotransferases are presently known in humans, and cDNAs have recently been cloned (Table 5). Four isoforms belong to the subfamily of phenol sulfotransferase (ST 1A2, ST 1A3, M-PST, EST) and one isoform belongs to the subfamily of hydroxysteroid sulfotransferases (hDHEAST). Two isoforms of phenol sulfotransferases, ST 1A2 and ST 1A3, are thermostable (previously thought to be only one enzyme: thermostable sulfotransferase in contrast to M-PST, which is relatively thermosensitive; Weinshilboum and Aksoy, 1994), whereas the thermosensitivity of HST (hDHEAST) is intermediate. Prototypical substrates of the thermostable sulfotransferases are 4-nitrophenol and other planar phenols, whereas the thermolabile sulfotransferase (M-PST) preferentially catalyzes sulfonation of dopamine and other catechols and phenolic monoamines. hDHEAST catalyzes sulfonation of dehydroepiandrosterone to dehydroepiandrosterone sulfate, the most abundantly circulating steroid in humans, which serves as a precursor for the formation of active androgens and estrogens. Plasma levels of dehydroepiandrosterone have been shown to be decreased in patients with prostatic cancer (Stahl et al. 1992).

Three cytosolic human sulfotransferase enzymes have been shown to be regulated by separate genetic polymorphisms: hDHEAST, hM-PST, and thermostable phenol sulfotransferase (TS PST) (the latter meaning ST 1A2 and/ or ST 1A3 isoforms, which share 96% amino acid identity; Yamazoe et al. 1994) and were not differentiated in the polymorphism study in which human platelet TS PST activity was determined (Weinshilboum and Aksay, 1994). hDHEAST activity was determined in 94 samples of human hepatic biopsy tissue (Aksoy et al. 1993; Weinshilbaum and Aksay 1994). A bimodal frequency distribution was obtained, with approximately 25% of the samples included in a high-activity subgroup, although the range in hDHEAST activity was not very wide (4.6-fold).

In contrast to hDHEAST, TS PST and hM-PST are expressed in human blood platelets. The activity of TS PST, but not of hM-PST has been shown to correlate with activity of this enzyme in human liver, jejunal mucosa and cerebral cortex (Young et al. 1985; Sundaram et al. 1989). For TS PST a trimodal frequency distribution of platelet enzyme activity (of 228 unrelated adults) was obtained (Weinshilboum and Aksoy 1994), with about 2%, 24%, and 74% of individuals in the high, intermediate and low activity subgroups, respectively (Van Loon and Weinshilboum 1984; Weinshilbaum and Aksoy

Table 5. Isoforms of human sulfotransferases

Sulfotransferase isoform	ST 1A2	ST 1A3	M-PST	EST	HST
Synonyms	hTSPST1 (human thermostable phenol sulfotransferase 1)	hTSPST2 human thermostable phenol sulfotransferase 2)	hTLPST (human thermosensitive phenol sulfotransferase)	hEST (human estrogen sulfotransferase)	hDHEAST human dehydro-epiandrosterone sulfotransferase)
Subfamily	Phenol sulfotransferases (PST)	PST	PST	PST	Hydroxysteroid sulfo-transferases (HST)
Chromosome	16p	16p	16p	4q	19q
Prototypical substrates	4-Nitrophenol Minoxidil	4-Nitrophenol Minoxidil	Dopamine 5-Hydroxytryptamine	β-Estradiol 17α-Ethinylestradiol	Dehydroepiandrosterone Pregnenolone
Polymorphisms	Frequency of low-activity allele: 0.86 Frequency of high-activity allele: 0.14	Frequency of low-activity allele: 0.86 Frequency of high-activity allee: 0.14	Low-activity allele: 0.92 High-activity allele: 0.08	No known Polymorphism	Low-activity: 75% High-activity: 25%

1994). These data were explained by a genetic polymorphism with gene frequencies of 0.14 for the high-activity allele and 0.86 for the low activity allele.

For hM-PST activity in human platelets, data from family studies were best explained by a genetic polymorphism with a high-activity allele frequency of 0.08 and a low-activity allele frequency of 0.92 (Price et al. 1988). However, no correlation of hM-PST activity in human platelets and other human tissues was observed. Thus, the hM-PST polymorphism observed in platelets is possibly of minor relevance for cancer susceptibility.

Although several studies have been performed, the molecular mechanisms of the sulfotransferase polymorphisms – to our knowledge – have not yet been discovered. In the hDHEAST gene of individuals from the slow sulfonation group, two point mutations, each resulting in an amino acid exchange (exon 2: Met-57→Tyr; exon 4: Glu-186→Val), were discovered (Wood et al. 1996). Transient expression of the respective cDNAs in COS-1 cells resulted in decreased expression of both hDHEAST enzymatic activity and the level of immunoreactive protein only when the Glu-186→Val variant was present. However, neither polymorphism was closely associated with enzyme activity in human liver samples. Thus, mechanisms other than the investigated genetic polymorphisms may additionally influence hDHEAST activity in human tissue.

To our knowledge no studies on sulfotransferase polymorphisms and human cancer risk have been published, although this seems to be a very promising field of research. A large number of environmental mutagens and carcinogens are activated by sulfotransferases (Table 6; from Glatt 1997). For example, methylene-briged polycyclic aromatic hydrocarbons, which are present in crude mineral oil and occur as environmental contaminants (Glatt et al. 1993; Adams et al. 1982), or the ketone derivates of bridged polyarenes, which are found in urban air, in emissions from wood and coal combustion and diesel exhausts (Glatt et al. 1993; Ramdahl, 1985), can be activated by sulfotransferases after hydroxylation by cytochrome P450. In addition, after hydroxylation in the liver, several heterocyclic amines formed during the cooking of meat and fish (e.g. PhIP or IQ; Table 6) are activated by sulfotransferases (Glatt 1997). In general, benzylic alcohols of polycyclic aromatic hydrocarbons are preferentially sulfonated by HST (Glatt et al. 1994), whereas human PSTs are preferentially responsible for the sulfation of aromatic hydroxylamines and hydroxamic acids (Glatt 1997). Thus, an increased cancer risk for the high-sulfonation subgroups of individuals exposed to the mentioned substances would not be unexpected, especially, since several animal and in vitro studies have shown an association between sulfonation activity and chemically induced cancer (for review see Burchell and Coughtrie 1997). For example, male rats, which have up to ten fold higher activities of sulfotransferases than female rats, are more susceptible to aromatic amines (requiring sulfonation for activation) than female rats. The carcinogenicity of aromatic amines to rats was significantly reduced by inhibitors of sulfotransferases (Miller 1994). Furthermore, a mouse strain with reduced capacity for

Table 6. Substances activated by various isoforms of human sulfotransferases. (From Glatt 1997)

Sulfotransferase isoform	Substances activated to mutagenic or DNA binding metabolites
Human thermostable phenol sulfotransferase	N-hydroxy-2-amino-1-methyl-6-phenylimidazo[4,5-b]pyridine (N-OH-PhIP) 1-Hydroxymethylpyrene 2-Hydroxymethylpyrene 2-Hydroxy-3-methylcholanthrene 7-Hydroxy-7,8,9,10-tetrahydrobenzo[a]pyrene
Human thermosensitive phenol sulfotransferase (hm-PST)	1-Hydroxymethylpyrene
Human estrogen sulfotransferase (hEST)	1-Hydroxymethylpyrene 7-Hydroxy-7,8,9,10-tetrahydrobenzo[a]pyrene
Hydroxysteroid sulfotransferase (hHST)	N-Hydroxy-2-acetylaminofluorene 9-Hydroxymethylanthracene 1-Hydroxymethylpyrene 2-Hydroxymethylpyrene 7-Hydroxymethyl-12-methylbenz[a]anthracene 1-Hydroxy-3-methylcholanthrene 2-Hydroxy-3-methylcholanthrene 4H-cyclopenta[def]chrysen4-ol 7-Hydroxy-7,8,9,10-tetrahydrobenzo[a]pyrene 1-Hydroxysafrole Hycanthone

PAPS synthesis (the rate limiting cofactor for sulfotransferase activity) was shown to be less susceptible to carcinogenesis initiated by aromatic amines. PAPS-dependent DNA binding of several N-hydroxy metabolites of carcinogenic arylamines and heterocyclic amines was examined using hepatic cytosols of 12 humans as an activating system (Chou et al. 1995). The extent of DNA binding significantly correlated with the levels of polymorphic thermostable PST activity. Furthermore, PAPS-dependent DNA binding of N-hydroxylated metabolites of heterocyclic amines was observed using colon cytosols, but not cytosols of the pancreas, larynx, or urinary bladder epithelium (Chou et al. 1995).

Although the tissue distribution of sulfotransferases in humans has only been studied to a limited extent, some examples of organ- and cell type-specific expression have been shown. A well known example of cell type-specific expression of sulfotransferase is the metabolic activation of the antihypertensive and hypertrichotic drug Minoxidil, which requires activation by sulfonation. Especially high activities of the sulfotransferase responsible for this reaction are expressed in the hair follicles, providing locally high concentrations of activated Minoxidil at the place of its hypertrichotic effect (Burchell and Coughtrie 1997; Baker et al. 1994). Furthermore, besides the liver, high levels of hHST have been observed in adrenals and in the endometrium

(Falany and Falany 1996), which therefore represent organs which might be especially sensitive to sulfotransferase-mediated carcinogenesis.

In conclusion studies on a possible association of sulfotransferase polymorphisms and cancer risk are urgently required.

References

Adams JD, LaVoie EJ, Hoffmann D (1982) Analysis of methylated polynuclear aromatic hydrocarbons by capillary gas chromatography. Influence of temperature on the pyrosynthesis of anthracene, phenanthrene and their methylated derivatives. J Chromatogr Sci 20:274–277

Agundez JA, Olivera M, Ladero JM, Rodriguez-Lescure A, Ledesma MC, Diaz-Rubio M, Meyer UA, Benitez J (1996) Increased risk for hepatocellular carcinoma in NAT2-slow acetylators and CYP2D6-rapid metabolizers. Pharmacogenetics 6:501–512

Ahmad H, Wilson DE, Fritz RR, Singh SV, Medh RD, Nagle GT, Awasthi YC, Kurosky A (1990) Primary and secondary analyses of glutathione S-transferase Pi from human placenta. Arch Biochem Biophys 287:398–408

Aksoy IA, Sochorova V, Weinshilboum RM (1993) Human liver dehydroepiandrosterone sulfotransferase: nature and extent of individual variation. Clin Pharmacol Ther 54:498–506

Alexandrie A-K, Sundberg MI, Seidegard J, Tornling G, Rannug A (1994) Genetic susceptibility to lung cancer with special emphasis on CYP 1A1 and GST M1: a study on host factors in relation to age at onset, gender and histological cancer types. Carcinogenesis 15:1785–1790

Ambrosone CB, Freudenheim JL, Graham S, Marshall JR, Vena JE, Brasure JR, Laughlin R, Nemoto T, Michalek AM, Harrington A, et al. (1995) Cytochrome P4501A1 and glutathione S-transferase (M1) genetic polymorphisms and postmenopausal breast cancer risk. Cancer Res 55:3483–3485

Ambrosone CB, Freudenheim JL, Graham S, Marshall JR, Vena JE, Brasure JR, Michalek AM, Laughlin R, Nemoto T, Gillenwater KA, Harrington AM, Shields PG (1996) Cigarette smoking, N-acetyltransferase 2 genetic polymorphisms, and breast cancer risk. JAMA 276:1511–1512

Anttila S, Hirvonen A, Vainio H, Husgafvel-Pursiainen K, Hayes JD, Ketterer B, (1993) Immunohistochemical localization of glutathione S-transferase in human lung. Cancer Res 53:5643–5648

Anwar WA, Abdel-Rahman SZ, El-Zein RA, Mostafa HM, Au WW (1996) Genetic polymorphisms of GSTM1, CYP2E1 and CYP2D6 in Egyptian bladder cancer patients. Carcinogenesis 17:1923–1929

Arand M, Mühlbauer R, Hengstler JG, Jäger E, Fuchs J, Winkler L, Oesch F (1996a) A multiplex polymerase chain reaction protocol for the simultaneous analysis of the glutathione S-transferase GSTM1 and GSTT1 polymorphisms. Anal Biochem 236:184–186

Arand M, Wagner H, Oesch F (1996b) Asp333, Asp495, and His523 form the catalytic triad of rat soluble epoxide hydrolase. J Biol Chem 271:4223–4229

Badawi AF, Stern SJ, Lang NP, Kadlubar FF (1996) Cytochrome P-450 and acetyltransferase expression as biomarkers of carcinogen DNA adduct levels and human cancer susceptibility. Prog Clin Biol Res 395:109–140

Baker CA, Uno H, Johnson GA (1994) Minoxidil sulfation in the hair follicle. Skin Pharmacol 7:335–339

Bartsch H, Rojas M, Alexander K, Camus A-M, Castegnaro C, Malaveille S, Antilla S, Hirvonen K, Husgafvel-Pursiainen E, Hietanen E, Vainio H (1995) Metabolic polymorphism affecting DNA binding and excretion of carcinogens in humans Pharmacogenetics 5:584–590

Beetham JK, Grant D, Arand M, Garbarino J, Kiyosue T, Pinot F, Oesch F, Belknap WR, Shinozaki K, Hammock BD (1995) Gene evolution of epoxide hydrolases and recommended nomenclature. DNA Cell Biol 14:61–71

Bell DA, Taylor JA, Paulson DF, Robertson CN, Mohler JL, Lucier GW (1993) Genetic risk and carcinogen exposure: a common inherited defect of the carcinogen-metabolism gene glutathione S-transferase M1 (GST M1) that increases susceptibility to bladder cancer. J Nat Cancer Inst 85:1159–1163

Bell DA, Badawi AF, Lang NP, Ilett KF, Kadlubar FF, Hirvonen A (1995) Polymorphism in the N-acetyltransferase 1 (NAT1) polyadenylation signal: association of NAT*10 allele with higher N-acetylation activity in bladder and colon tissue. Cancer Res 55:5226–5229

Blum M, Grant DM, McBridge OW, Heim M (1990) Human arylamine N-acetyltransferase genes: Isolation, chromosomal localization, and functional expression. DNA Cell Biol 9:193–203

Brockmöller J, Kerb R, Drakoulis N, Nitz M, Roots I (1993) Genotype and phenotype of glutathione S-transferase class μ isoenzymes μ and φ in lung cancer patients and controls. Cancer Res 53:1004–1011

Brockmöller J, Kerb R, Drakoulis N, Staffeldt B, Roots I (1994) Glutathione S-transferase M1 and its variants A and B as host factors of bladder cancer susceptibility: a case-control study. Cancer Res 54:4103–4111

Brockmöller J, Cascorbi I, Kerb R, Roots I (1996a) Combined analysis of inherited polymorphisms in arylamine N-acetyltransferase 2, glutathione S-transferases M1 and T1, microsomal epoxide hydrolase, and cytochrome P450 enzymes as modulators of bladder cancer risk. Cancer Res 56:3915–3925

Brockmöller J, Kaiser R, Kerb R, Cascorbi I, Jaeger V, Roots I (1996b) Polymorphic enzymes of xenobiotic metabolism as modulators of acquired p53 mutations in bladder cancer. Pharmacogenetics 6:535–545

Brüning T, Lammert M, Kempkes M, Thier R, Golka K, Bolt HM (1997) Influence of polymorphisms of GSTM1 and GSTT1 for risk of renal cell cancer in workers with long-term high occupational exposure to trichloroethene. Arch Toxicol 71:596–599

Buehler BA, Delimont D, VanWaes M, Finnell RH (1990) Prenatal prediction of risk of the fetal hydantoin syndrome. N Engl J Med 322:1567–1572

Burchell B, Coughtrie MWH (1997) Genetic and environmental factors associated with variation of human xenobiotic glucuronidation and sulfation. Environ Health Perspect 105:739–747

Cartwright RA (1984) Epidemiological studies on N-acetylation and C-center ring oxidation in neoplasia. In: Omenn GS, Gelboin HV (eds) Genetic variability in responses to chemical exposure. Cold Spring Harbor Laboratory New York, pp 359–369

Cascorbi I, Brockmöller J, Mrozikiewicz PM, Bauer S, Loddenkemper R, Roots I (1996) Homozygous rapid arylamine N-acetyltransferase (NAT2) genotype as a susceptibility factor for lung cancer. Cancer Res 56:3961–3966

Chen CJ, Yu MW, Liaw YF, Wang LW, Chiamprasert S, Matin F, Hirvonen A, Bell DA (1996) Chronic hepatitis B carriers with null genotypes of glutathione S-transferase M1 and T1 polymorphisms who are exposed to aflatoxin are at increased risk of hepatocellular carcinoma. Am J Hum Genet 59:128–134

Chen CL, Liu Q, Pui CH, Rivera GK, Sandlund JT, Ribeiro R, Evans WE, Relling MV (1997) Higher frequency of glutathione S-transferase deletions in black children with acute lymphoblastic leukemia. Blood 89:1701–1707

Chen H, Sandler DP, Taylor JA, Shore DL, Liu E, Bloomfield CD, Bell DA (1996) Increased risk for myelodysplastic syndromes in individuals with glutathione transferase theta 1 (GSTT1) gene defect. Lancet 347:295–297

Chenevix-Trench G, Young J, Coggan M, Board P (1995) Glutathione S-transferase M1 and T1 polymorphisms: susceptibility to colon cancer and age of onset. Carcinogenesis 16:1655–1657

Chou HC, Lang NP, Kadlubar FF (1995) Metabolic activation of N-hydroxy arylamines and N-hydroxy heterocyclic amines by human sulfotransferases. Cancer Res 55:525–529

Coutelle C, Ward PJ, Fleury B, Quattrocchi P, Chambrin H, Iron A, Couzigou P, Cassaigne A (1997) Laryngeal and oropharyngeal cancer, and alcohol dehydrogenase 3 and glutathione S-transferase M1 polymorphisms. Hum-Genet 99:319–325

Daly AK, Cholerton S, Gregory W, Idle JR (1993) Metabolic polymorphisms. Pharmacol Ther 57:129–160

Deakin M, Eider J, Hendricksen C, Peckham D, Baldwin D, Pantin C, Wild N, Leopard P, Bell D, Jones P, Duncan H, Brannigan K, Alldersen J, Fryer AA, Strange RC (1996) Glutathione S-transferase GSTT1 genotype and susceptibility to cancer: studies of interactions with GSTM1 in lung, oral, gastric and colorectal cancers. Carcinogenesis 17:881–884

Dekant W, Vamvakas S (1993) Glutathione-dependent bioactivation of xenobiotics. Xenobiotica 23:873–887

Dipple A (1995) DNA adducts of chemical carcinogens. Carcinogenesis 16:437–441

Elexpuru-Camiruaga J, Buxton N, Kandula V, Dias PS, Campbell D, McIntosh J, Broome J, Jones P, Inskip A, Alldersea J et al (1995) Susceptibility to astrocytoma and meningioma: influence of allelism at glutathione S-transferase (GSTT1 and GSTM1) and cytochrome P-450 (CYP2D6) loci. Cancer Res 55:4237–4239

Esteller M, Garcia A, Martinez-Palones JM, Xercavins J, Reventos J (1997) Susceptibility to endometrial cancer: influence of allelism at p53, glutathione S-transferase (GSTM1 and GSTT1) and cytochrome P-450 (CYP1A1) loci. Br J Cancer 75:1385–1388

Evans DA (1968) Genetic variations in the acetylation of isoniazid and other drugs. Ann N Y Acad Sci 151:723–733

Falany JL, Falany CN (1996) Regulation of estrogen sulfotransferase in human endometrial adenocarcinoma cells by progesterone. Endocrinology 137:1395–1401

Feng Y, Wagner RJ, Fretland AJ, Becker WK, Cooley AM, Pretlow TP, Lee KJ, Hei DW (1996) Acetylator genotype (NAT2)-dependent formation of aberrant crypts in congenic Syrian hamsters administered 3,2′-dimethyl-4-aminobiphenyl. Cancer Res. 56:527–531

Fost U, Tornqvist M, Leutbrecher M, Granath F, Hallier E, Ehrenberg L (1995) Effects of variation in detoxification rate on dose monitoring through adducts. Hum Exp Toxicol 14:201–203

Fryer AA, Zhao L, Alldersea J, Boggild MD, Perrett CW, Clayton RN, Jones PW, Strange RC (1993) The glutathione S-transferases: polymerase chain reaction studies on the frequency of the GSTM1-0 genotype in patients with pituitary adenomas. Carcinogenesis 14:563–566

Gaedigk A, Spielberg SP, Grant DM (1994) Characterization of the microsomal epoxide hydrolase gene in patients with anticonvulsant adverse drug reactions. Pharmacogenetics 4:142–153

Garcia-Closas M, Kelsey KT, Wiencke JK, Xu X, Wain JC, Christiani DC (1997) A case-control study of cytochrome P450 1A1, glutathione S-transferase M1, cigarette smoking and lung cancer susceptibility. 8:544–553

Garcia-Saez I, Parraga A, Phillips MF, Mantle TJ, Coll M (1994) Molecular structure of 1.8 Å of mouse liver class pi glutathione S-transferase complex with S-(p-nitrobenzyl)glutathione and other inhibitors. J Mol Biol 237:298–314

Glatt H (1997) Bioactivation of mutagens via sulfation. FASEB J 11:314–321

Glatt H, Henschler R, Frank H, Seidel A, ChengXi Y, Abu-Shqara E, Harvey RG (1993) Sulfotransferase-mediated mutagenicity of 1-hydroxymethylpyrene and 4H-cyclopenta[def]chrysen-4-ol and its enhancement by chloride anions. Carcinogenesis 14:599–602

Glatt H, Pauly K, Frank H, Seidel A, Oesch F, Harvey RG, Werle-Schneider G (1994) Substance dependent sex differences in the activation of benzylic alcohols to mutagens by hepatic sulfotransferases of the rat. Carcinogenesis 15:2605–2611

Glatt H, Christoph S, Czich A, Pauly K, Schwierzok A, Seidel A, Coughtrie MWH, Doehmer J, Falany CN, Phillips DH, Yamazoe Y, Bartsch I (1996) Rat and human sulfotransferases expressed in Ames's Salmonella typhimurium strains and Chinese hamster V79 cells for the activation of mutagens. In: Hengstler JG, Oesch F (eds) Control mechanisms of carcinogenesis. Mainz, pp 98–115 (publishing by editors)

Golka K, Prior V, Blaszkewicz M, Cascorbi I, Schops W, Kierfeld G, Roots I, Bolt HM (1996) Occupational history and genetic N-acetyltransferase polymorphism in urothelial cancer patients of Leverkusen, Germany Scand J Work Environ Health 22:332–338

Gonzalez FJ, Idle JR (1994) Pharmacogenetic phenotyping and genotyping: present status and future potential. Clin Pharmacokinet 26:59–70

Grant DM, Josephy PD, Lord HL, Morrison LD (1992) Salmonella typhimurium strains expressing human arylamines N-acetyltransferases: metabolism and mutagenic activation of arylamines. Cancer Res 52:3961–3964

Green VJ, Pirmohamed M, Kitteringham NR, Gaedigk A, Grant DM, Boxer M, Burchell B, Park BK (1995) Genetic analysis of microsomal epoxide hydrolase in patients with carbamazepine hypersensitivity. Biochem Pharmacol 50:1353–1359

Guengerich FP (1996) Metabolic control of carcinogens. In: Hengstler JG, Oesch F (eds) Control mechanisms of carcinogenesis. Publishing House of the Editors, Mainz, pp 12–35

Guengerich FP, Johnson WW, Y-F Ueng, Yamazaki H, Shimada T (1996) Involvement of cytochrome P450 glutathione S-transferase, and epoxide hydrolase in the metabolism of aflatoxin B1 and relevance to risk of human liver cancer. Environ Health Perspect 104:557–562

Hallier E, Langhof T, Dannappel D, Leutbrecher M, Schröder K, Goergens HW, Müller A, Bolt H (1993) Polymorphism of glutathione conjugation of methyl bromide, ethylene oxide and dichloromethane in human blood: influence on the induction of sister chromatid exchanges (SCE) in lymphocytes. Arch Toxicol 67:173–178

Hand PA, Inskip A, Gilford J, Alldersea J, Elexpuru-Camiruaga J, Hayes JD, Jones PW, Strange RC, Fryer AA (1996) Allelism at the glutathione S-transferase GSTM3 locus: interactions with GSTM1 and GSTT1 as risk factors for astrocytoma. Carcinogenesis 17:1919–1922

Harries LW, Stubbins MJ, Forman D, Howard GCW, Wolf CR (1997) Identification of genetic polymorphism at the glutathione S-transferase Pi locus and association with susceptibility to bladder, testicular and prostate cancer. Carcinogenesis 18:641–644

Harrison DJ, Cantlay AM, Rae F, Lamb D, Smith CA (1997) Frequency of glutathione S-transferase M1 deletion in smokers with emphysema and lung cancer. Hum Exp Toxicol 16:356–360

Hassett C, Aicher L, Sidhu JS, Omiecinski CJ (1994) Human microsomal epoxide hydrolase: genetic polymorphism and functional expression in vitro of amino acid variants. Hum Mol Genet 3:412–428

Hassett C, Lin J, Carty CL, Laurenzana EM, Omiecinski CJ (1997) Human hepatic microsomal epoxide hydrolase: comparative analysis of polymorphic expression. Arch Biochem Biophys 337:275–283

Hayes JD, Pulford DJ (1995) The glutathione S-transferase supergene family: regulation of GST* and the contribution of the enzyme to cancer chemoprotection and drug resistance. Crit Rev Biochem Mol Biol 30:445–600

Heagerty AHM, Fitzgerald D, Smith A, Bowers B, Jones P, Fryer AA, Zhao L, Alldersea J, Strange RC (1994) Glutathione S-transferase GST M1 phenotypes and protection against cutaneous tumours. Lancet 343:266–268

Heckbert SR, Weiss NS, Hornung SK, Eaton DL, Motusky AG (1992) Glutathione S-transferase and epoxide hydrolase activity in human leukocytes in relation to risk of lung cancer and other smoking-related cancers. J Natl Cancer Inst 84:414–422

Hein DW, Rustan TD, Ferguson RJ, Doll MA, Gray K (1994) Metabolic activation of aromatic and heterocyclic N-hydroxyarylamines by wild-type and mutant recombinant human NAT1 and NAT2 acetyltransferases. Arch Toxicol 68:129–133

Hengstler JG, Fuchs J, Oesch F (1992) DNA strand breaks and DNA cross-links in peripheral mononuclear blood cells of ovarian cancer patients during chemotherapy with cyclophosphamide/carboplatin. Cancer Res 52:5622–5626

Hengstler JG, Kett A, Arand M, Oesch B, Oesch F, Knapstein PG, Tanner B (1998a) Glutathione S-transferase T1 and M1 gene defects in ovarian carcinoma. Cancer Lett (in press)

Hengstler JG, Böttger T, Tanner B, Dietrich B, Henrich M, Knapstein PG, Junginger T, Oesch F (1998b) Resistance factors in colon cancer tissue and the adjacent normal tissue: glutathione S-transferases α and π, glutathione, and aldehyde dehydrogenase. Cancer Lett (in press)

Herrero ME, Arand M, Hengstler JG, Oesch F (1997) Recombinant expression of human microsomal epoxide hydrolase protects V79 Chinese hamster cells from styrene oxide-induced but not from ethylene oxide-induced DNA strand breaks. Environ Molecul Mutag 30:429–439

Hickman D, Sim E (1991) N-Acetyltransferase polymorphism. Comparison of phenotype and genotype in humans. Biochem Pharmacol 42:1007–1014

Hirvonen A, Nylund L, Kociba P, Husgafvel-Pursiainen K, Vainio H (1994) Modulation of urinary mutagenicity by genetically determined carcinogen metabolism in smokers. Carcinogenesis 15:813–815

Hirvonen A, Pelin K, Tammilehto L, Karjalainen A, Mattson K, Linnainmaa K (1995) Inherited GSTM1 and NAT2 defects as concurrent risk modifiers in asbestos-related human malignant mesothelioma. Cancer Res 55:2981–2983

Hirvonen A, Saarikoski ST, Linnainmaa K, Koskinen K, Husgafvel-Pursiainen K, Mattson K, Vainio H (1996) Glutathione S-transferase and N-acetyltransferase genotypes and asbestos-associated pulmonary disorders. J Natl Cancer Inst 88:1853–1856

Holler R, Arand M, Mecky A, Oesch F, Friedberg T (1997) The membrane anchor of microsomal epoxide hydrolase from human, rat, and rabbit displays an unexpected membrane topology. Biochem Biophys Res Commun 236:754–759

Hsieh LL, Huang RC, Yu MW, Chen CJ, Liaw YF (1996) L-myc, GST M1 genetic polymorphism and hepatocellular carcinoma risk among chronic hepatitis B carriers. Cancer Lett 103:171–176

Hu X, O'Donnell R, Srivastava SK, Xia H, Zimniak P, Nanduri B, Bleicher RJ, Awasthi S, Awasthi YC, Ji X, Singh SV (1997a) Active site architecture of polymorphic forms of human glutathione S-transferase P1-1 accounts for their enantioselectivity and disparate activity in the glutathione conjugation of 7beta, 8alpha-dihydroxy-9alpha, 10alpha-oxy-7,8,9,10-tetrahydrobenzo[a]pyrene. Biochem. Biophys Res Commun 235:424–428

Hu X, Ji X, Srivastava SK, Xia H, Awasthi S, Nanduri B, Awasthi YC, Zimniak P, Singh SV (1997b) Mechanism of differential catalytic efficiency of two polymorphic forms of human glutathione S-transferase P1-1 in the glutathione conjugation of carcinogenic diol epoxide of chrysene. Arch Biochem Biophys 345:32–38

Izawa I, Ali-Osman F (1993) Structure of glutathione S-transferase Pi gene cloned from a malignant glioma cell line (Abstr). Proc Ann Meet Assoc Cancer Res 34:A2030

Jahnke V, Strange R, Matthias C, Fryer A (1997) Glutathione S-transferase and cytochrome P450 genotypes as risk factors for laryngeal carcinoma. Eur Arch Otorhinolaryngol Suppl 1:147–149

Johnson WW, Yamazaki H, Shimada T, Ueng Y-F, Guengerich FP (1997) Aflatoxin B1 8,9-epoxide hydrolysis in the presence of rat and human epoxide hydrolase. Chem Res Toxicol 10:672–676

Kadlubar FF, Badawi AF (1995) Genetic susceptibility and carcinogen-DNA adduct formation in human urinary bladder carcinogenesis. Toxicol Lett 82/83:627–632

Karakaya AE, Cok I, Sardas S, Gogus OS (1989) N-Acetyltransferase phenotype of patients with bladder cancer. Hum Toxicol 5:333–335

Katoh T, Inatomi H, Nagaoka A, Sugita A (1995) Cytochrome P4501A1 gene polymorphism and homozygous deletion of the glutathione S-transferase M1 gene in urothelial cancer patients. Carcinogenesis 16:655–657

Katoh T, Nagata N, Kuroda Y, Itoh H, Kawahara A, Kuroki N, Ookuma R, Bell DA (1996) Glutathione S-transferase M1 (GSTM1) and T1 (GSTT1) genetic polymorphism and susceptibility to gastric and colorectal adenocarcinoma. Carcinogenesis 17:1855–1859

Kawajiri K, Nakachi K, Imai K, Watanabe J, Hayashi S (1993) The CYP1A1 gene and cancer susceptibility. Crit Rev Oncol Hematol 14:77–87

Kelsey KT, Spitz MR, Zuo ZF, Wiencke JK (1997a) Polymorphisms in the glutathione S-transferase class mu and theta genes interact and increase susceptibility to lung cancer in minority populations. Cancer Causes Control 8:554–559

Kelsey KT, Hankinson SE, Colditz GA, Springer K, Garcia-Closas M, Spiegelman D, Manson JE, Garland M, Stampfer MJ, Willett WC, Speizer FE, Hunter DJ (1997b) Glutathione S-transferase class mu deletion polymorphism and breast cancer: results from prevalent versus incident cases. Cancer Epidemiol Biomarkers Prev 6:511–515

Kempkes M, Wiebel FA, Golka K, Heitmann P, Bolt HM (1996a) Comparative genotyping and phenotyping of glutathione S-transferase GST T1. Arch Toxicol 70:306–309

Kempkes M, Golka K, Reich S, Reckwitz T, Bolt (1996b) Glutathione S-transferase GSTM1 and GSTT1 null genotypes as potential risk factors for urothelial cancer of the bladder. Arch Toxicol 71:123–126

Kerdar RS, Fasshauer I, Probst M, Blum M, Meyer UA, Wild D (1993) ^{32}P-postlabelling studies on the DNA adducts of the food mutagens/carcinogens IQ and PhIP-adduct formation in a chemical system, and by rat and human metabolism. IARC Sci Publ 124:173–179

Kihara M, Kihara M, Noda K (1995a) Risk of smoking for squamous and small cell carcinomas of the lung modulated by combinations of CYP 1A1 and GST M1 gene polymorphisms in a Japanese population. Carcinogenesis 16:2331–2336

Kihara M, Noda K, Kihara M (1995b) Distribution of GST M1 null genotype in relation to gender, age and smoking status in Japanese lung cancer patients. Pharmacogenetics 5:74–79

Kihara M, Kihara M, Kubota A, Furukawa M, Kimura H (1997) GSTM1 gene polymorphism as a possible marker for susceptibility to head and neck cancers among Japanese smokers. Cancer Lett 112:257–262

Kiyohara C, Hirohata T (1994) A role of hydrocarbon hydroxylase inducibility in susceptibility to lung carcinogenesis. Jpn J Hyg 48:1027–1036

Kroetz DL, McFarland LV, Kerr BM, Levy RH (1990) Distribution of microsomal epoxide hydrolase (mEH) activity in healthy Caucasian subjects. Clin Pharmacol Ther 47:160

Lacourciere GM, Armstrong RN (1994) Microsomal and soluble epoxide hydrolases are members of the same family of C-X bond hydrolase enzymes. Chem Res Toxicol 7:121–124

Lancaster JM, Brownlee HA, Bell DA, Futreal A, Marks JR, Berchuck A, Wiseman RW, Taylor JA (1996) Microsomal epoxide hydrolase polymorphism as a risk factor for ovarian cancer. Mol Carcinog 17:160–162

Lear JT, Smith AG, Heagerty AH, Bowers B, Jones PW, Gilford J, Alldersea J, Strange RC, Fryer AA (1997) Truncal site and detoxifying enzyme polymorphisms significantly reduce time to presentation of further primary cutaneous basal cell carcinoma. Carcinogenesis 18:1499–1503

Lin HJ, Han C-Y, Bernstein DA, Hsiao W, Lin BK, Hardy S (1994) Ethnic distribution of the glutathione transferase Mu 1-1 (GSTM1) null genotype in 1473 individuals and application to bladder cancer susceptibility. Carcinogenesis 15:1077–1081

Lin HJ, Probst-Hensch M, Ingles SA, Han C, Lin BK, Lee DB, Frankl HD, Lee ER, Longnecker MP, Haile RW (1995) Glutathione S-transferase (GST M1) null genotype, smoking, and prevalence of colorectal adenomas. Cancer Res 55:1224–1226

London SJ, Daly AK, Cooper J, Navidi WC, Carpenter CL, Idle JR (1995) Polymorphism of glutathione S-transferase M1 and lung cancer risk among African-Americans and Caucasians in Los Angeles County, California. J Natl Cancer Inst 87:1246–1253

MacLeod S, Sinha R, Kadlubar FF, Lang NP (1997) Polymorphisms of CYP1A1 and GSTM1 influence the in vivo function of CYP1A2. Mutat Res 376:135–142

Martinez C, Agundez JA, Olivera M, Martin R, Ladero JM, Benitez J (1995) Lung cancer and mutations at the polymorphic NAT2 gene locus. Pharmacogenetics 5:207–214

McGlynn KA, Rosvold EA, Lustbader ED, Hu Y, Clapper ML, Zhou T, Wild C, Xia X-L, Baffoe-Bonnie A, Ofori-Adjei D, Chen G-C, London WT, Sheen F-M, Buetow KH (1995) Susceptibility to hepatocellular carcinoma is associated with genetic variation in the enzymatic detoxification of aflatoxin B$_1$. Proc Natl Acad Sci USA 92:2384–2387

McWilliams JE, Sanderson BJ, Harris EL, Richert-Boe KE, Henner-WD (1995) Glutathione S-transferase M1 (GSTM1) deficiency and lung cancer risk. Cancer Epidemiol Biomarkers Prev 4:589–594

Medina JF, Wetterholm A, Radmark O, Shapiro R, Haeggstrom JZ, Vallee BL, Samuelsson B (1991) Leukotriene A4 hydrolase: determination of the three zinc-binding ligands by site-directed mutagenesis and zinc analysis. Proc Natl Acad Sci USA 88:7620–7624

Mertes I, Fleischmann R, Glatt HR, Oesch F (1985) Interindividual variations in the activities of cytosolic and microsomal epoxide hydrolase in human liver. Carcinogenesis 6:219–223

Miller JA (1994) Sulfonation in chemical carcinogenesis – history and present status. Chem Biol Interact 92:329–341

Minchin RF, Reeves PT, Teitel CH, McManus ME, Mojarabbi B, Ilett KF, Kadlubar FF (1992) N- and O-acetylation of aromatic and heterocyclic amine carcinogens by human monomorphic and polymorphic acetyltransferases expressed in COS-1 cells. Biochem. Biophys Res Commun 185:839–844

Moreira A, Martins G, Monteiro MJ, Alves M, Dias J, DaCosta JD, Melo MJ, Matias D, Costa A, Cristovao M, Rueff J, Monteiro C (1996) Glutathione S-transferase mu polymorphism and susceptibility to lung cancer in the Portuguese population. Teratogenesis Carcinog Mutagen 16:269–274

Morita S, Yano M, Shiozaki H, Tsujinaka T, Ebisui C, Morimoto T, Kishibuti M et al (1997) CYP1A1, CYP2E1 and GSTM1 polymorphisms are not associated with susceptibility to squamous-cell carcinoma of the esophagus. Int J Cancer 71:192–195

Nakajima T, Elovaara E, Anttila S, Hirvonen A, Camus A-M, Hayes JD, Ketterer B, Vainio H (1995) Expression and polymorphism of glutathione S-transferase in human lungs: risk factors in smoking-related lung cancer. Carcinogenesis 16:707–711

Nazar-Stewart V, Motulsky AG, Eaton DL, White E, Hornung SK, Long ZT, Stapelton P, Weiss NS (1993) The glutathione S-transferase μ polymorphism as a marker for susceptibility to lung carcinoma. Cancer Res 53:2313–2318

Nebert DW (1991) Identification of genetic differences in drug metabolism: prediction of individual risk of toxicity or cancer. Hepatology 14:398–401

Nebert DW, McKinnon RA, Puga A (1996) Human drug-metabolizing polymorphisms: effects on risk of toxicology and cancer. DNA Cell Biol 15:273–280

Nerurkar PV, Schutt HA, Anderson LM, Riggs CW, Snyderwine EG, Thorgeirsson SS, Weber WW, Rice JM, Levy GN (1995) DNA adducts of 2-amino-3-methylimidazo[4,5-f]quinoline (IQ) in colon, bladder, and kidney of congenic mice differing in Ah responsiveness and N-acetyltransferase genotype. Cancer Res 55:3043–3049

Nimura Y, Yokoyama S, Fujimori M, Aoki T, Adachi W, Nasu T, He M, Ping YM, Iida F (1997) Genotyping of the CYP1A1 and GSTM1 genes in esophageal carcinoma patients with special reference to smoking. Cancer 80:852–857

Oesch F (1988) Antimutagenesis by shift in monooxygenase isoenzymes and induction of microsomal epoxide hydrolase. Mutat Res 202:335–342

Oesch F, Timms CW, Walker CH, Guenther TM, Sparrow A, Watabe T, Wolf CR (1984) Existance of multiple forms of microsomal epoxide hydrolases with radically different substrate specificities. Carcinogenesis 5:7–9

Oesch F, Fuchs J, Arand M, Gebhard S, Hallier A, Oesch-Bartlomowicz B, Jung D, Tanner B, Bolm-Audorff U, Hiltl G, Bienfait G, Konietzko J, Hengstler JG (1997) Möglichkeiten und Grenzen der alkalischen Filterelution zum Biomonitoring gentoxischer Belastungen. In: Bundesanstalt für Arbeitsschutz und Arbeitsmedizin (ed) Molekulare Marker bei beruflich verursachten Tumoren. Bundesanstalt für Arbeitsschutz, Berlin

Okkels H, Sigsgaard T, Wolf H, Autrup H (1996) Glutathione S-transferase (as a risk factor in bladder tumours. Pharmacogenetics 6:251–256

Okkels H, Sigsgaard T, Wolf H, Autrup H (1997) Arylamine N-acetyltransferase μ (NAT1) and 2 (NAT2) polymorphisms in susceptibility to bladder cancer: the influence of smoking. Cancer Epidemiol Biomarkers Prev 6:225–231

Pemble S, Schroeder KR, Spencer SR, Meyer DJ, Hallier E, Bolt HM, Ketterer B, Taylor JB (1994) Human glutathione S-transferase theta (GSTT1): cDNA cloning and the characterization of a genetic polymorphism. Biochem J 300:271–276

Perrett CW, Clayton RN, Pistorello M, Boscaro M, Scanarini M, Bates AS, Buckley N, Jones P, Fryer AA, Gilford J et al (1995) GSTM1 and CYP2D6 genotype frequencies in patients with pituitary tumours: effects on p53 and ras. Carcinogenesis 16:1643–1645

Peter H, Deutschmann S, Reichel C, Hallier E (1989) Metabolism of methyl chloride by human erythrocytes. Arch Toxicol 63:351–355

Preudhomme C, Nisse C, Hebbar M, Vanrumbeke M, Brizard A, Lai JL, Fenaux P (1997) Glutathione S-transferase theta 1 gene defects in myelodysplastic syndromes and their correlation with karyotype and exposure to potential carcinogens. Leukemia 11:1580–1582

Price RA, Cox NJ, Spielman RS, Van Loon J, Maidak BL, Weinshilboum RM (1988) Inheritance of human platelet thermolabile phenol sulfotransferase (TL PST) activity. Genet Epidemiol 5:1–15

Probst-Hensch NM, Haile RW, Li DS, Sakamoto GT, Louie AD, Lin BK, Frankl HD, Lee ER, Lin HL (1996) Lack of association between the polyadenylation polymorphism in the NAT1 (acetyltransferase 1) gene and colorectal adenomas. Carcinogenesis 17:2125–2129

Ramdahl T (1985) Polycyclic aromatic ketones in source emissions and ambient air. In: Cooke M, Dennis AJ (eds) Polynuclear aromatic hydrocarbons: mechanisms, methods and metabolism. Battelle, Columbus, OH, pp 1075–1087

Rebbeck TR (1997) Molecular epidemiology of the human glutathione S-transferase genotypes GST M1 and GST T1 in cancer susceptibility. Cancer Epidemiol Biomarkers Prev 6:733–743

Roberts-Thomson IC, Ryan P, Khoo KK, Hart WJ, McMichael AJ, Butler RN (1996) Diet, acetylator phenotype, and risk of colorectal neoplasia. Lancet 347:1372–1374

Ross RK, Jones PA, Yu MC (1996) Bladder cancer epidemiology and pathogenesis. Semin Oncol 23:536–545

Rothman N, Hayes RB, Zenser TV, DeMarini DM, Bi W, Hirvonen A, Talaska G, Bhatnagar VK, Caporaso NE, Brooks LR, Lakshmi VM, Feng P, Kashyap SK, You X, Eischen BT, Kashyap R, Shelton ML, Hsu FF, Jaeger M, Parikh DJ, Davis BB, Yin S, Bell DA (1996) The glutathione S-transferase M1 (GSTM1) null genotype and benzidine-associated bladder cancer, urine mutagenicity, and exfoliated urothelial cell DNA adducts. Cancer Epidemiol. Biomarkers Prev 5:979–983

Ryberg D, Skaug V, Hewer A, Phillips DH, Harries LW, Wolf CR, Ogreid D, Ulvik A, Vu P, Haugen A (1997) Genotypes of glutathione transferase M1 and P1 and their significance for lung DNA adduct levels and cancer risk. Carcinogenesis 18:1285–1289

Sabbioni G, Skipper PL, Büchi G, Tannenbaum SR (1987) Isolation and characterization of the major serum albumin adduct formed by aflatoxin B_1 in vivo in rats. Carcinogenesis 8:819–824

Sadrieh N, Davis CD, Snyderwine EG (1996) N-acetyltransferase expression and metabolic activation of the food-derived heterocyclic amines in the mammary gland. Cancer Res 56:2683–2687

Sarhanis P, Redman C, Perrett C, Brannigan K, Clayton RN, Hand P, Musgrove C, Suarez V, Jones P, Fryer AA, Farrell WE, Strange RC (1996) Epithelial ovarian cancer: influence of polymorphism at the glutathione S-transferase GSTM1 and GSTT1 loci on p53 expression. Br J Cancer 74:1757–1761

Schröder KR, Wiebel FA, Reich S, Dannappel D, Bolt HM, Hallier E (1995) Glutathione-S-transferase (GST) theta polymorphism influences background SCE rate. Arch Toxicol 69:505–507

Schröder KR, Hallier E, Meyer DJ, Wiebel FA, Muller AM, Bolt HM (1996) Purification and characterization of a new glutathione S-transferase, class theta, from human erythrocytes. Arch Toxicol 70:559–566

Seidegard J, Ekström G (1997) The role of human glutathione transferases and epoxide hydrolases in the metabolism of xenobiotics. Environ Health Perspect 105:791–799

Seidegard J, DePierre JW, Pero RW (1984) Measurement and characterization of membrane-bound and soluble epoxide hydrolase activities in resting mononuclear leucocytes from human blood. Cancer Res 44:3654–3660

Seidegard J, Pero RW, Miller DG, Beattie EJ (1986) A glutathione transferase in human leucocytes as a marker for the susceptibility to lung cancer. Carcinogenesis 7:751–753

Seidegard J, Vorachek WR, Pero RW, Pearson WR (1988) Hereditary difference in the expression of the human glutathione transferase active on trans-stilbene oxide are due to a gene deletion. Proc Natl Acad Sci USA 85:7203–7207

Seidegard J, Pero RW, Markowitz MM, Roush G, Miller DG, Beattie EJ (1990) Isoenzymes of glutathione transferase (class μ) as a marker for the susceptibility to lung cancer: a follow up study. Carcinogenesis 11:33–36

Silverman DT, Hartge P, Morrison AS et al (1992) Epidemiology of bladder cancer. Hematol Oncol Clin North Am 6:1–30

Sinha R, Rothman N, Brown ED, Mark SD, Hoover RN, Caporaso NE, Levander OA, Knize MG, Lang NP, Kadlubar FF (1994) Pan-fried meat containing high levels of heterocyclic aromatic amines but low levels of polycyclic aromatic hydrocarbons induces cytochrome P4501A2 activity in humans. Cancer Res 54:6154–6159

Smith CAD, Harrison DJ (1997) Association between polymorphism in gene for microsomal epoxide hydrolase and susceptibility to emphysema. Lancet 350:630–633

Sorsa M, Osterman-Golkar S, Peltonen K, Saarikoski ST, Sram R (1996) Assessment of exposure to butadiene in the process industry. Toxicology 113:77–83

Stahl F, Schnorr D, Pilz C, Dorner G (1992) Dehydroepiandrosterone (DHEA) levels in patients with prostatic cancer, heart diseases and under surgery stress. Exp Clin Endocrinol 92:68–70

Sundaram RS, Van Loon JA, Tucker R, Weinshilboum RM (1989) Sulfation pharmacogenetics: correlation of human platelet and small intestinal phenol sulfotransferase. Clin Pharmacol Ther 46:501–509

Tanner B, Hengstler JG, Dietrich B, Henrich M, Steinberg P, Weikel W, Meinert R, Kaina B, Oesch F, Knapstein PG (1997) Glutathione, glutathione S-transferase α and π, and aldehyde dehydrogenase content in relationship to drug resistance in ovarian cancer. Gynecol Oncol 65:54–62

Thier R, Pemble SE, Kramer H, Taylor JB, Guengerich FP, Ketterer B (1996) Human glutathione S-transferase T1-1 enhances mutagenicity of 1,2-dibromoethane, dibromomethane and 1,2,3,4-diepoxybutane in *Salmonella typhimurium*. Carcinogenesis 17:163–166

To-Figueras J, Gene M, Gomez-Catalan J, Galan C, Firvida J, Fuentes M, Rodamilans M, Huguet E, Estape J, Corbella J (1996) Glutathione-S-transferase M1 and codon 72 p53 polymorphisms in a northwestern Mediterranean population and their relation to lung cancer susceptibility. Cancer Epidemiol Biomarkers Prev 5:337–342

To-Figueras J, Gene M, Gomez-Catalan J, Galan MC, Fuentes M, Ramon JM, Rodamilans M, Huguet E, Corbella J (1997) Glutathione S-transferase M1 and T1 polymorphisms and lung cancer risk among Northwestern Mediterraneans. Carcinogenesis 18:1529–1533

Trizna Z, Clayman GL, Spitz MR, Briggs KL, Goepfert H (1995) Glutathione S-transferase genotypes as risk factors for head and neck cancer. Am J Surg 170:499–501

Turesky R, Lang NP, Butler MA, Teitel CH, Kadlubar FF (1991) Metabolic activation of carcinogenic heterocyclic aromatic amines by human liver and colon. Carcinogenesis 12:1839–1845

Van Loon JA, Weinshilboum RM (1984) Human platelet phenol sulfotransferase: familial variation in the thermal stability of the TS form. Biochem Genet 22:997–1014

Vatsis KP, Martelli KJ, Weber WW (1991) Diverse point mutations in the human gene for polymorphic N-acetyltransferase. Proc Natl Acad Sci USA 88:6333–6337

Vaury C, Laine R, Noguiez P, DeCoppet P, Jaulitz C, Praz F, Pompon D, Amor-Gueret M (1995) Human glutathione S-transferase M1 null genotype is associated with a high inducibility of cytochrome P450 1A1 gene transcription. Cancer Res 55:5520–5523

Vineis P, McMichael A (1996) Interplay between heterocyclic amines in cooked meat and metabolic phenotype in the etiology of colon cancer. Cancer Causes Control 7:479–478

Warwick A, Sarhanis P, Redman C, Pemble S, Taylor JB, Ketterer B, Jones P, Alldersea J, Gilford J, Yengi L et al (1994) Theta class glutathione S-transferase GSTT1 genotypes and susceptibility to cervical neoplasia: interactions with GSTM1, CYP2D6 and smoking. Carcinogenesis 15:2841–2845

Weber WW, Hein DW (1985) N-Acetylation pharmacogenetics. Pharmacol Rev 37:25–79

Weinshilboum R, Aksoy I (1994) Sulfation pharmacogenetics in humans. Sulfation and sulfotransferases 1: Sulfotransferase molecular biology: cDNAs and genes. Chem Biol Interact 92:233–246

Weinshilboum RM, Otterness DM, Aksoy IA, Wood TC, Her C, Raftogianis RB (1997) FASEB J 11:3–14

Wiencke JK, Pemble S, Ketterer B, Kelsey KT (1995) Gene deletion of glutathione S-transferase theta: correlation with induced genetic damage and potential role in endogenous mutagenesis. Cancer Epidemiol Biomarkers Prev 4:253–259

Wiencke JK, Wrensch MR, Mike R, Zuo Z, Kelsey KT (1997) Population-based study of glutathione S-transferase mu gene deletion in adult glioma cases and controls. Carcinogenesis 18:1431–1433

Wild D, Feser W, Michel S, Lord HL, Josephy PD (1995) Metabolic activation of heterocyclic aromatic amines catalyzed by human arylamine N-acetyltransferase isozymes (NAT1 and NAT2) expressed in *Salmonella typhimurium.* Carcinogenesis 16:643–648

Wood TC, Her C, Aksoy I, Otterness DM, Weinshilboum RM (1996) Human dehydroepiandrosterone sulfotransferase pharmacogenetics: quantitative Western analysis and gene sequence polymorphisms. J Steroid Biochem Molec Biol 59:467–478

Wu RW, Tucker JD, Sorensen KJ, Thompson LH, Felton JS (1997) Differential effects of acetyltransferase expression on the genotoxicity of heterocyclic amines in CHO cells. Mutat Res 390:93–103

Yamazoe Y, Nagata K, Ozawa S, Kato R (1994) Structural similarity and diversity of sulfotransferases. Chem Biol Interact 92:107–117

Yanagawa Y, Sawada M, Deguchi T, Gonzalez FJ, Kamataki T (1994) Stable expression of human CYP1A2 and N-acetyltransferases in Chinese hamster CHL cells: mutagenic activation of 2-amino-3-methylimidazo[4,5-f]quinoline and 2-amino-3,8-dimethylimidazo[4,5-f]quinoxaline. Cancer Res 54:3422–3427

Yengi L, Inskip A, Gilford J, Alldersea J, Bailey L, Smith A, Lear JT, Heagerty AH, Bowers B, Hand P, Hayes JD, Jones PW, Strange RC, Fryer AA (1996) Polymorphism at the glutathione S-transferase locus GSTM3: interaction with cytochrome P450 and glutathione S-transferase genotypes as risk factors for multiple cutaneous basal cell carcinoma. Cancer Res 56:1974–1979

Young WF, Laws ER, Sharbrough FW, Weinshilboum RM (1985) Human phenol sulfotransferase: correlation of brain and platelet activities. J Neurochem 44:1131–1137

Yu MW, Gladek-Yarborough A, Chiamprasert S, Santella RM, Liaw YF, Chen CJ (1995) Cytochrome P450 2E1 and glutathione S-transferase M1 polymorphisms and susceptibility to hepatocellular carcinoma. Gastroenterology 109:1266–1273

Zhong S, Howie AF, Ketterer B, Taylor J, Hayes JD, Beckett GJ, Wathen CG, Wolf CR, Spurr NK (1991) Glutathione S-transferase μ locus: use of genotyping and phenotyping assays to assess association with lung cancer susceptibility. Carcinogenesis 12:1533–1537

Zhong S, Wyllie AH, Barnes D, Wolf CR, Spurr NK (1993) Relationship between GSTM1 genetic polymorphism and susceptibility to bladder, breast and colon cancer. Carcinogenesis 14:1821–1824

Impact of Adduct Determination
on the Assessment of Cancer Susceptibility

H. Bartsch, M. Rojas, K. Alexandrov, and A. Risch

German Cancer Research Center (DKFZ), Division of Toxicology
and Cancer Risk Factors, Im Neuenheimer Feld 280, 69120 Heidelberg, Germany

Abstract

The characterization of genetic determinants for cancer susceptibility is important for understanding disease pathogenesis and for preventive measures. There is growing evidence that a group of predisposing polymorphic genes exists, such as those involved in carcinogen metabolism and repair, which may increase cancer in certain environmentally exposed subjects, even those exposed only to low levels of carcinogens. In developing preventive strategies, it is therefore necessary to identify these vulnerable members in our society, particularly those suffering from an unfortunate combination of high carcinogen exposure, cancer-predisposing genes and lack of protective (dietary) factors. Thus, molecular epidemiology faces the difficult task of analyzing carcinogen-exposed individuals for a combination of genotypes associated with cancer susceptibility. Once identified, combinations of cancer-predisposing genes can then be used as intermediate risk markers rather than taking cancer as an endpoint. In case-control studies, simultaneous measurements were carried out in each subject to determine exposure/early effect markers, e.g. polycyclic aromatic hydrocarbons (PAH)-DNA adducts, and susceptibility markers, e.g. genetic polymorphism, in drug-metabolizing enzymes related to cytochrome P450 1A1 *(CYP1A1)* and glutathione *S*-transferase *(GSTM1)* genes. The genotype dependence of human lung (+)-*anti*-benzo[*a*]pyrene diol-epoxide (BPDE)-DNA adducts in lung cancer patients was examined. BPDE-DNA adduct levels in bronchial tissue of smokers with high pulmonary *CYP1A1* inducibility (by immunohistochemistry) and *GSTM1* inactive were ~100-fold higher than in subjects with an active *GSTM1* at similar smoking dose. Further genetic analyses confirmed that the combination of *CYP1A1* homozygous mutants and *GSTM1* inactive leads to high levels of BPDE-DNA adducts in human lung of smokers and white blood cells of PAH-exposed coke oven workers. Thus, BPDE-DNA adduct levels resulting from the "at risk" genotype combinations may serve as markers to identify high-risk subjects among smokers and individuals occupationally and/or environmentally exposed to PAH.

Recent Results in Cancer Research, Vol. 154
© Springer-Verlag Berlin · Heidelberg 1998

Introduction

Past efforts in analytical epidemiology and more recent molecular, human genetic studies identified two types of "at risk" populations: one consisting of individuals with high carcinogen exposure, such as smokers or occupationally exposed workers, and the other consisting of carriers of mutated cancer-determining genes that confer a very high cancer risk (Caporaso and Goldstein 1995). However, there is growing evidence that a third group of predisposing polymorphic genes exists, for example those involved in carcinogen metabolism and repair, which increase cancer in certain environmentally exposed subjects, even those exposed only to low levels of carcinogens (Vineis et al. 1994; Vineis 1997). In developing preventive strategies it would therefore be necessary to identify vulnerable members in our society, in particular those suffering from very unfortunate combinations of carcinogen exposure, predisposing genes and lack of protective dietary factors.

Individual cancer susceptibility to environmental carcinogens must result from several host factors including the individual's genotype or phenotype for a number of carcinogen-activating and -detoxifying enzymes. Given their great number, their variability in expression and the complexity of chemical exposures, assessment of a single polymorphic enzyme or genotype may not be sufficient (Bartsch and Hietanen 1996). The difficult task now is to analyze carcinogen-exposed individuals for a combination of genotypes associated with cancer susceptibility. Once identified, combinations of cancer-predisposing genes can then be used as intermediate risk markers rather than taking cancer itself as an endpoint. For these reasons we are carrying out, within case-control studies, simultaneous measurements in each subject to determine carcinogen exposure using early effect markers such as polycyclic aromatic hydrocarbons (PAH)-DNA adduct levels and susceptibility markers related to genetic polymorphism in drug-metabolizing enzymes. With this approach we aim at better defining gene-environment interactions and providing knowledge that should facilitate the identification of high-risk subjects within carcinogen-exposed populations. Two of the authors' current studies on environmentally induced lung cancer, one related to cigarette smoking and the other to PAH-exposed coke oven workers, are briefly summarized. The literature cited is not exhaustive, and the reader is referred to review articles published earlier (Bartsch and Hietanen 1996; Bartsch 1996; Bartsch et al. 1995).

Materials and Methods

Normal lung tissue was obtained from untreated lung cancer patients undergoing surgery. Samples were frozen immediately and stored at $-80\,^\circ$C until DNA isolation. Blood samples from male coke oven workers were obtained during the summer of 1995 in Houillères du Bassin de Lorraine, France. Occupational exposure in the year of blood sampling ranged from <0.15 to

$\geq$4 µg/m^3 of benzo[*a*]pyrene (BP). Workers were exposed for 6–8 working hours per day for at least 4–6 months prior to blood collection. Workers with other relevant and occupational exposures were excluded from the study. White blood cells (WBCs) were prepared on Ficoll and frozen before DNA extraction. All samples were coded prior to molecular analysis.

DNA was extracted from nontumorous tissue using proteinase K/RNAse digestion and a modified phenol extraction procedure (Alexandrov et al. 1992). The DNA from WBCs was isolated as described (Rojas et al. 1995). 0.2 to 1 mg DNA was used for analysis of BP-tetrols, allowing quantification of (+)-*anti*-benzo[*a*]pyrene diol-epoxide (BPDE)-DNA adducts. High performance liquid chromatography analysis of BP-tetrols combined with fluorimetric detection (HPLC-FD) was carried out as described (Alexandrov et al. 1992; Rojas et al. 1994). Using 1 mg of DNA, this assay can detect $\geq$0.2 BPDE-DNA adducts per 10^8 nucleotides (nt). The HPLC-FD runs were qualitatively reproducible, and variability between the two assays was <5%. All BP metabolites used as standards in this study were obtained from the NCI Carcinogen Standard Repository (Midwest Research Institute, Kansas City, MO, USA). PCR/RFLP based analysis of *CYP1A1* gene polymorphisms and *GSTM1* gene deletion was analyzed as described (Cascorbi et al. 1996; Brockmöller et al. 1993). An allele carrying only a T to C transition 1194 bp downstream of exon 7 in the 3′-flanking region, leading to a *MspI* restriction site *(m1)*, was termed *2A. An allele with *m1* plus a mutation in exon 7 leading to an Ile/Val exchange at codon 462 *(m2)* due to an A to G transition at nt 4889 was termed *2B. The corresponding deficient phenotype of *GSTM1*0/*0* genotype is termed *GSTM1* null phenotype. The "*GSTM1* active" genotype summarizes the following allele configurations: *GSTM1*A/*A, GSTM1*A/*0, GSTM1*B/*B, GSTM1*B/*0* and *GSTM1*A/*B.*

Results and Discussion

Role of Metabolism and PAH-DNA Adducts in Lung Carcinogenesis and Disease susceptibility

Cigarette smoking is the strongest risk factor for lung cancer, but drug-metabolizing enzymes, which often display genetic polymorphism and convert lung carcinogens from occupational environment or tobacco into DNA-binding metabolites in target cells, can modulate intermediate effect markers, e.g., DNA adducts, and ultimately the cancer risk. Table 1 summarizes some of the published evidence that bulky PAH-derived DNA adducts are significant in the onset of lung carcinogenesis in smokers. Having developed a sensitive and specific method for BPDE-DNA adduct detection in human lung tissue and WBCs (Rojas et al. 1994), the aims of our ongoing studies are: (1) to identify specific genotype combinations that lead to high BPDE-DNA adduct levels in smokers and PAH-exposed workers and (2) to use the characterized markers for early detection of individuals susceptible to lung cancer. Within

Table 1. Bulky (PAH) DNA adducts in smokers: significance in human lung carcinogenesis

- Present in all target organs of tobacco carcinogenesis.
- Linear relation to total smoking dose.
- Higher in "at risk" (lung cancer) genotypes *(CYP1A1, GSTM1)*.
- Patients with high adduct levels developed lung carcinoma after lower smoking dose/shorter (susceptible individuals).
- High prevalence of GC→TA mutations in p53 tumor suppressor gene in smokers' lung carcinoma, compatible with BPDE-induced mutational specificity; coincidence of BPDE-adduct-related and mutational hotspots in p53

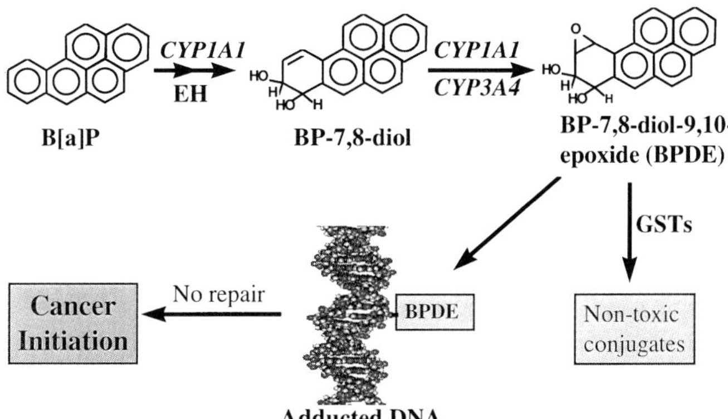

Fig. 1. Principal metabolic pathways of BP in human lung, leading to the formation of the ultimate carcinogenic metabolite BPDE which reacts with DNA, if not detoxified by glutathione *S*-transferases (GSTs); the resulting DNA adducts lead to the initiation of lung carcinogenesis

the complex DNA adduct pattern found in smokers' lungs, we concentrated on the polycyclic aromatic hydrocarbon BP, because it is an important carcinogenic constituent in tobacco smoke, air pollution and occupational environment. The mechanism by which BP interacts with DNA, activates oncogenes and initiates carcinogenic processes involves the formation of one of the enantiomeric BP diol-epoxides (BPDE). The biologically most active enantiomer is (+)-*anti*-BPDE, a major ultimate carcinogen which can now be quantified by our HPLC-FD technique (see below).

In human lung, cytochrome P450 1A1-related catalytic activity is one of the enzymes that convert polycyclic PAH into DNA-binding metabolites as shown for BP (Fig. 1). For *CYP1A1*-related enzyme activity in human lung, BP-3-hydroxylase (AHH) is a marker. Glutathione *S*-transferases (GSTs), including *GSTM1* in the liver and *GSTM3* in the lung, detoxify the reactive diol-epoxide intermediates (Fig. 1). Our previous studies revealed a dramatic impact of tobacco smoke on carcinogen-metabolizing enzymes in the human lung (Bartsch 1996). Recent smoking strongly and significantly induced phase I and phase II drug-metabolizing enzymes in a coordinated fashion.

Induction of the *CYP1A1*-related enzyme was up to sevenfold higher, whereas glutathione *S*-transferases were significantly repressed. Surprising was the long-lasting nature of this enzyme modulation, as the enzyme activities fell to the basal levels found in nonsmokers only after several weeks. This is probably due to tar deposition in the lungs of smokers and a slow release of PAH-type enzyme inducers. Therefore, individuals who smoke a sufficient number of cigarettes a day would have these PAH-activating enzymes induced and the detoxifying pathways by glutathione *S*-transferases repressed for life. Variations in these enzymes due to genetic polymorphism would therefore greatly affect the lung tissue dose of DNA-reactive tobacco carcinogens. In the same study a significant increase in *CYP1A1*-related enzyme activity in lung was noted only in lung cancer patients who were recent smokers, but not in smoking patients with nonmalignant pulmonary diseases (Bartsch 1996). These results from earlier work suggest that PAH present in tobacco smoke induce pulmonary *CYP1A1* gene expression only in certain individuals. As a consequence, the generation of DNA-reactive metabolites from tobacco carcinogens in lung target cells should be affected by polymorphic genes whose products are involved in PAH activation and detoxifying reactions.

Correlation Between Pulmonary PAH-DNA Adduct Levels and Lung CYP1A1-Related Activity: Effect of Enzyme Polymorphism

We examined whether a correlation exists between the *CYP1A1*-related catalytic activity in the lung of smokers and the level of PAH-DNA adducts that are thought to be critical at the onset of lung carcinogenesis. Initially, we used the sensitive method of ^{32}P-postlabelling for detecting tobacco smoke-associated DNA adducts. Then, because of its low specificity, an improved analytical method was developed to quantitate BPDE after binding to cellular DNA in humans (Alexandrov et al. 1992). The assay was validated for human lung tissue and later modified to analyze peripheral WBC DNA (Rojas et al. 1994). In brief, the method consists of HPLC-FD for quantifying BPDE adducts via formation of tetrols that are released after acid hydrolysis of DNA. With this assay it is possible to quantify the most important, biologically reactive (+)-*anti*-BPDE via the corresponding BP-tetrol, among the other less active enantiomers. The ^{32}P-postlabelling assay and the HPLC-FD method were then applied to lung parenchyma of smokers to determine the level of DNA adducts; in the same lung samples microsomal *CYP1A1*-related enzyme (AHH) activity was measured. A positive, highly significant correlation was found between pulmonary enzyme activity and the level of BPDE-DNA adducts (Table 2). The levels of total bulky PAH-DNA adducts were also correlated, but less strongly. Surprisingly, the BPDE-DNA adducts alone accounted for over 20% of the total bulky adducts in smokers' lungs. These positive correlations explain why variation in inducibility or genetic polymorphism of *CYP1A1*-related enzyme activity is a modifier of lung cancer risk in smokers

Table 2. Comparisons of BPDE-DNA adducts (determined by HPLC-FD) and of total bulky DNA adducts (by ^{32}P-postlabelling) with *CYP1A1*-related enzyme activity in smokers' lungs. (Data extracted from Alexandrov et al. 1992)

- *CYP1A1*-related enzyme (lung AHH) activity and level of BPDE-DNA adducts were correlated ($r = 0.91$; $p < 0.001$, $n = 13$).
- Levels of BPDE adducts and of total bulky DNA adducts (determined by ^{32}P-postlabelling) were correlated ($r = 0.78$; $p < 0.02$; $n = 13$).
- BPDE-DNA adducts accounted for over 20% of bulky DNA adducts in smokers' lungs.

and also implicate *CYP1A1* in the formation and binding of BPDE to lung DNA in smokers.

The regulation of *CYP1A1* expression is complex and also involves transcriptional control elements regulating enzyme induction which have not fully been characterized at the molecular level. Therefore, a genotype/phenotype approach was applied to examine the BPDE-DNA adduct levels in lung cancer tissue from patients with high *CYP1A1* inducibility (cf. Bartsch 1996). This phenotype was measured by immunohistochemical staining with a monoclonal antibody while the *GSTM1* genotype was determined by PCR. Smokers with similar cigarette consumption had a 100-fold higher BPDE-DNA adduct level in bronchial tissue when they were *GSTM1* inactive and highly inducible for *CYP1A1*, than found in controls. This large difference was not seen in parenchymal tissue.

Although *GSTM1* is not expressed in human lung, a *GSTM3* activity is found which seems to be co-regulated with the *GSTM1* form (Nakajima et al. 1995). Thus, individuals with the *GSTM1* null genotype suffer from impaired detoxification of tobacco carcinogens both qualitatively because of the absence of *GSTM1* in the body and low expression of *GSTM3* in the lung, and quantitatively because of the overall lower glutathione S-transferase activity. This effect of *GSTM1* null on lung PAH adduct levels was also seen in a Finnish cohort of lung cancer patients (Bartsch and Hietanen 1996). In current smokers the *GSTM1* gene deletion resulted in 10% increase in total bulky DNA adducts in lung, whereas even in ex-smokers a 2.5-fold excess of bulky DNA adducts was observed. This increase in DNA adduct levels is compatible with results from a meta-analysis of lung cancer patients with *GSTM1* deficiency whereby in smokers the relative risk increases to 1.4 for lung cancer of all major histological subtypes. This increased risk would account for 17% of all new lung cancers annually being caused in smokers because of the high prevalence of the *GSTM1* null genotype that occurs in about 50% of Caucasians (McWilliams et al. 1995).

A recent study in human cell lines revealed that *GSTM1* deletion is associated with high inducibility by 2,3,7,8-Tetrachlorodibenzo-p-dioxin of the *CYP1A1* gene transcription (Vaury et al. 1995). Although the underlying mechanism is not fully understood, this observation in vitro and our data on genotype dependence of PAH adduct levels in humans further underline the major importance of *CYP1A1/GSTM1* as risk modifiers of tobacco-associated

DNA damage and lung cancer. The latter was supported by case-control studies in Japanese populations (see below).

BPDE-DNA Adducts in White Blood Cells of PAH-Exposed Coke Oven Workers

Due to the precision of the HPLC-FD method, the level of BPDE-DNA adducts could be determined in WBCs from PAH-exposed coke oven workers. The specific aim was to see whether smoking enhances the binding of PAH to DNA and whether *CYP1A1/GSTM1* genotype combinations act as DNA-adduct modifiers.

Groups of coke oven workers exposed to PAH and nonexposed controls, each group including smokers and nonsmokers, were investigated (Rojas et al. 1995). The BPDE-DNA levels in WBCs of workers was 15 times higher than in those from nonexposed controls. However, the most important finding was that smoking increased the adduct levels in PAH-exposed workers, leading to a 200-fold interindividual variation in smoking workers, which was only sixfold in nonsmoking workers. The enhancing effect of smoking on DNA-adduct levels in WBCs from PAH-exposed workers was confirmed recently (Van Schooten et al. 1995).

The increased levels and high variability of BPDE-DNA adducts in smoking workers suggest genetic variations in PAH metabolism and DNA-adduct formation. As the same synergistic effects may occur in the lung, this would provide an explanation for the enhancing effect of smoking in PAH-associated occupational lung cancer risk. Recent studies showed that DNA-adduct levels in WBCs of smokers are correlated with adduct levels in lung tissue of lung cancer patients (Tang et al. 1995; Wiencke et al. 1995). The results from our study on coke oven workers suggest that the increment of DNA damage arising from occupational exposure to PAH is relatively small, but is greatly increased by smoking and genetic predisposition. The latter is now supported by the observed BPDE-DNA adduct dependence in WBCs as related to specific genotype combinations of *CYP1A1* and *GSTM1* (see below).

Association Between *CYP1A1, GSTM1*0/*0* Genotype, BPDE-DNA Adducts and Risk for Smoking- or Occupation-Related Lung Cancer

In Japanese populations, a significant correlation between susceptibility to lung cancer and homozygosity for the *CYP1A1 MspI* allele *(*2A/*2A)* was reported (Kawajiri et al. 1990; Nakachi et al. 1991, 1993). Hayashi et al. (1992) found exon 7 mutation *(m2)* to be associated with squamous cell and small cell lung cancer. Case-control studies revealed that Japanese individuals with the susceptible *CYP1A1(*2A/*2A* or **2B/*2B)* genotype combined with *GSTM1*0/*0* were at remarkably higher risk, particularly for Kreyberg I type and squamous cell lung carcinoma, at a low-dose level of cigarette smoking (Hayashi et al. 1992; Kihara et al. 1995). Individuals having homozygous

CYP1A1(MspI/MspI) were found to be relatively resistant to tobacco-related lung cancers when combined with *GSTM1* active, but were highly susceptible when combined with *GSTM1*0/*0* leading to a seven to eightfold increased risk (Kihara et al. 1995). Interestingly, lung cancer patients with the "at risk" *CYP1A1(*2A/*2A or *2B/*2B)* genotype when combined with a deficient genotype *GSTM1*0/*0* had remarkably shortened survivals, whereas the longest survival was seen in patients with the wild-type combination *CYP1A1*1/*1* and *GSTM1* active (Goto et al. 1996). Similar observations were made previously on the shortened survival time of lung cancer patients with a high expression of *CYP1A1* (induced AHH activity) in the lung (Bartsch et al. 1990). Although, homozygous carriers of the *MspI*-mutation of *CYP1A1* are very rare among Caucasians (<1%) (Cascorbi et al. 1996), a recent Scandinavian study found the combined *CYP1A1(MspI)* and *GSTM1*0/*0* genotype significantly overrepresented in patients with squamous cell carcinoma (Alexandrie et al. 1994).

Taken together, these studies suggest a genetic basis for the association of high *CYP1A1* metabolic activity and *GSTM1*0/*0* genotypes with increased lung cancer incidence, but the underlying molecular mechanisms regulating this effect are still not well understood. For these reasons the levels of BPDE-DNA adducts were analyzed by HPLC-FD in non-tumorous lung tissues from 20 lung cancer patients and WBCs from 20 PAH-exposed coke oven workers, all current tobacco smokers. *CYP1A1* mutations and *GSTM1* deletion polymorphisms in each subject were analyzed in genomic DNA by PCR/RFLP. The following results were obtained (Rojas et al., 1998): Independently of the *CYP1A1* genotype, all samples in the two groups with nondetectable adducts (<0.2 per 10^8 nt) were of *GSTM1* active genotype, and the 17 samples with detectable adducts ($\geq$0.2 per 10^8 nt) in the two groups were *GSTM1*0/*0*. The difference in adduct levels between *GSTM1*0/*0* and *GSTM1* active genotype was highly significant ($p<0.00005$). Among GSTM1-deficient individuals ($n=17$), a subgroup of 14 subjects with *CYP1A1*1/*1* (wild type, $n=7$) or heterozygous genotype *(*1/*2A or *1/*2B, $n=7$) showed low levels of BPDE-DNA-adducts (range: 0.2–1.3 per 10^8 nt), whereas three subjects with the rare combination *CYP1A1*2A/*2A or *2A/*2B* and *GSTM1*0/*0* showed significantly higher adduct levels (median: 17.4 adducts/10^8 nt, range 1.9–44; $p=0.017$). Therefore, combination of homozygous mutated *CYP1A1* and *GSTM1*0/*0* genotypes lead, at a similar or even lower smoking dose, to a stronger increase of BPDE-DNA adduct levels than found in subjects with *CYP1A1* and *GSTM1* wild type (Fig. 2).

In conclusion, our results showed a clear effect of the combination of *CYP1A1* and *GSTM1* genotypes on the formation of BPDE-DNA adducts in human lung and WBCs. Using BP as a reference carcinogen and a specific, sensitive detection method for its DNA-bound metabolite, we conclude that: (1) subjects with *GSTM1* active genotype did not show any detectable BPDE-DNA-adducts, (2) those with *CYP1A1*1/*1* or heterozygous for *CYP1A1*2A* or *2B* and with *GSTM1*0/*0* combination showed low levels of BPDE-DNA-adduct formation, and (3) those with *CYP1A1*2A/*2A* mutant allele from the

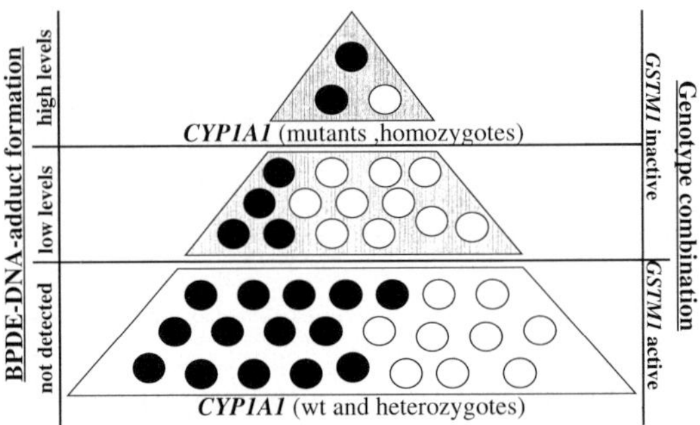

Fig. 2. Classification of *CYP1A1/GSTM1* genotype combinations into three groups with low, intermediate and high levels of BPDE adducts; the data was compiled for lung parenchyma from individual smoking lung cancer patients (*filled circles*) and for WBC from PAH-exposed coke oven workers (*open circles*) (Rojas et al., 1998). Smokers with the rare combination of mutated *CYP1A1* (homozygotes) and *GSTM1* inactive had highest PAH-DNA adduct levels and consequently were shown to be at higher lung cancer risk. (From Kawajiri et al. 1990; Nakachi et al. 1991, 1993; Hayashi et al. 1992; Kihara et al. 1995; Alexandrie et al. 1994)

*GSTM1*0/*0* group showed the highest BPDE-DNA-adduct levels. These preliminary but consistent results in the two study groups demonstrated that the combination of *CYP1A1*2A/*2A* and *GSTM1*0/*0* modulates the level of BPDE-DNA adducts in human lung and WBCs; they provide a mechanistic understanding of previous epidemiological studies that correlated these at risk genotypes in Japanese individuals with both increased smoking-related lung cancers and shortened survival of lung cancer patients. Our findings are also consistent with the prevalence of G:C→T:A transversion mutations in the p53 tumor suppressor gene found in lung tumors, suggestive of PAH-related mutational damage, which occurs more frequently in persons who are *GSTM1*0/*0* (Ryberg et al. 1994). Furthermore, the coincidence of mutational hotspots in p53 and BPDE-related adduct hotspots suggests that BPDE and structurally related PAH diol-epoxides are involved in the transformation of human lung tissue in smokers (Denissenko et al. 1996).

The continued examination of the role of BPDE-DNA adducts resulting from the *GSTM1* and *CYP1A1* polymorphisms and their interaction with other susceptibility markers, e.g., mutagen sensitivity and impaired DNA-repair capacity (Hsu 1987), may help to identify high-risk subjects among smokers and subjects occupationally and/or environmentally exposed to PAH.

Acknowledgements. We acknowledge the collaboration and contributions during various phases of our studies by G. Auburtin and L. Mayer from the Institut National de l'Environment Industriel et des Risques, Verneuil en Hallate, France, I. Cascorbi, J. Brockmöller and I. Roots from the University Clinic Charité, Humboldt University, Berlin, Germany, and H. Vainio, S. Anttila and K. Husgafvel-Pursiainen from the Institute of Occupational Health, Helsinki, Finland. We thank Mrs. G. Bielefeldt for skilled secretarial assistance.

References

Alexandrie AK, Sundberg MI, Seidegard J, Tornling G, Ranung A (1994) Genetic susceptibility to lung cancer with special emphasis on *CYP1A1* and *GSTM1*: a study on host factors in relation to age at onset, gender and histological cancer types. Carcinogenesis 15:1785–1790

Alexandrov K, Rojas M, Geneste O, Castegnaro M, Camus AM, Petruzzelli S, Giuntini C, Bartsch H (1992) An improved fluorometric assay for dosimetry of benzo[a]pyrene diol-epoxide-DNA adducts in smoker's lung: comparison with total bulky adducts and aryl hydrocarbon hydroxylase activity. Cancer Res 52:6248–6253

Bartsch H (1996) DNA adducts in human carcinogenesis: etiological relevance and structureactivity relationship. Mutat Res 40:67–79

Bartsch H, Hietanen E (1996) The role of individual susceptibility in cancer burden related to environmental exposure. Environ Health Perspect 104 (Suppl 3):569–577

Bartsch H, Hietanen E, Petruzzelli S, Giuntini C, Saracci R, Mussi A, Angeletti CA (1990) Possible prognostic value of pulmonary *Ah*-locus-linked enzymes in patients with tobacco-related lung cancer. Int J Cancer 46:185–188

Bartsch H, Rojas M, Alexandrov K, Camus A-M, Castegnaro M, Malaveille C, Anttila S, Hirvonen K, Husgafvel-Pursiainen K, Hietanen E, Vainio H (1995) Metabolic polymorphism effecting DNA binding and excretion of carcinogens in humans. Pharmacogenetics 5:S84–S90

Brockmöller J, Kerb R, Drakoulis N, Nitz M, Roots I (1993) Genotype and phenotype of glutathione *S*-transferase class μ isoenzymes in lung cancer patients and controls. Cancer Res 53:1004–1011

Caporaso N, Goldstein A (1995) Cancer genes: single and susceptibility: exposing the difference. Pharmacogenetics 5:59–63

Cascorbi I, Brockmöller J, Roots I (1996) A C4887A polymorphism in exon 7 of human *CYP1A1*: population frequency, mutation linkages, and impact on lung cancer susceptibility. Cancer Res 56:4965–4969

Denissenko MF, Pao A, Tang MS, Pfeifer GP (1996) Preferential formation of benzo[a]pyrene adducts at lung cancer mutational hotspots in p53. Science 274:430–432

Goto M, Yoneda S, Yamamoto M, Kawajiri K (1996) Prognostic significance of germ line polymorphisms of the *CYP1A1* and glutathione *S*-transferase genes in patients with non-small cell lung cancer. Cancer Res 6:3725–3730

Hayashi SI, Watanabe J, Kawajiri K (1992) High susceptibility to lung cancer analyzed in terms of combined genotypes of P4501A1 and Mu-class glutathione *S*-transferase genes. Jpn J Cancer Res 83:866–870

Hsu TC (1987) Genetic predisposition to cancer with special reference to mutagen sensitivity. In vitro Cellular and Developmental Biology 23:591–603

Kawajiri K, Nakachi K, Imai K, Yoshii A, Shinoda N, Watanabe J (1990) Identification of genetically high risk individuals to lung cancer by DNA polymorphism of the cytochrome P4501A1 gene. FEBS Lett 263:131–133

Kihara M, Kihara M, Noda K (1995) Risk of smoking for squamous and small cell carcinomas of the lung modulated by combinations of *CYP1A1* and *GSTM1* gene polymorphisms in a Japanese population. Carcinogenesis 16:2331–2336

McWilliams JE, Sanderson BJS, Harris EL, Richert-Boe KE, Henner WD (1995) Glutathione *S*-transferase M1 (GSTM1) deficiency and lung cancer risk. Cancer Epidemiol Biomarkers Prev 4:589–594

Nakachi K, Imai K, Hayashi S-I, Watanabe J, Kawajiri K (1991) Genetic susceptibility to squamous cell carcinoma of the lung in relation to cigarette smoking dose. Cancer Res 51:5177–5180

Nakachi K, Imai K, Hayashi S-I, Kawajiri K (1993) Polymorphisms of the *CYP1A1* and glutathione *S*-transferase genes associated with susceptibility to lung cancer in relation to cigarette dose in a Japanese population. Cancer Res 53:2994–2999

Nakajima T, Elovaara E, Anttila S, Hirvonen A, Camus A-M, Hayes JD, Ketterer B, Vainio H (1995) Expression and polymorphism of glutathione S-transferase in human lungs: risk factors in smoking-related lung cancer. Carcinogenesis 16:707–711

Rojas M, Alexandrov K, van Schooten F-J, Hillebrand M, Kriek E, Bartsch H (1994) Validation of a new fluorometric assay for benzo[a]pyrene diolepoxide-DNA adducts in human white blood cells: comparison with ^{32}P-postlabeling and ELISA. Carcinogenesis 15:557–560

Rojas M, Alexandrov K, Auburtin G, Wastiaux-Denamur A, Mayer L, Mahieu B, Sebastien P, Bartsch H (1995) Anti-benzo[a]pyrene diolepoxide-DNA adduct levels in peripheral mononuclear cells from coke oven workers and the enhancing effect of smoking. Carcinogenesis 6:1373–1376

Rojas M, Alexandrov K, Cascorbi I, Brockmöller J, Likhachev A, Pozharisski K, Bouvier G, Auburtin G, Mayer L, Koop-Schneider A, Roots I, Bartsch H (1998) High benzo[a]pyrene diol-epoxide DNA adduct levels in lung and blood cells from subjects with combined CYP1A1 MspI/MspI-GSTM1*0/*0 genotypes. Pharmacogenetics 8:109–118

Ryberg D, Kure E, Lystad S, Skaug V, Stangeland L, Mercy I, Børresen A-L, Haugen A (1994) p53 mutations in lung tumors: relationship to putative susceptibility markers for cancer. Cancer Res 54:1551–1555

Tang D, Santella RM, Blackwood AM, Young T-L, Mayer J, Jaretzki A, Grantham S, Tsai W-Y, Perera FP (1995) A molecular epidemiological case-control study of lung cancer. Cancer Epidemiol Biomarkers Prev 4:341–346

Van Schooten FJ, Jongeneelen FJ, Hillebrand MJX, van Leeuwen FE, de Loof AJA, Dijkmans APG, van Rooij JGM, den Engelse L, Kriek E (1995) Polycyclic aromatic hydrocarbon-DNA adducts in white blood cell DNA and 1-hydroxypyrene in the urine from aluminum workers: relation with job category and synergistic effect of smoking. Cancer Epidemiol Biomarkers Prev 4:69–77

Vaury C, Laine R, Noguiez P, de Coppet P, Jaulin C, Praz F, Pompon D, Amor-Guéret M (1995) Human glutathione S-transferase M1 null genotype is associated with a high inducibility of cytochrome P450 1A1 gene transcription. Cancer Res 55:5520–5523

Vineis P (1997) Molecular epidemiology: low-dose carcinogens and genetic susceptibility. Int J Cancer 71:1–3

Vineis P, Bartsch H, Caporaso N, Harrington AM, Kadlubar FF, Landi MT, Malaveille C, Shields PG, Skipper P, Talaska G, Tannenbaum SR (1994) Genetically based N-acetyltransferase metabolic polymorphism and low-level environmental exposure to carcinogens. Nature 369:154–156

Wiencke JK, Kelsey KT, Varkonyi A, Semey K, Wain JC, Mark E, Christiani DC (1995) Correlation of DNA adducts in blood mononuclear cells with tobacco carcinogen-induced damage in human lung. Cancer Res 55:4910–4914

Mutation Spectra Resulting from Carcinogenic Exposure: From Model Systems to Cancer-Related Genes

E. Dogliotti[1], P. Hainaut[2], T. Hernandez[2], M. D'Errico[1], and D. M. DeMarini[3]

[1] Laboratory of Comparative Toxicology and Ecotoxicology,
 Viale Regina Elena 299, 00161, Rome, Italy
[2] International Agency for Research on Cancer, 150 cours Albert-Thomas,
 69372 Lyon Cedex 08, France
[3] Environmental Carcinogenesis Division, U.S. Environmental Protection Agency,
 Research Triangle Park, North Carolina 27711, USA

Abstract

The events leading to cancer are complex and interactive. Alteration of cancer genes, such as the tumor suppressor gene *p53*, plays a central role in this process. Analysis of the frequency, type and site of mutations in important cancer-related genes may provide clues to the identification of etiological factors and sources of exposure. In this chapter we have selected a few examples of environmental human carcinogens and have attempted to use the knowledge of their mechanisms of mutagenesis, as derived from in vitro cell systems, as a key to understanding the complexity of p53 mutation spectra in tumors arising at the putative target organ. The analysis will focus on environmental exposure to UV radiation. The examples of tobacco smoke, dietary aflatoxin and vinyl chloride will be also briefly discussed.

Background

The interpretation of mutation spectra is influenced and complicated by a series of factors. A mutagen will generally introduce a variety of lesions with different mutagenic potential. The primary sequence of the target gene is one of the factors affecting the site-specificity of the lesion, while cell metabolism reflects another layer of complexity. Mutations are also affected by the efficiency of repair as well as by the replicative bypass machinery and the DNA polymerase insertion preference. Finally, biological selection of mutations will introduce another "filter" by confining the detectable mutations to those genetic alterations that, for example, produce a functionally altered gene product. The mutation spectrum is, therefore, the product of the probability patterns of all these sequential steps of mutagenesis: damage, repair, polymerase misreading and biological selection.

Recent Results in Cancer Research, Vol. 154
© Springer-Verlag Berlin · Heidelberg 1998

How to Interpret Mutation Spectra?

In Vitro Cell Systems: Mutation Spectra in Reporter Genes

In the last decade considerable efforts have been directed towards the molecular analysis of gene mutations after exposure to physical and chemical agents. Mutation spectra have been analyzed either in intrachromosomal or in extrachromosomal (carried by episomic vectors) selectable genes in both prokaryotic and eukaryotic cell systems. The information that can be derived from a mutation spectrum relates to the type and position of the mutations. First, the type of mutation is the end-product of the type of lesion induced and of the host cell's strategy to cope with that specific DNA modification. Second, it is well known that interaction of a carcinogen with DNA is sequence-specific and that the efficiency and specificity of both DNA repair and trans-lesion bypass may be affected by the sequences surrounding the lesion. Moreover, two cellular mechanisms can introduce strand asymmetry in mutation distribution: transcription-coupled excision repair (Hanawalt 1994) and DNA replication machinery.

Besides these carcinogen and host cell variables, the distribution of mutations along any gene reflects the functional domains of the protein. The drawback of any selective mutation assay (often based on resistance to the toxic effects of drugs) is that mutation analysis is confined to those genetic alterations that produce a functionally altered gene product. Proteins are surprisingly tolerant of amino acid substitutions. In the 1980s Miller (1983) studying the *lac* repressor, found that about one half of all substitutions (1500 at 142 positions) were phenotypically silent. This phenomenon, which is called "protein filter", may drastically affect the mutation distribution. An example is given in the study by Palombo et al. (1992a) in which alkylation damage-induced mutations in the *gpt* gene carried by a shuttle vector were selected by nonphenotypic methods and compared with mutations detected by traditional phenotypic assays. By analysis of *gpt* mutation spectra obtained either in bacteria (Richardson et al. 1987, 1988) or mammalian cells (Palombo et al. 1992b; Basic-Zaninovic et al. 1995) after treatment with alkylating agents, a striking unbalance for mutations at 5'GG3' sequences was observed between the two strands. For example, G > A transition mutations were often described at G_{128} on the nontranscribed DNA strand but not at G_{124}, which presents the same flanking bases but is located on the transcribed DNA strand (Fig. 1). Non-phenotypic selection of induced mutations within this sequence (Palombo et al. 1992a) revealed that in fact mutations could be induced on both sites but only the G_{128} > A base change drastically affected the functionality of the GPT protein and, therefore, was detected by the phenotypic assay while G_{124} > A mutation was functionally silent.

The effects of all these variables on mutation spectra have been investigated using in vitro experimental cell systems. Here we review these data for a selected number of environmental carcinogens obtained either in bacterial systems, in particular in *Salmonella typhimurium*, or in mammalian cells.

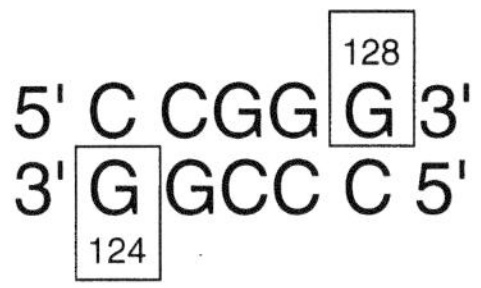

mutation	aa change	growth in MATG	GPT activity (U/mg)
G_{124}>A	Pro-Ser	–	13.2
G_{128}>A	Gly>Asp	+	N.D.
wild-type		–	13.8

Fig. 1. Effect of the "protein filter" on mutation spectrum. Top: Sequence of the NciI site of the *gpt* gene carried by an EBV-derived shuttle vector. The top strand is the non transcribed DNA strand. Mutations arising within this sequence after cell treatment with an alkylating agent were selected by a nonphenotypic assay, the RFLP/PCR. Bottom: The properties – ability of growth in selective medium containing 6-thioguanine (MATG) and xanthine-phosphoribosyltransferase (GPT) activity – of *E. coli gpt⁻* cells transformed with plasmids containing these mutations are indicated. The nucleotide position of the *gpt* mutation is indicated (data from Palombo et al. 1992 a)

This knowledge is the basis for the correct interpretation of tumor-specific mutation spectra.

Mutation Spectra in Cancer-Related Genes: The Example of the P53 Gene

The p53 tumor suppressor gene encodes a nuclear phosphoprotein with cancer-inhibiting properties. The development of human cancer often involves inactivation of this suppressor function through several mechanisms, including gene deletions, point mutations or silencing of the p53 protein by binding to viral or cellular proteins. These mutations frequently arise somatically. However, p53 mutations may also be inherited in several families with a predisposition to multiple cancers, as in the Li-Fraumeni syndrome. Loss of alleles at the p53 locus (on 17p13) is commonly observed in many forms of cancer. Point mutations are scattered over more than 250 codons and are common in many forms of human cancer. In this respect, the p53 gene differs from other tumor suppressor genes such as Rb, APC and p16 MTS-1, which are frequently inactivated by deletion or nonsense mutations, and from the oncogenes of the *ras* family, which are activated by mutations at a small number of well-defined codons (Harris 1996 a).

Since the identification of somatic, tumor-specific, missense p53 mutations in 1989, about 570 different p53 mutations have been identified in more than 8000 individual tumors. Analysis of these mutations reveals clues about the etiology and the molecular pathogenesis of human cancer (Harris 1996 b, Greenblatt et al. 1994). A database of these mutations was initiated by M. Hollstein and C.C. Harris in 1990 to provide a tool to classify, sort, retrieve, compare and analyze these mutations in order to generate hypotheses on the natural history of human cancer. This database is maintained at the International Agency for Research on Cancer and is available at URL http://www.iarc.fr/p53/homepage.htm (Hainaut et al. 1998). The diversity of p53 mutations provides a valuable tool to identify sources of cancer-causing mutation in the human setting.

The p53 gene is located on chromosome 17p13 and has 11 exons encoding a protein of 393 aminoacid residues within a chromosomal domain of about 20 kilobases. The p53 protein is a multifunctional transcription factor that plays a role in the control of cell cycle progression, DNA integrity and cell survival in cells exposed to DNA-damaging agents. Typically, DNA damage induces a rapid and transient nuclear accumulation and activation of the p53 protein, resulting in the *trans*-activation of target genes, including the cyclin kinase inhibitor p21waf-1 (a negative regulator of cell cycle progression) and the regulator of apoptosis bax-1 (a dominant-negative inhibitor of bcl-2). The p53 protein also interacts with several key proteins regulating DNA replication, transcription and repair, and some of its suppressor functions may involve transcription-independent pathways. Mutation of p53 impairs the DNA-binding and *trans*-activating properties of p53 and prevents growth arrest or apoptosis under conditions in which p53-competent cells are normally suppressed. Thus, inactivation of p53 provides a selective advantage for the clonal expansion of preneoplastic or neoplastic cells. In addition, some mutants may exert an oncogenic activity of their own. The molecular basis for this "gain-of-function" phenotype is still unclear (reviewed in Levine 1997).

Analysis of the p53 mutation database reveals that 91.2% of reported mutations fall within the DNA-binding domain (residues 102-292) (Fig. 2). This particular distribution may reflect a bias since many studies are limited to the central portion of the protein (exons 4–9). Taking into account studies that have covered all coding exons (2–11), the proportion of mutations in the central domain is still very high (84%). This high proportion may be explained by: (1) the importance of DNA-binding as an essential functional property of p53, and (2) the particular structure of this protein domain, which can be unfolded by amino acid substitutions at many different sites. The DNA-binding domain of p53 differs from those of other known DNA-binding proteins (Cho et al. 1994). It is made of two distorted, anti-parallel β sheets that form a scaffold supporting a DNA-binding surface made of non-contiguous loops and helixes. These loops and helixes are kept in the correct orientation by the binding of a zinc atom. About 30% of all known mutations affect residues that make important contacts with DNA, such as Arg-248 (the most important contact in the minor groove of target DNA), Arg-273 (which contacts the DNA phosphate backbone) or Arg-282 (which binds in the major groove). Other frequently mutated residues, such as Arg-175 and Arg-249, are not in direct contact with DNA but their mutation alters the architecture of the whole DNA-binding surface. These various mutants are not functionally equivalent and differ by their biological properties in ex-

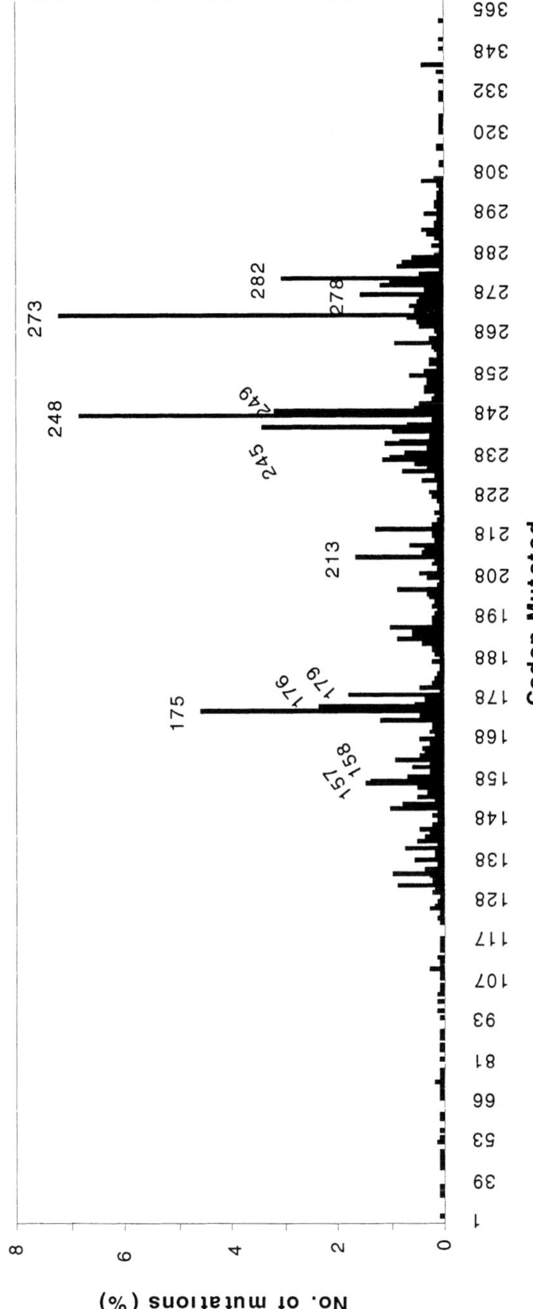

Fig. 2. Distribution of p53 gene mutations in human cancers. The data are derived from the July 1997 version of the IARC p53 database

perimental systems (Ory et al. 1994). Thus, the occurrence of particular mutants in cancer is strongly influenced by a protein filter selecting mutant proteins with particular functional properties. It is now emerging that specific mutant proteins may have different consequences on the progression and prognosis of cancer. For example, mutation at Arg-175 carries a particularly poor prognosis in colon cancer (Goh et al. 1995), whereas mutations at codon 248 are an indicator of poor response to treatment by doxorubicyn in breast cancer (Aas et al. 1996).

Analysis of Mutation Spectra Induced by Selected Carcinogens

Ultraviolet Light

The carcinogenicity of sunlight to the skin has been recognized for over 100 years (Unna 1894), and hundreds of studies on UV-induced mutation spectra have been conducted in experimental systems. However, most of these studies have used germicidal lamps that emit UVC wavelengths in the range of 180-280 nm, especially monochromatic light at 254 nm (International Agency for Research on Cancer 1992). The relevance of these wavelengths to sunlight-associated human skin cancer is questionable considering that UV wavelengths < 280 nm (i.e., UVC) are absorbed almost completely by the earth's atmosphere, and, therefore, only a negligible amount of UVC reaches the surface of the earth (Madronich 1993).

As described elsewhere in this chapter, the mutation spectrum of simulated sunlight in mammalian cells (Drobetsky et al. 1994) is different from that produced by UVC (250–280 nm). This suggests that results from UVC studies may have limited relevance to results produced by sunlight itself, which is a complex array of wavelengths and radiations.

Bacterial Cell Systems

Mutagenesis studies in *Salmonella* of filtered fluorescent light have shown that wavelengths > 375 nm are not mutagenic (Hartman et al. 1991) and that wavelengths < 335 nm from sunlight account for most of the mutagenicity of sunlight in *Salmonella* (De Flora et al. 1990). Considering that only negligible amounts of sunlight at wavelengths < 280 nm penetrate the earth's atmosphere, the likely range of wavelengths accounting for sunlight-induced mutations and skin cancer are 280–335 nm (UVB).

One study has been performed in which mutation spectra were determined in *Salmonella* cells exposed to full sunlight (DeMarini et al. 1995 a). In this case, $\sim 10\%$ of the solar radiation was in the UVABC range, with 50–60 times more of these emissions being in the UVA relative to UVB range; $< 0.08\%$ of the total emissions were in the UVC range. The strains used contained the base substitution allele His-G46, which consists of a TCCC target that can be reverted by either single base substitutions involving the middle two Cs or by tandem (primarily double base) mutations involving any of the four nucleotides.

The mutagenic potency and mutation spectrum varied depending on the DNA repair capacity of the cells. In wild-type cells, or those containing the pKM101 plasmid, which confers the SOS response, sunlight produced only a two- to three-fold increase in the mutant yield relative to control cells; however, in a strain containing the nucleotide-excision repair (NER) mutation *f*uvrB (TA1535), sunlight induced a 19-fold increase in mutant yield. Sunlight induced a tenfold increase in mutant yield in strain TA98, which contains both the pKM101 plasmid and the *f*uvrB mutation.

In a wild-type strain, sunlight induced only a ~twofold increase in transitions and transversions (relative to spontaneous levels) in the absence of pKM101; the addition of the plasmid had little effect. However, in the NER-deficient strain TA1535, sunlight induced a tenfold increase in transversions (GC>TA) and a 20-fold increase in transitions (GC>AT). In strain TA98 (*f*uvrB, pKM101), sunlight induced only an ~twofold increase in transversions but a 24-fold increase in transitions, indicating that, in a *f*uvrB background, the plasmid reduced the production of transversions but had little effect on the production of transitions.

In terms of the proportion of transitions and transversions recovered in these strains, sunlight induced equal proportions of these two classes of mutations in excision repair-proficient cells; however, sunlight induced more transitions relative to transversions in excision repair-deficient cells. The plasmid had no influence on the proportions of sunlight-induced transitions and transversions. In terms of site specificity, sunlight induced single base transversions equally at either of the middle two Cs of the TCCC target. However, sunlight induced single base transitions (C>T) preferentially at the first C (TCCC) in strain TA1535 (*f*uvrB); transitions were induced equally between the middle two Cs in the other strains.

The single base mutations in this study were determined by probe hybridization; the remaining mutants (probe-negative) are considered to contain multiple (tandem) mutations. Thus, in excision repair-proficient cells, sunlight induced an eightfold increase in presumptive multiple mutations; the addition of the plasmid increased this only slightly to ninefold. However, sunlight induced a 20-fold increase in presumptive multiple mutations in strain TA1535 (*f*uvrB) and a 38-fold increase in this class of mutation in TA98 (*f*uvrB, pKM101). Thus, sunlight increased the yield of presumptive multiple mutations more than any other class of mutation. In general, almost 5% of the sunlight induced mutations were multiple mutations.

DNA sequence analysis of one of the mutants containing a presumptive multiple mutation confirmed the presence of a multiple (triple) mutation (TCCC>TTTT). DNA sequence analysis of other mutants containing presumptive multiple mutations induced by light from a tanning salon bed showed that 83% were tandem CC>TT transitions (DeMarini et al. 1995a). A study with 254 nm UV at the His-G46 allele also found induction of a high percentage (64%) of CC>TT transitions (Koch et al. 1994). Similar findings were obtained for fluorescent light in *Salmonella* (DeMarini et al. 1995a; Cebula et al. 1995). For various types of UV radiation in bacteria, yeast, and mammalian cells, excision repair deficiency increases the frequency of transitions and multiple mutations and reduces the frequency of transversions.

Although different wavelengths preferentially produce different lesions, such as thymine glycol, alkali labile sites, DNA-protein cross-links, etc., two lesions appear to be especially important for UV mutagenesis: cyclobutane pyrimidine dimers (CPD) and (6-4) photoproducts (6-4 PP). CPD and 6-4 PP account for 85% and 10% of the UV lesions in double stranded DNA respectively. In bacteria TC, TCC, CC, and CCC are hotspots for UV-induced transitions and both CPD and 6-4 PP are important premutagenic lesions at these sites (see DeMarini et al. 1995a). Thus, the TCCC sequence of the His-G46 allele may present an ideal target for the formation of UV-induced photoproducts and subsequent mutagenesis.

Neighboring DNA sequence and the resulting local DNA conformation may also play a critical role in the ability of UV-induced lesions to form at these sites and may influence the accessibility of such lesions to DNA repair enzymes. Runs of pyrimidines may adopt different conformations than that of B-DNA, such as bent, triple helix, and A-DNA (Mei and Barton 1988), and this may be promoted further by the presence of photoproducts. Consequently, DNA repair may be inhibited, and such sites may be prone to misincorporation by DNA polymerase followed by elongation (Sage et al. 1992), especially in the presence of the pKM101 plasmid.

Studies have shown that UVC-induced photolesions are repaired selectively on the transcribed strand in bacteria and that, consequently, most UVC-induced mutations occur at sites where the pyrimidine run is on the nontranscribed strand (Hanawalt 1991; Terleth et al. 1991; Oller et al. 1992), as it is at the His-G46 allele of *Salmonella*. As discussed previously by Oller et al. (1992), the question of which strand produces mutations (due to photolesions on that strand) depends on the rate of repair of one strand relative to the other.

Although a detailed understanding of the mechanism underlying the sunlight-induced mutation spectra in *Salmonella* reviewed above is lacking, some general features can be inferred from studies with UVB and UVC. In NER-proficient strains, the majority of mutations may have been produced during the filling of excision repair gaps, perhaps when repair of a lesion in one strand encountered a lesion in the opposite strand, resulting in misrepair. In *fuvrB* strains, the mutations may have been produced later, when DNA replication resumed. In this situation, mutations may have occurred either at the replication fork (misreplication) or during the filling of the daughter strand gaps that were created when DNA replication was blocked at photolesions and reinitiated downstream from the lesion. A possible mechanism for fixation of a photolesion into a $C > T$ transition implies that the bypass of a totally noncoding lesion occurs via insertion of an A ("A rule") across from the lesion. This would result in the $C > T$ transition only since photolesions involving T residues would not result in mutations, due to the insertion of the correct base (A) opposite the T. Furthermore, it has been hypothesized that the high frequency of cytosine deamination of PyPy lesions can be responsible for the observed C > T transitions (according to the A rule) (Tessman et al. 1992). The presence of the pKM101 plasmid presumably facilitated trans-lesion synthesis past pyrimidine photoproducts, and this bypass was mutagenic primarily via misincorporation of dAMP opposite a cytosine (or uracil) in the dimer.

Mammalian Cell Systems

In eukaryotic cells UVC light-induced mutation spectra have been widely studied either at the level of endogenous genes, such as *aprt*, *dhfr* and *hprt*, or using shuttle vectors that carry reporter genes (Vrieling et al. 1989; Dorado et al. 1991; McGregor et al. 1991; Bourre et al. 1989; Hsia et al. 1989; Brash et al. 1987; Seidman et al. 1987). As in the case of bacterial spectra, C > T transitions predominated and tandem mutations constituted almost 10% of all mutations. As previously reported for bacteria, most C > T transitions occurred at TC and CC sites on the 3′ side or within a short run of pyrimidines. By applying the A rule, the prediction is that, also in mammalian cells, T <> T are not mutagenic and T <> C, C <> T and C <> C are the major premutagenic lesions.

Mutation specificity of UVC (254 nm), UVB (290–320 nm), UVA (350–400 nm) and broad-spectrum simulated sunlight (SSL) (310–1100 nm) was analyzed and compared in the *aprt* gene of NER-proficient and -deficient CHO cells (Dobretsky et al. 1994, 1995; Sage et al. 1996). The data revealed that AT > TG transversions, a rare class of mutation in spontaneous and induced

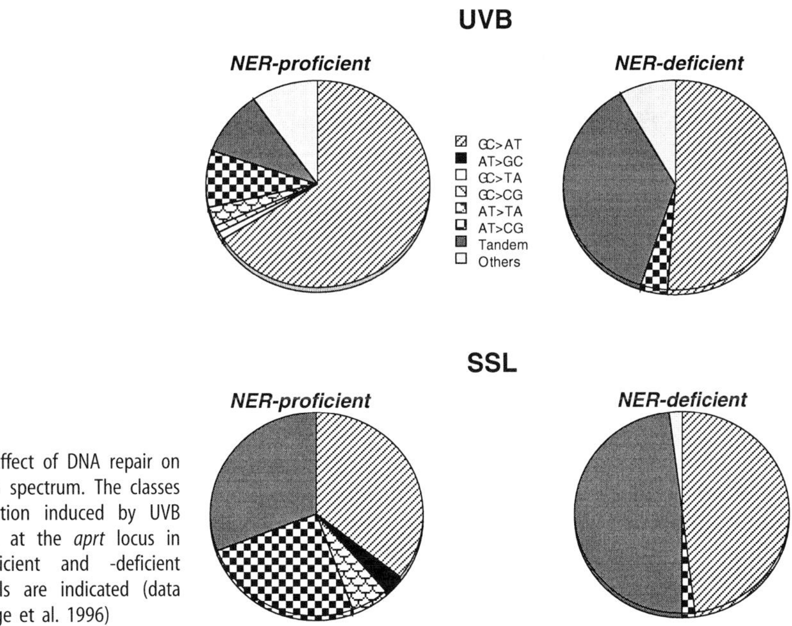

Fig. 3. Effect of DNA repair on mutation spectrum. The classes of mutation induced by UVB and SSL at the *aprt* locus in NER-proficient and -deficient CHO cells are indicated (data from Sage et al. 1996)

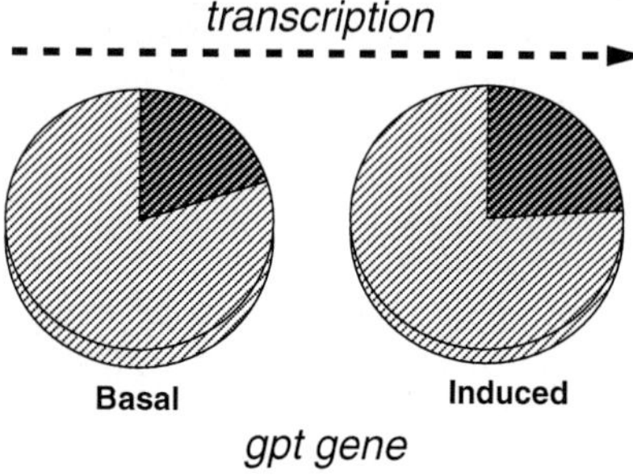

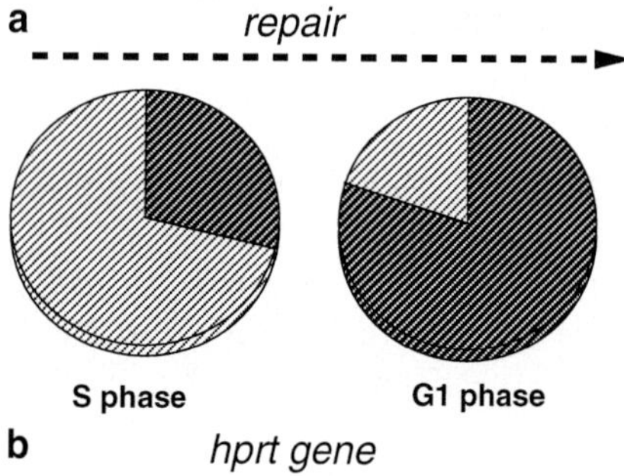

Fig. 4. Effects of DNA transcription and repair on mutation distribution. **a** Distribution of UV-induced base substitutions on the transcribed and non transcribed strand of the *gpt* gene as a function of the transcriptional activity of the gene (data from Basic-Zaninovic et al. 1995). **b** Distribution of UV-induced base substitutions on the transcribed and non transcribed strand of the *hprt* gene in human fibroblasts irradiated in G_1- and S-phase (data from McGregor et al. 1991)

spectra, constituted a high proportion (up to 50%) of mutations in UVA-exposed cells. This mutation event comprised also a significant part of the SSL-induced mutations (25%) while it was rarely detected after UVB or UVC exposure (5%–9% of the total mutants). Therefore the mutagenic specificity of SSL indicates that, besides the UVB component, UVA also plays a significant role in solar mutagenesis. When UV mutation specificity was investigated in NER-deficient cells (Sage et al. 1996) (Fig. 3) the mutation spectrum of both UVB and SSL showed a marked increase in tandem CC>TT transitions relative to NER-proficient cells. Moreover, the T>G transversion class disappeared from the SSL spectrum that could be entirely accounted for by the UVB-induced mutations.

As in the case of bacteria, the occurrence of preferential repair of the transcribed strand (Mellon et al. 1986, 1987) is expected to lead to the accumulation of UV-induced mutations on the nontranscribed strand of active genes. In general, this expectation has been borne out experimentally (Vrieling et al. 1989, 1991; Menichini et al. 1991). However, in the case of exponentially growing human cells, no strand bias in favor of the nontranscribed DNA strand was reported for UV-induced mutations in the highly transcribed *gpt* gene carried by an episomic shuttle vector (Baisc-Zaninovic et al. 1995). In contrast, the majority of UV-induced mutations were located on the transcribed *gpt* strand (Fig. 4A). It is important to recall that human cells repair efficiently both strands of active genes (Mellon et al. 1987), although the transcribed strand is repaired faster than the nontranscribed strand. By 24 h post-irradiation time, no difference between the two strands was detected by gene-specific repair assay. It might well be that the rate of strand-specific repair is not sufficient to leave its "fingerprint" on mutation distribution. In agreement with this hypothesis, the expected accumulation of mutations on the nontranscribed DNA strand of the *hprt* gene of human fibroblasts was only detected when G_1-synchronized cells were irradiated (McGregor et al. 1991) (Fig. 4B). This finding clearly indicates that if sufficient time is provided for transcription associated repair to occur, mutation distribution is indeed biased also in human cells. In the case of S-phase irradiated human fibroblasts the majority of *hprt* mutations were located on the transcribed strand (Fig. 4B). This strand asymmetry which was also observed with the *gpt* gene is likely to reflect the "protein filter" (see above).

UV-induced mutation spectra were also studied in several NER-defective human syndromes complementations groups. In UV-treated xeroderma pigmentosum (XP) A cells (Dorado et al. 1991; McGregor et al. 1991), although the type of mutations were very similar to those observed in repair proficient cells, an unexpected bias towards mutations on the transcribed strand was detected. The occurrence of this phenomenon was also reported in repair-defective rodent cells (Sage et al. 1996; Vrieling et al. 1992). In the absence of NER, the repair of the transcribed strand via alternative pathways might be preferentially inhibited ultimately favoring mutation due to lesions on the transcribed strand. UV-induced mutation spectra were also studied in defective cell lines by introducing UV-irradiated shuttle vector molecules into cells. The SV40-derived shuttle vector pZ189 (Seidman et al. 1987), which carries the *sup*F gene as a target for mutations, was used to investigate UV mutagenesis in XP variant (XP-V) cells (Wang et al. 1991). Cells isolated from XP-V have a nearly normal rate of NER of UV-induced DNA damage and are slightly more sensitive than normal cells to the cytotoxic effect of UV radiation. However, they show a significantly higher sensitivity than normal cells to the mutagenic effect of UV light. Sequence analysis showed that in XP-V cells 28% of the mutations involved AT base pairs, while in normal cells this value was only 11%. The type of mutations induced strongly suggests that these cells are defective in the process that leads to the preferential insertion of dAMP opposite UV photolesions. The UV-induced mutation frequency and type were also analyzed in XP-D and trichothiodystrophy (TTD) cell lines using a shuttle vector system, pR2, carrying the target lacZ' gene (Marionnet et al. 1995). XP-D and TTD/XP-D cells are mutated in the same gene, ERCC2, but the mutations differ by their pathological consequences. Whereas XP-D patients develop early skin tumors, TTD patients are not prone to early cancers. The UV mutation frequency was significantly higher in both defective cell lines than in normal cells. TTD cells presented more rearrangements (16%) than normal cells and XP-D cells exhibited a twofold higher rate of multiple mutations than normal cells. The types of mutations

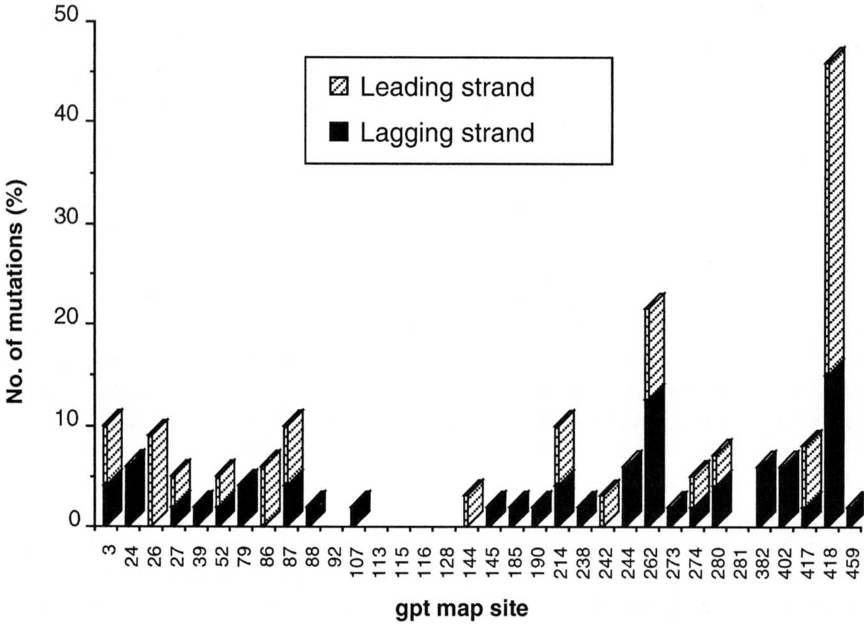

Fig. 5. Distribution of UV-induced base pair substitutions in the leading and lagging strands of the *gpt* gene carried by an EBV-derived shuttle vector (data from Calcagnile et al. 1996)

in TTD were, however, more similar to those in normal cells than those found in XP-D cells. A difference in the processing of UV-induced mutations might explain some of the differences between these two syndromes.

Sequence- and strand-specificity of mutation distribution can also be affected by the insertion preference of the replicative DNA polymerase/s. The question of whether the asymmetric nature of the replication complex might lead to differences in error rates for leading and lagging strand replication of UV-irradiated DNA was addressed using a cell-free SV40 origin-dependent replication mutagenesis assay (Thomas and Kunkel 1993) as well as by using an EBV-derived shuttle vector system (Calcagnile et al. 1996). In the latter case (Fig. 5) two human cell lines were constructed that contain the same episomic shuttle vector but with an opposite orientation of the marker gene relative to the EBV-oriP. Both studies showed that, although the overall error rate during replicative bypass was the same, the fidelity of leading and lagging strand trans-lesion synthesis varied by sequence context and position.

Mutation Spectra in the p53 Gene: UV Exposure and Non-melanoma Skin Cancers

Strong experimental and epidemiological evidence links UV irradiation to the development of human non-melanoma skin cancer (NMSC). Mutations in the p53 gene are common in these cancers (in contrast with malignant melanoma, in which p53 mutations are rarely observed in primary tumors). The

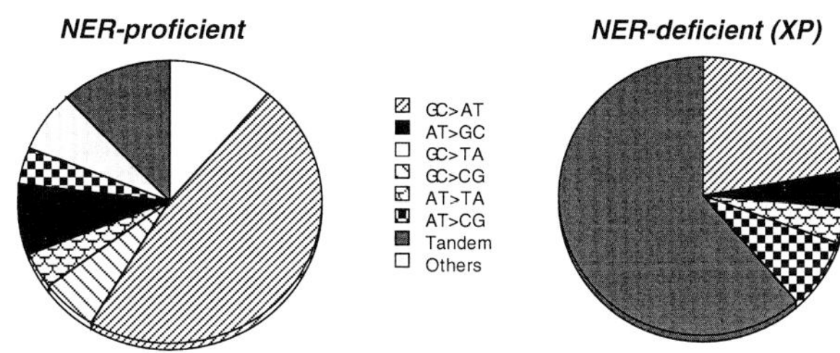

Fig. 6. Effect of DNA repair on p53 mutation spectrum in human skin cancer. The classes of mutation found in the p53 gene of skin tumors from normal subjects (data from IARC database) and XP patients (data from Dumaz et al. 1993) are indicated

mutation spectrum in NMSC is characterized by frequent C>T transitions and, more specifically, by a high frequency of tandem CC>TT transitions, which represent 9% of the mutations in squamous cell carcinomas and 12% in basal cell cancers (Greenblatt et al. 1994; Sage et al. 1996). Both types of mutations are consistent with the mutagenic action of UV in vitro. Although C>T transitions are common in all tumor types, tandem CC>TT transitions are exceptional in internal malignancies (only two cases are reported in primary internal malignancies, one in lung cancer and one in breast cancer). Further evidence for a direct link between these mutations and UV comes from the analysis of skin tumors from DNA repair-deficient XP patients, which show a particularly high frequency of tandem CC>TT transitions (Dumaz et al. 1993) (Fig. 6). It is interesting to recall that the same drastic increase in the relative percentage of CC>TT tandem mutations was reported in NER-deficient mammalian cells exposed to UVB or SSL (Sage et al. 1996) (see above). Mutations at dipyrimidines have also been observed in normal, sun-exposed skin of skin cancer patients from Australia, suggesting that they occur at a very early stage of skin carcinogenesis (Nakazawa et al. 1994). Studies in basal cell carcinoma show that tandem dipyrimidine transitions are preferentially detected in cancers developing from regions of the skin exposed to sunlight, whereas tumors arising from less exposed areas show mostly transversions (Gailani et al. 1996; Matsumura et al. 1996). These data also implicate agents different than UVB in the etiology of skin cancer. In experimental skin cancer induced in mice, distinct types of p53 mutations are observed in tumors induced by UVB and by PUVA (8-methylpsoralen+UVA) (Nataraj et al. 1996).

The distribution of mutations in skin cancers (Fig. 7) shows striking differences when compared with most other types of cancers (Fig. 2). Three factors may be involved in the generation of such a particular mutation distribution: (1) targeting of specific bases by UV light, (2) inefficient DNA repair at specific positions and (3) selection of forms of mutant p53 with functional specificity for skin carcinogenesis. There is no evidence for the latter interpretation; however, there is experimental evidence of slow repair of UV-induced lesions at several sites that are commonly mutated in skin cancers, including codons 177, 196 and 278 (Tornaletti and Pfeifer 1994). When the distribution of the UV-induced p53 mutations is analyzed an almost even distribution of the mutations over the two strands is detected. Using human di-

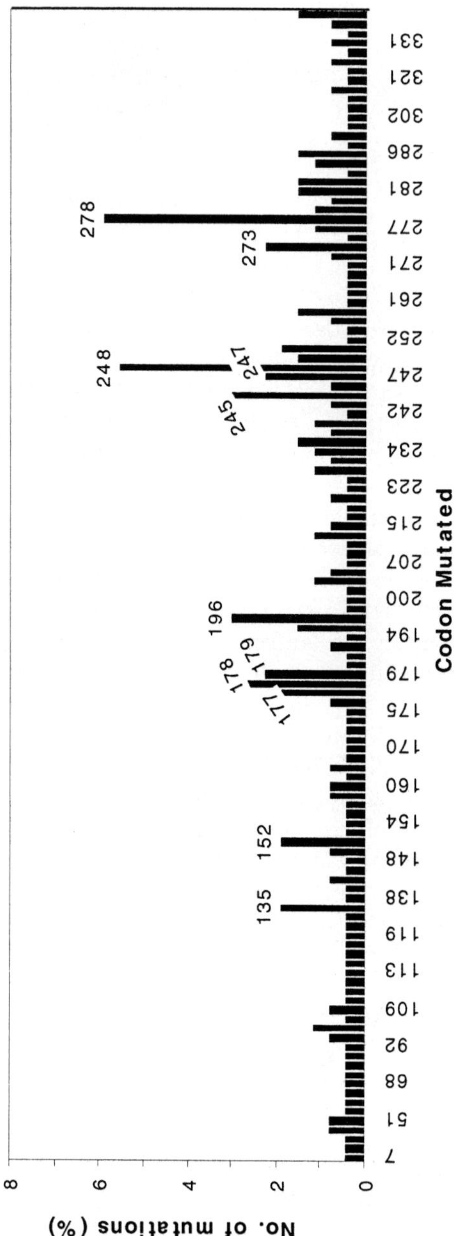

Fig. 7. Distribution of p53 gene mutations in human skin cancers. The data are derived from the July 1997 version of the IARC p53 database

ploid skin fibroblast as a model, Tornaletti and Pfeifer (1994) have shown that the average repair rate of UV-induced cyclobutane pyrimidine dimers in p53 exons 5–9 was slower than in the control, housekeeping gene PGK1 (encoding phosphoglycerate kinase) and that the transcribed strand of p53 was more rapidly repaired than the nontranscribed strand. However, as in the case of the reporter *gpt* and *hprt* genes of UV-treated human cells (see above), the difference in strand-specific repair might not be sufficient to leave its fingerprint on mutation distribution. When the analysis is confined only to tandem CC>TT transitions in NMSC they are all located on the coding (nontranscribed) strand, suggesting that transcription-coupled repair might act preferentially on these lesions. Also, half of the CC>TT transitions observed in NMSC are within CpG sequences, suggesting that spontaneous deamination of 5-methylcytosine may contribute to enhance the mutation rate at such sequences. Finally, it cannot be excluded that UV may more efficiently target specific bases than others. In a recent study, Denissenko et al. (1997) have shown that absorption of near-UV light by 5-methylcytosine is five- to ten-fold higher than by cytosine, suggesting that solar UV light could preferentially affect methylated cytosine.

Tobacco Smoke

Bacterial Systems

The mutagenicity and carcinogenicity of tobacco smoke have been studied extensively, revealing that a variety of mutagenic polycyclic aromatic hydrocarbons (PAHs), aromatic amines, nitrosamines, etc., are present and likely to play a role in the induction of smoking-associated cancer (International Agency for Research on Cancer 1986). The mutation spectra of these and many other single compounds found in tobacco smoke have been determined in a variety of systems. However, the mutation spectrum of tobacco smoke itself (cigarette smoke condensate, CSC) in the presence of metabolic activation (S9) has been determined only in *Salmonella* at both frameshift (His-D3052) and base-substitution (His-G46) alleles (DeMarini et al. 1995b). At the frameshift allele, CSC induced exclusively a hotspot, 2-base deletion of GC or CG within the hotspot sequence CGCGCGCG. At the base substitution allele, CSC induced primarily (80%) GC>TA transversions; the remaining ~20% of the mutations were GC>AT transitions. Approximately 80% of the single base substitutions were at the middle of the CCC target sequence of the base substitution allele. How do these results compare to those produced by some model single compounds that represent the primary chemical classes responsible for the mutagenic and carcinogenic activity of CSC? Decades of bioassay-directed chemical fractionation studies have shown that most of the carcinogenic activity of CSC in mouse skin resides in the neutral fraction (which contains, for example, PAHs), whereas most of the mutagenic activity of CSC at the frameshift allele in *Salmonella* resides in the basic and weakly acidic fractions (which contains for example, aromatic amines) (International Agency for Research on Cancer 1986). PAHs have been implicated as a primary chemical class responsible for smoking-associated lung cancer, and aromatic amines have been most strongly associated with smoking-associated bladder cancer (International Agency for Research on Cancer 1986). Comparisons of the mutation spectra produced by chemicals in these classes to that of CSC in a variety of *Salmonella* strains have confirmed the important contribution of these compounds to the mutagenic activity of CSC (DeMarini et al. 1995b). For example, the pKM101 plasmid (conferring the SOS response, see above) had the same effect on the mutagenic activity of CSC as on that of a heterocyclic amine food mutagen present in CSC (Glu-P-1), i.e., the plasmid had no effect on the ability of the two agents to revert the frameshift allele, but the plasmid was required by both agents to revert the base substitution allele. Likewise, both agents were more potent at the frameshift than at the base substitution allele, whereas the opposite was true for the aromatic amine 4-aminobiphenyl (4AB) (Levine et al. 1994) and the PAH benzo[a]pyrene (BP) (Koch et al. 1994; DeMarini et al. 1994). At the frameshift allele, only Glu-P-1 and the model aromatic amine 2-acetylaminofluorene (2AAF) (Shetton and DeMarini 1995) induced the same mutation spectrum as CSC, i.e., only the 2-base, hotspot deletion. Thus, the frameshift specificity of CSC was similar to that of the heterocyclic amine Glu-P-1. This is consistent with studies showing that the frameshift activity of CSC resides in the basic fraction, which contains aromatic amines. The results at the base substitution allele indicated that the base substitution specificity of CSC shares features of the mutation spectra induced by BP as well as by the aromatic amines 4AB, Glu-P-1, and 2AAF. For example, CSC and all of the single compounds induced primarily GC>TA transversions, and most of the mutations were in the middle of the CCC target sequence of the base substitution allele (His-G46). One difference, however, was the induction of GC>CG transversions by BP but not by CSC.

The mechanisms by which BP, 2AAF, Glu-P-1, and 4AB induce mutation in *Salmonella* and other systems have been described previously, and similar mechanisms could be postulated for related chemical mutagens in CSC (Koch et al. 1994; DeMarini et al. 1994, 1995b; Shelton and DeMarini 1995; Levine et al. 1994). For all of these compounds, metabolic activation (S9) is required for bacterial mutagenesis, and metabolites of these compounds are the ultimate mutagenic forms that are responsible for the observed mutation spectra.

Mutagenic and carcinogenic nitrosamines, such as 4-(methylnitrosamino)-1-(3-pyridyl)-1-butanone (NNK), are also present in cigarette smoke. NNK induces predominantly either GC>TA transversions or GC>AT transitions, depending on the experimental system being used (Wynder and Hoffmann 1994). However, there are no experimental studies that implicate NNK or the other N-nitrosamines in tobacco smoke as bladder carcinogens in laboratory animals (Hoffmann et al. 1994). The contribution of NNK to the observed mutation spectrum of CSC is unclear at this time.

Mammalian Cell Systems

Among the PAHs present in cigarette smoke and implicated as causative agents in the development of lung cancer, BP is by far the best studied in mammalian cells. The metabolite of BP, $(\pm)$-7β, 8α-dyhydroxy-9α, 10α-epoxy-7,8,9,10-tetrahydrobenzo(α)pyrene (BPDE), reacts with DNA and forms predominantly covalent (+) trans adducts at the N^2 position of guanine (Singer and Grunberger 1983). BPDE-induced mutation spectra have been analyzed in several endogeneous genes (Mazur and Glickman 1998; Carothers and Grunberger 1990; Yang et al. 1991) of mammalian cells as well as in bacterial genes carried by shuttle vectors (Yang et al. 1987). In every case the majority of mutations were base pair substitutions involving G:C base pairs mainly GC > TA transversions and the distribution of mutations was not random. Determination of the distribution of mutations induced in the *hprt* gene of G_1-synchronized repair-proficient human cells as compared to S-phase cells showed that the base substitutions located at guanine residues on the transcribed DNA strand decreased when the cells were allowed to repair before the onset of DNA replication (Chen et al. 1990). These results predicted that BPDE-induced adducts were preferentially repaired from the transcribed strand of the active *hprt* gene, and Chen et al. (1992) showed that indeed this was the case. The analysis of BPDE adducts and repair rate at nucleotide level (Wei et al. 1995; McGregor et al. 1997) along exon 3 of the *hprt* gene revealed that at least three factors play a role in the formation of mutation hotspots: sequence context dependent binding of the mutagen to DNA, site-specific rates of excision repair and the ability of adducts to block replication and transcription. The complex interplay of several factors in determining mutation specificity was also shown by lesion-specific mutagenesis studies. The DNA polymerase insertion preference opposite (+) and (–)-BPDE-N^2-dG adducts incorporated in a single-stranded shuttle vector was strongly influenced by host cell, sequence context and chirality when trans-lesion synthesis occurred either in *Escherichia coli* or simian kidney cells. Targeted BPDE adduct formation seems also to be the main determinant of lung cancer p53 mutation hotspots (Denissenko et al. 1996) (see below).

N-nitrosoamines are quantitatively the major carcinogens present in unburnt tobacco. They are expected to alkylate DNA in vivo. For example, chronic treatment of rats with NNK induces in the tumor target tissues O^6-methylguanine, O^4-methylthymidine and 7-methylguanine (Hecht et al. 1986). In agreement with the known premutagenic properties of O^6-methylguanine (Ellison et al. 1989), NNK-treatment of CYP2A6 transfected CHO cells showed a predominance of GC > AT transitions (Tiano et al. 1985). As stated above, the precise contribution of NNK-induced mutations to CSC mutation spectrum is open to question.

Table 1. Mutation spectra of p53 in human lung and bladder cancer

Mutation type %	Tumor type (number of cases)							
	Lung			Bladder				All
	Total ($n=834$)	Smoker ($n=186$)	Nonsmoker ($n=36$)	Total ($n=311$)	Smoker ($n=61$)	Nonsmoker ($n=43$)	ARY[a] ($n=27$)	($n=6609$)
AT > CG	3	3	6	3	2	–	–	4
AT > GC	8	8	–	10	10	9	15	11
AT > TA	4	3	3	4	2	5	4	5
GC > AT	17	22	28	33	34	42	63	19
GC > AT (CpG)	10	7	17	15	13	12	–	24
GC > CG	12	9	31	14	18	21	4	8
GC > TA	33	36	11	12	15	9	11	16
Other	13	13	6	10	6	2	4	13

[a] Workers exposed to aromatic amines.

Mutation Spectra in the p53 Gene:
Lung and Bladder Cancers as Examples of Tumors Related to Exposure to Tobacco Smoke

Smoking is a major risk factor in many cancers, including cancers of the oral cavity, squamous cell carcinoma of the esophagus, lung cancer and bladder cancer. In these pathologies, the prevalence of p53 mutations is generally higher in smokers than in nonsmokers, at least in regions of the world where epidemiological evidence points to tobacco as the major risk factor (Montesano et al. 1996; Kondo et al. 1996; Brennan et al. 1995). In addition, the spectrum of p53 mutations varies from one pathology to the other. In lung cancers (Table 1), the dominant mutation type is G > T transversions, a typical signature of BPDE. In squamous cell carcinoma of the esophagus, G > T transversions are comparatively rare (12%) and the predominant types of mutations are transitions or transversions at A:T base pairs (31%), and G:C transitions at non-CpG sequences (22%). A similar spectrum is observed in squamous cell carcinomas of the oral cavity. In both of these cancers, the combined consumption of tobacco and alcohol is considered to be a cumulative risk factor. This mutation spectrum is consistent with a role of nitrosamines (G:C transitions) and of some metabolites of ethanol, such as acetaldehyde (mutations at A:T bases) (Montesano et al. 1996). In bladder cancer (Table 1), the mutation spectrum is dominated by mutations at G:C base pairs (75%, including 28% of transitions at non-CpG). The major tobacco carcinogen(s) in these tumors are thought to be aromatic amines such as 4AB, an agent which is considered to cause G > T and G > C transversions (Vineis et al. 1996; Essigmann and Wood 1993). Interestingly, this high frequency of mutations at G:C base pairs is found in bladder cancer of workers occupationally exposed to aromatic amines as well as in bladder cancer of nonoccupationally exposed individuals (Table 1). Although the number of cases with occupational exposure is small, these patients may have a higher frequency of G:C transversions. These observations support the notion that the carcinogens involved are identical in both groups (Taylor et al. 1996; Sorlie et al. 1998). Bladder cancer also shows a unique, distinct mutation distribution, with specific hotspots at several codons in exon 8, including 280 and 285. It is not known whether these hotspots represent preferential targeting by a specific carcinogen rather than functional selection of particular mutants.

Analysis of the G>T transversions found in lung cancers from smokers reveals interesting clues about how specific base targeting and bioselection cooperate to generate tumor-specific mutation spectra. First, these mutations show a very strong strand bias, 94% of them being located on the nontranscribed strand. Second, the most frequently mutated codons in lung cancer are 157, 158, 248 and 273. Codon 157 and 158 are rarely mutated in all other types of cancer and these codons may be considered as a hotspot specific to lung cancer. In contrast, mutations at codons 248 and 273 are common in most types of cancer (Fig. 2). Experimental evidence shows that codons 157, 248 and 273 are among the preferential sites for BPDE-DNA adduct formation in bronchial cells exposed to BPDE (Denissenko et al. 1996). Interestingly, mutations at codons 248 and 273 in lung cancers are different from those in other cancers. In breast or colon cancers, codon 248 and 273 are almost exclusively mutated by C>T transitions at a CpG dinucleotide, a type of mutation that may be interpreted as the result of an endogenous mutation event. In contrast, in lung cancers, about half of the mutations at these two codons are G>T transversions, in agreement with the notion that BPDE may target these codons. Recent evidence also indicates that BPDE adducts form preferentially at G bases adjacent to 5-methylcytosine (Denissenko et al. 1997). This observation provides a good example of how bioselection, methylation, specific targeting by environmental mutagens and inefficient repair all concur to the definition of a specific mutation profile.

Aflatoxin B$_1$

Bacterial Systems

In the base substitution strain TA100 of *Salmonella*, aflatoxin B$_1$ (AFB$_1$) induced predominantly (84%–86%) GC>TA transversions, with a substantial preference (8:1) for the middle C relative to the first C of the CCC target of the His-G46 allele (Koch et al. 1994). As in *Salmonella*, AFB$_1$ induced predominantly (89%) GC>TA transversions in the *E. coli lacI* gene (Foster et al. 1983). In contrast, AFB$_1$ induced GC>TA transversions and GC>AT transitions at nearly equal frequencies in the M13-borne *lacZ* target (Sambamurti et al. 1988). AFB$_1$ is metabolized to a highly reactive electrophile, AFB$_1$-8,9-oxide, that reacts almost exclusively at the N^7 position of guanine (Croy et al.

1978; Lin et al. 1977). The preferential insertion of adenines opposite AFB_1-N^7-guanine-directed apurinic sites has been postulated to account for the mutation spectrum of AFB_1 (Foster et al. 1983). Recent evidence (Bailey et al. 1996) questions this mechanism and point to the adduct as the premutagenic lesion in AFB_1-treated cells.

AFB_1 induced most (76%–78%) of its GC>TA transversions in *Salmonella* TA100 at the middle position of the CCC/GGG target (Koch et al. 1994). This site specificity, observed for AFB_1 at the His-G46 allele, likely reflects preferential adduct formation at the middle guanine of the CCC/GGG target. For example, AFB_1-induced mutations have been recovered primarily at runs of Gs in forward mutation targets, including 5′-GpG doublets where the 3′ second guanine is most often altered. Formation of AFB_1-N7-guanine is nonrandom, and in most cases the second guanine in contiguous doublets and triplets of Gs is favored for modification (Meunch et al. 1983; Benasutti et al. 1988).

Mammalian Cell Systems

AFB_1 is carcinogenic in many animal species and mutagenic in cells in culture. The mutagenic spectrum was analyzed in repair-proficient and -deficient human cells by using a shuttle vector plasmid containing the *supF* marker gene (Levy et al. 1992). Base pair substitutions, one-half of which were GC>TA transversions, predominated the spectrum. As compared to normal cells, DNA repair-deficient fibroblasts showed a higher frequency of mutations, a unique induction of tandem mutations at GG sites and different mutation hotspots. Mutation rate, type and distribution are therefore affected by the efficiency of repair. The mutation spectrum of AFB_1 in exon 3 of the *hprt* gene in B-lymphoblasts (Cariello et al. 1994) showed one strong mutation hotspot that contained 10%–17% of all mutations induced. This frequent mutation event was a GC>TA transversion located within a run of six Gs. This internal G is also a hotspot for other mutagens suggesting that, in this sequence context, this residue becomes highly prone to chemical modification and/or hardly accessible to repair enzymes.

A striking mutation hotspot has also been described for the p53 gene at codon 249 in hepatocellular carcinomas (HCC) from regions with food contamination with AFB_1 (see below). To gain insight into this mechanism AFB_1-induced mutagenesis of p53 codons 247–250 was analyzed in human HCC cells HepG2 cells (Aguilar et al. 1993) and in CYP450-expressing human liver cell lines (Mace et al. 1997). A high frequency of G>T transversions at codon 249 (AGG>AGT) was indeed observed. However, other dominant mutations at neighboring bases were also detected indicating that, besides the induction of AFB_1-specific mutations, the mutant serine 249 p53 protein should play per se an important role in the development of HCC (see below).

Mutation Spectra in the p53 Gene: Exposure to Aflatoxin B₁ and Hepatocellular Carcinoma

The most spectacular example of an obvious relationship between a specific environmental mutagen and a specific mutation profile is that of AFB_1 in HCC. This profile is observed in regions of the world where this type of cancer is associated with high exposure to AFB_1 and chronic infection by hepatitis B virus (HBV), such as China or central Africa (reviewed in Montesano et al. 1998). This profile is dominated by a high frequency of $G>T$ transversion at codon 249 (AGG>AGT, Arg>Ser). This mutation is also occasionally observed in other types of cancers (it represents 2.1% of all p53 mutations, 65% or which are in HCC). Critical review of the data from geographic areas with high, moderate of low exposure to AFB_1 reveals a clear correlation between the level of food contamination by AFB_1 and the prevalence of this particular mutation (Montesano et al. 1998). Experimentally, AFB_1 has been shown to bind to codon 249 as well as to other codons in p53 cDNA. Why mutations at codon 249 are almost exclusively selected in HCC within the context of exposure to both AFB_1 and HBV is not understood at present. Experimentally, the Arg>Ser mutant at codon 249 has strong dominant-negative properties in cultured hepatic cells, suggesting that this mutant may be particularly deleterious in liver cells (Ponchel et al. 1994; Forrester et al. 1995).

Vinyl Chloride

Bacterial Systems

As reviewed and demonstrated by Basu et al. (1993), vinyl chloride (VC) and other agents that form etheno adducts produce primarily $GC>AT$ transitions. This has been confirmed recently with chloromalonaldehyde at the base substitution allele His-G46 in *Salmonella* (Knasmuller et al. 1996). An etheno adduct on cytosine appears to be the primary lesion; however, etheno adducts on adenine are also formed and are weakly mutagenic.

Mammalian Cell Systems

The mutagenic potential of the ultimate carcinogenic form of VC, 2-chloroacetaldehyde (CAA), was analyzed in human cells using a shuttle vector containing the *supF* gene (Matsuda et al. 1995). More than half of the single base pair substitutions were GC>AT transitions. The majority of the mutations involved G:C bp in 5′AAGG3′ or 5′CCTT3′ sequences. The mutagenic specificity of two exocyclic DNA adducts produced by chloroethylene oxide and CAA, which are both reactive metabolites of VC, was investigated by performing single-lesion mutagenesis with a single-stranded shuttle vector transfected into COS cells (Moriya et al. 1994; Pandya and Moriya 1996). 1, N^6-ethenodeoxyadenosine was highly mutagenic and induced primarily $A>G$ transitions (Pandya and Moriya 1996). 3, N^4-ethenodeoxycytidine displayed comparable mutagenic potency and produced both $C>T$ transitions and $C>A$ transversions (Moriya et al. 1994) .

Mutation Spectra of the p53 Gene:
Exposure to Vinyl Chloride and Angiosarcoma of the Liver

There is preliminary evidence of a specific mutation spectrum in patients with angiosarcoma of the liver (ASL) associated with occupational exposure to VC. Mutations of p53 are apparently rare in ASL. In 21 ASL patients with ASL not associated to exposure to VC, Soini et al. (1995) have reported only two mutations. In six patients with occupational exposure to VC, Hollstein et al. (1994) have found three mutations, and all of them are AT > TA transversions, a type of mutation which is very rare in all other types of cancer (they represent 2.8 % of all mutations, with a maximum of 8.9% in squamous cell carcinoma of the esophagus). In contrast, the two mutations found in patients with other exposures (including thorotrast) were both G > A transitions (Soini et al. 1995). A majority of AT > TA mutations were also detected in ASL of rats experimentally exposed to VC (Barbin et al. 1997). In addition, serum anti-p53 antibodies have been found in ASL patients and in some workers with occupational exposure to VC (Trivers et al. 1995). It remains to be determined whether detection of these antibodies may be useful in identifying individuals at high risk of ASL.

Conclusions

Molecular epidemiology stems from the crossing-over of laboratory studies and classical cancer epidemiology, with the aim of exploiting molecular end-

Table 2. Mutation spectra of p53 in human cancers

Carcinogen exposure	Tumor type (number of cases)			
Mutation type (%)	Skin (279) Sunlight	HCC (393) AFB$_1$	Lung (834) BPDE	All (6609)
AT > CG	4	3	3	4
AT > GC	8	12	8	11
AT > TA	5	15	4	5
GC > AT	31	11	17	19
GC > AT (CpG)	13	9	10	24
GC > CG	6	6	12	8
GC > TA	11	36	33	16
Other	11	7	13	13
CC > TT	10	–	0.1	1

points to improve cancer risk assessment. In this review, we have discussed the best characterized examples of human cancers in which the p53 mutation profile reflects the impact of environmental mutagens and DNA repair processes. The nature and the position of p53 mutations in the tumor are indeed expected on the basis of the mechanisms of mutagenesis of the environmental carcinogen as known from in vitro systems (Table 2). However, in most tumors, the mutation profiles are complex and there is little direct evidence that a suspected mutagen is indeed causing the mutations observed. This may of course reflect the fact that cancer is a complex process involving interactions between multiple factors of endogenous and exogenous origin. As a result of this complexity, the contribution of a single risk factor to the generation of a tumor-specific mutation spectrum may be difficult, if not impossible, to assess in many situations. However, additional factors other than the inherent complexity of the cancer process may contribute to blurr the picture provided by tumor-specific mutation spectra. In particular, it is important to remember that a significant potential limitation of mutational spectra is that various chemicals from different chemical classes can often produce similar mutation spectra (DeMarini 1998). For example, PAHs, aromatic amines, and nitroarenes all produce primarily GC > TA transversions in most organisms and targets in which they have been tested. Consequently, it is almost impossible to look at a mutation spectrum that contains predominantly GC > TA transversions and infer which class of chemical, let alone which individual compound, produced the observed mutation. Because of this overlap in mutational specificity, caution must be exercised to avoid over-interpretation of mutation spectra in oncogenes or tumor suppressor genes.

Another important concern that we have attempted to illustrate in this review is that the correct interpretation of tumor-specific mutation spectra requires a good and detailed understanding of the molecular mechanisms that are responsible for the formation, escape from repair mechanisms and biological selection of these mutations. In the future, we believe that it will be necessary to develop research on mutation spectra in two parallel directions: (1) experimental analysis of the mechanisms of mutagenicity using reporter systems as close as possible to the human context, and (2) well-defined molecular epidemiological studies to reveal subtle differences in mutation patterns using exposure cohorts matched for various parameters that could influence the mutation spectrum (such as age, sex, ethnic origin, etc.).

References

Aas T, Borresen AL, Geisler S et al (1996) Specific p53 mutations are associated with de novo resistance to doxorubicin in breast cancer patients. Nat Med 2:811–814

Aguilar F, Hussain SP, Cerutti P (1993) Aflatoxin B1 induces the transversion of G > T in codon 249 of the p53 tumor suppressor gene in human hepatocytes. Proc Natl Acad Sci USA 90:8586–8590

Bailey EA, Iyer RS, Stone MP, Harris TM, Essigmann JM (1996) Mutational properties of the primary aflatoxin B1-DNA adduct. Proc Natl Acad Sci USA 93:1535–1539

Barbin A, Froment O, Boivin S et al (1997) p53 gene mutation pattern in rat liver tumors induced by vinyl chloride. Cancer Res 57:1695–1698

Basic-Zaninovic T, Meschini R, Calcagnile AS et al (1995) Strand bias of UV-induced mutations in a transcriptionally active gene in human cells. Mol Carcinog 14:214–225

Basu AK, Wood ML, Niedernhofer LJ, Ramos LA, Essigmann JM (1993) Mutagenic and genotoxic effects of three vinyl-induced DNA lesions: 1,N6-ethenoadenine, 3,N4-ethenocytosine, and 4-amino-5-(imidazol-2-yl)imidazole. Biochemsitry 32:12793–12801

Benasutti M, Ejadi S, Whitlow MD, Loechler EL (1988) Mapping the binding site of aflatoxin B1 in DNA: systematic analysis of the reactivity of aflatoxin B1 with guanines in different DNA sequences. Biochemistry 27:472–481

Bourre F, Benoit A, Sarasin A (1989) Respective roles of pyrimidine dimer and pyrimidine (6-4) pyrimidione photoproducts in UV mutagenesis of simian virus 40 DNA in mammalian cells. J Virol 63:4520–4524

Brash DE, Seetharam S, Kraemer KH, Seidman MM, Bredberg A (1987) Photoproduct frequency is not the major determinant of UV base substitution hot spots or cold spots in human cells. Proc Natl Acad Sci USA 84:3782–3786

Brennan JA, Boyle JO, Koch WM et al (1995) Association between cigarette smoking and mutation of the p53 gene in squamous-cell carcinoma of the head and neck. N Engl J Med 332:712–717

Calcagnile A, Basic-Zaninovic T, Palombo F, Dogliotti E (1996) Misincorporation rate and type on the leading and lagging strands of UV-damaged DNA. Nucleic Acids Res 24:3005–3009

Cariello NF, Cui L, Skopek TR (1994) In vitro mutatinal spectrum of aflatoxin B1 in the human hypoxanthine guanine phosphoribosyltransferase gene. Cancer Res 54:4436–4441

Carothers AM, Grunberger D (1990) DNA base changes in benzo(a)pyrene diol epoxide-induced dihydrofolate reductase mutants of Chinese hamster overy cells. Carcinogenesis 11:189–192

Cebula TA, Henrikson EN, Hartman PE, Biggley WH (1995) Reversion profiles of coolwhite fluorescent light compared with far ultraviolet light: homologies and differences. Photochem Photobiol 61:353–359

Chen R-H, Maher VM, McCormick JJ (1990) Effect of excision repair by diploid human fibroplasts on the kinds and locations of mutations induced by (±)-7b,8a-dyhdroxy-9a,10a-epoxy-7,8,9,10-tetrahydrobenzo(a)pyrene in the coding region of the HPRT gene. Proc Natl Acad Sci USA 87:8680–8684

Chen RH, Maher VM, Brouwer J, De Putte PV, McCormick JJ (1992) Preferential repair and strand-specific reapir of benzo(a)pyrene diol epoxide adducts in the HPRT gene of diploid human fibroblasts. Proc Natl Acad Sci USA 89:5413–5417

Cho Y, Gorina S, Jeffrey PD, Pavletich NP (1994) Crystal structure of a p53 tumor suppressor-DNA complex: understanding tumorigenic mutations. Science 265:346–355

Croy RG, Essigman JM, Rheinhold VN, Wogan GN (1978) Identification of the principle aflatoxin B1-DNA adduct formed in vivo in rat liver. Proc Natl Acad Sci USA 75:1745–1749

De Flora S, Camoirano A, Izzotti A, Bennicelli C (1990) Potent genotoxicity of halogen lamps, compared to fluorescent light and sunlight. Carcinogenesis 11:2171–2177

DeMarini DM (1998) Mutation spectra of complex mixtures. Mutat Res (in press)

DeMarini DM, Shelton ML, Bell DA (1994) Mutation spectra in Salmonella of complex mixtures: comparison of urban air to benzo[a]pyrene. Environ Mol Mutagen 24:262–275

DeMarini DM, Shelton ML, Stankowski LF jr (1995a) Mutation spectra in Salmonella of sunlight, white fluorescent light, and light from tanning salon beds: induction of tandem mutations and role of DNA repair. Mutat Res 327:131–149

DeMarini DM, Shelton ML, Levine JG (1995b) Mutation spectrum of cigarette smoke condensate in Salmonella: comparison to mutations in smoking-associated tumors. Carcinogenesis 16:2535–2542

Denissenko MF, Pao A, Tang M, Pfeifer GP (1996) Preferential formation of benzo(a)pyrene adducts at lung cancer mutational hotspots in p53. Science 274:430–432

Denissenko MF, Chen JX, Tang MS, Pfeifer GP (1997) Cytosine methylation determines hot spots of DNA damage in the human p53 gene. Proc Natl Acad Sci USA 94:3893–3898

Dorado G, Steingrimsdottir H, Arlett CF, Lehmann AF (1991) Molecular analysis of ultraviolet-induced mutations in a Xeroderma pigmentosum cell line. J Mol Biol 217:217–222

Drobetsky EA, Moustacchi E, Glickman BW, Sage E (1994) The mutational specificity of simulated sunlight at the aprt locus in rodent cells. Carcinogenesis 15:1577–1583

Drobetsky EA, Turcotte J, Chateauneuf A (1995) A role for ultraviolet-A in solar mutagenesis. Proc Natl Acad Sci USA 92:2350–2354

Dumaz N, Drougard A, Sarasin A, Daya-Grosjean L (1993) Specific UV-induced mutation spectrum in the p53 gene of skin tumors from DNA-repair-deficient xeroderma pigmentosum patients. Proc Natl Acad Sci USA 90:10529–10533

Ellison KS, Dogliotti E, Connors TD, Basu AK, Essigmann JM (1989) Site-specific mutagenesis by O^6-alkylguanines located in the chromosomes of mammalian cells. influence of the mammalian O^6-alkylguanine-DNA alkyltransferase. Proc Natl Acad Sci USA 86:8620–8624

Essigmann JM, Wood M (1993) The relationship between chemical structures and mutagenic specificites of the DNA lesions formed by chemical and physical mutagens. Toxciol Lett 67:29–39

Forrester K, Lupold SE, Ott VL et al (1995) Effects of p53 mutants on wild-type p53-mediated transactivation are cell type dependent. Oncogene 10:2103-2111

Foster PL, Eisenstadt E, Míller JH (1983) Base substitution mutations induced by metabolically activated Aflatoxin B1. Proc Natl Acad Sci USA 80:2695–2698

Gailani MR, Leffell DJ, Ziegler A, Gross EG, Brash DE, Bale AE (1996) Relationship between sunlight exposure and a key genetic alteration in basal cell carcinoma. J Natl Cancer Inst 88:349–354

Goh HS, Yao J, Smith DR (1995) p53 point mutation and survival in colorectal cancer patients. Cancer Res 55:5217–5521

Greenblatt MS, Bennett WP, Hollstein M, Harris CC (1994) Mutations in the p53 tumor suppressor gene: clues to cancer etiology and molecular pathogenesis. Cancer Res 54:4855–4878

Hainaut P, Hernandez T, Rodriguez-Tome P et al (1998) IARC database of p53 gene somatic mutation in human tumors and cell lines: revised formats, updated compilation and new tools for mutation visualisation future prospects. Nucleic Acids Res (in press)

Hanawalt PC (1991) Heterogeneity of DNA repair at the gene level. Mutat Res 247:203–211

Hanawalt PC (1994) Transcription-coupled repair and human disease. Science 266:1957–1958

Harris CC (1996a) p53 tumor suppressor gene: from the basic research laboratory to the clinic – an abridged historical perspective. Carcinogenesis 17:1187–1198

Harris CC (1996b) The 1995 Walter Hubert Lecture-Molecular epidemiology of human cancer: insights from the mutational analysis of the p53 tumor-suppressor gene. Br J Cancer 73:261–269

Hartman Z, Hartman PE, McDermott WL (1991) Mutagenicity of coolwhite fluorescent light for Salmonella. Mutat Res 260:25–38

Hecht SS, Trushin N, Castonguay A, Rivenson A (1986) Comparative tumorigenicity and DNA methylation in F344 rats by 4-(methylnitrosoamino)-1-(3-pyridyl)-1-butanone and N-nitrosodimethylamine. Cancer Res 46:498–502

Hoffmann D, Brunnemann KD, Prokopczyk B, Djordjevic MV (1994) Tobacco-specific N-nitrosamine and area-derived N-nitrosamines: chemistry, biochemistry, carcinogenicity, and relevance to humans. J Toxicol Environ Health 41:1–52

Hollstein M, Marion MJ, Lehman T et al (1994) p53 mutations at A:T base pairs in angiosarcomas of vinyl chloride-exposed factory workers. Carcinogenesis 15:1–3

Hsia HC, Lebkowski JS, Leong P-M, Calos MP, Miller JH (1989) Comparison of ultraviolet irradiation-induced mutagenesis of the lacI gene in Escherichia coli and in human 293 cells. J Mol Biol 205:103–113

International Agency for Research on Cancer (1986) Tobacco smoking. IARC Monogr Eval Carcinog Risks Chem Hum 38

International Agency for Research on Cancer (1992) Solar and ultraviolet radiation. IARC Monogr Eval Carcinog Risks Hum 55

Knasmuller S, Zohrer E, Kronberg L, Kundi M, Franzen F, Schulte-Hermann R (1996) Mutational spectra of Salmonella typhimurium revertrans induced by chlorohydroxyfuranones, byproducts of chlorine disinfection of drinking water. Chem Res Toxciol 9:374–381

Koch WH, Henrikson EN, Kupchella E, Cebula TA (1994) Salmonella typhimurium strain TA100 differentiates several classes of carcinogens and mutagens by base substitution specificity. Carcinogenesis 15:79–88

Kondo K, Tsuzuki H, Sasa M, Sumitomo M, Uyama T, Monden Y (1996) A dose-response relationship between the frequency of p53 mutations and tobacco consumption in lung cancer patients. J Surg Oncol 61:20–26

Levine AJ (1997) p53, the cellular gatekeeper for growth and division. Cell 88:323–331

Levine JG, Schaaper RM, DeMarini DM (1994) Complex frameshift mutations mediated by plasmid pKM101: mutational mechanisms deduced from 4-aminobiophenyl-induced mutation spectra in Salmonella. Genetics 136:731–746

Levy DD, Groopman JD, Lim SE, Seidman MM, Kraemer KH (1992) Sequence specificity of Alfatoxin B1-induced mutations in a plasmid replicated in Xeroderma Pgimentosum and DNA repair proficient human cells. Cancer Res 52:5668–5673

Lin JK, Miller JA, Miller EC (1977) 2,3-dihydro-2-(guan-7-yl)-3-hydroxy-aflatoxin B1, a major hydrolysis product of aflatoxin B1-DNA or irbosomal RNA adducts formed in hepatic microsome mediated reactions in rat liver in vivo. Cancer Res 37:4430–4438

Mace K, Aguilar F, Wang J-S et al (1997) Aflatoxin B1-induced DNA adduct formation and p53 mutations in CYPP450-expressing human liver cell lines. Carcinogenesis 18:1291–1297

Madronich S (1993) The atmosphere and UV-B radiation at ground level. In: Young AR, Moan J, Nultsch W (eds) Environmental UV photobiology. Plenum, New York, pp 1–39

Marionnet C, Benoit A, Benhamou S, Sarasin A, Stary A (199%) Characteristics of UV-induced mutation spectra in human XP-D/ERCC2 gene-mutated Xerdoderma Pigmentosum and Trichothiodystrophy cells. J Mol Biol 252:550–562

Mtasuda T, Yagi T, Kawanishi M, Matsui S, Takebe H (1995) Molecular analysis of mutations induced by 2-chloroacetaldeyde, the ultimate carcinogenic form of vinyl chloride, in human cells using shuttle vectors. Carcinogenesis 16:2389–2394

Matsumura Y, Nishigori C, Yagi T, Imamura S, Takebe H (1996) Characterization of p53 gene mutations in basal-cell caricnomas: Comparison between sun-exposed and less-exposed skin areas. Int J Cancer 65:778–780

Mazur M, Glickman BW (1988) Sequence specificity of mutations induced by benzo(a)pyrene-7,8-diol-9,10-epoxide at endogeneous *aprt* gene in CHO cells. Somat Cell Mol Genet 14:383–400

McGregor WG, Chen R-H, Lukash L, Maher VM, McCormick JJ (1991) Cell cycle-dependent strand bias for UV-induced mutations in the transcribed strand of excision repair-proficient human fibroblasts but not in repair-deficient cells. Mol Cell Biol 11:1927–1934

McGregor WG, Wei D, Chen R-H, Maher VM, McCormick JJ (1997) Relationship between adduct formation, rates of excision repair and the cytotoxic and mutagenic effects of structurally-related polycyclic aromatic carcinogens. Mutat Res 376:143–152

Mei HY, Barton JK (1988) Tris(tetramethyl-phenanthroline)(ruthenium(II): a chiral probe that cleaves A-DNA conformation. Proc Natl Acad Sci USA 85:1339–1343

Mellon I, Bohr VA, Smith CA, Hanawalt PC (1986) Preferential DNA repair of an active gene in human cells. Proc Natl Acad Sci USA 83:8878–8882

Mellon I, Spivak G, Hanawalt PC (1987) Selective removal of transcription-blocking DNA damage from the transcribed strand of the mammalian DHFR gene. Cell 51:241–249

Menichini P, Vrieling H, van Zeeland AA (1991) Strand specific mutation spectra in repair proficient and repair deficient hamster cells. Mutat Res 251:143–155

Meunch KF, Misra RP, Humayun MZ (1983) Sequence specificity in aflatoxin B1-DNA interactions. Proc Natl Acad Sci USA 80:6–10

Miller JH (1983) Mutational specificty in bacteria. Annu Rev Genet 17:215–238

Montesano R, Hollstein M, Hainaut P (1996) Genetic alterations in esophageal cancer and their relevance to etiology and pathogenesis: a review. Int J Cancer 69:225–235

Montesano R, Hainaut P, Wild C (1998) Hepatocellular carcinoma: from the gene to public health. J Natl cancer Inst (in press)

Moriya M, Zhang W, Johnson F, Grollman AP (1994) Mutagenic potency of exocyclic DNA adducts: marked differences betweeen Escherichia coli and simian kidney cells. Proc Natl Acad Sci USA 91:11899–11903

Nakazawa H, English D, Randell PL et al (1994) UV and skin cancer: specific p53 gene mutations in normal skin as a biologically relevant exposure measurement. Proc Natl Acad Sci USA 91:360–364

Nataraj AJ, Black HS, Ananthaswamy HN (!996) signature p53 mutation at DNA crosslinking sites in methoxypsoralen and ultraviolet A (PUVA)-induced murine skin cancers. Proc Natl Acad Sci USA 93:7961–7965

Oller AR, Fijalkowska IJ, Dunn RL, Schaaper RM (1992) Transcription-repair coupling determines the strandness of ultraviolet mutagenesis in Escherichia coli. Proc Natl Acad Sci USA 89:11036–11040

Ory K, Legros Y, Auguin C, Soussi T (1994) Analysis of the most representative tumour derived p53 mutants reevals that changes in protein conformation are not correlated with loss of transactivation or inhibition of cell proliferation. EMBO J 13:3496–3504

Palombo F, Bignami M, Dogliotti E (1992a) Non-phenotypic selection of N-methyl-N-nitrosourea-induced mutations in human cells. Nucleic Acids Res 20:1349–1354

Palombo F, Kohfeldt E, Calcagnile A, Nehls P, Dogliotti E (1992b) N-methyl-N-nitrosourea-induced mutations in human cells. Effects of the transcriptional activity of the target gene. J Mol Biol 223:587–594

Pandya GA, Moriya M (1996) 1,N6-ethenodeoxyadenosine, a DNA adduct highly mutagenic in mammalian cells. Biochemistry 35:11487–11492

Ponchel F, Puisieux A, Tabone E et al (1994) Hepatocarcinoma-specific mutant p53-249ser induces mitotic activity but has no effect of transforming growth factor β 1-mediated apoptosis. Cancer Res 54:2064–2068

Richardson KK, Richardson FC, Crosby RM, Swenberg JA, Skopek TR (1987) DNA base changes and alkylation following in vivo exposure of Escherichia coli to N-methyl-N-nitrosourea or N-ethyl-N-nitrosourea. Proc Natl Acad Sci UA 84:344–348

Richardson KK, Crosby RM, Skopek TR (1988) Mutation spectra of N-ethyl-N'-nitro-N-nitrosoguanidine and 1-(2-hydroxyethyl)-1-nitrosourea in Escherichia coli. Mol Gen Genet 214:460–466

Sage E, Cramb E, Glickman BW (1992) The distribution of UV damage in the lacI gene of Escherichia coli: correlation with mutation spectrum. Mutat Res 269:285–299

Sage E, Lamolet B, Brulay E, Moustacchi E, Chateauneuf A, Drobetsky EA (1996) Mutagenic specificity of solar UV light in nucleotide excision repair-deficient rodent cells. Proc Natl Acad Sci USA 93:176–180

Sambamurti K, Callahan J, Luo X, Perkins CP, Jacobsen JS, Humayun MZ (1988) Mechanisms of mutagenesis by a bulky DNA lesion at the guanine N7 position. Genetics 120:863–873

Seidman MM, Bredberg A, Seetharam S, Kraemer KH (1987) Multiple point mutations in a shuttle vector propagated in huamn cells: evidence for an error-prone DNA polymerase activity. Proc Natl Acad Sci USA 84:4944–4948

Shelton ML, DeMarini DM (1995) Mutagenicity and mutation spectra of 2-acetylaminofluorene at frameshift and base-subsitution alleles in four DNA reapir backgrounds of Salmonella. Mutat Res 327:75–86

Singer B, Grunberger B (1983) The molecular biology of mutagens and carcinogens. Plenum, New York

Soini Y, Walsh JA, Ishak KG, Bennett WP (1995) p53 mutations in primary hepatic angiosarcomas not associated with vinyl chloride exposure. Carcinogenesis 16:2879–2881

Sorlie T, Martel-Planche G, Hainaut P et al (1998) Analysis of p53, p16MTS-1, p21waf-1 and H-RAS in archived bladder tumors from workers exposed to aromatic amines. B J Cancer (in press)

Taylor JA, Li Y, He M et al (1996) p53 mutations in bladder tumors from arylamineexposed workers. Cancer Res 56:294–298

Terleth C, van de Putte P, Brouwer J (1991) New insights in DNA rapair: preferential repair of transcriptionally active DNA. Mutagenesis 6:103–111

Tessman I, Liu S-K, Kennedy MA (1992) Mechanisms of SOS mutagenesis of UV-irradiated DNA: mostly eror-free processing of deaminated cytosine. Proc Natl Acad Sci USA 89:1159–1163

Thomas DC, Kunkel TA (1993) Replication of UV-irradiated DNA in human cell extracts: evidence for mutagenic bypass of pyrimidine dimers. Proc Natl Acad Sci USA 90:7744–7748

Tiano HF, Wang R-L, Hosokawa M, Crespi C, Tindall KR, Langenbach R (1995) Human CYP2A6 activation of 4-(methylnitrosoamino)-1-(3-pyridyl)-1-butanone (NNK): mutational specificity in the gpt gene of AS52 cells. Carcinogenesis 15:2859–2866

Tornaletti S, Pfeifer GP (1994) Slow repair of pyrimidine dimers at p53 mutation hotspots in skin cancer. Science 263:1436–1438

Trivers GE, Cawley HL, Debnedetti VM et al (1995) Anti-p53 antibodies in sera of workers occupationally exposed to vinyl chloride. J Natl Cancer Inst 87:1400–1407

Unna P (1894) Histopathologie der Hautkrankheiten. Hirschwald, Berlin

Vineis P, Talaska G, Malaveille C et al (1996) DNA addcuts in urothelial cells: relationship with biomarkers of exposures to arylamines and polycyclic aromatic hydrocarbons from tobacco smoke. Int J Cancer 65:314–316

Vrieling H, van Rooijen ML, Groen NA et al (1989) DNA strand specificity for UV-induced mutations in mammalian cells. Mol Cell Biol 9:1277–1283

Vrieling H, Venema, van Rooyen M-L et al (1991) Strand specificity for UV-induced DNA repair and mutations in the Chinese Hamster HPRT gene. Nucleic Acids Res 19:2411–2415

Vrieling H, Zhang LH, van Zeeland AA, Zdzienicka M (1992) UV-induced *hprt* mutations ina UV-sensitive hamster celle line from complementation group 3 are biased towards the transcribed strand. Mutat Res 274:147–155

Wang Y-C, Maher VM, McCormik JJ (1991) Xeroderma Pigmentosum variant cells are less likely than normal cells to incorporate dAMP opposite photoproducts during replication of UV-irradiated plasmids. Proc Natl Acad Sci USA 88:7810–7814

Wei D, Maher VM, McCormick JJ (1995) Site-specific rates of excision repair of benzo(a)pyrene diol epoxide adducts in the hypoxhantine phosphoribosyltransferase gene of human fibroblasts: correlation with mutation spectra. Proc Natl Acad Sci USA 92:2204–2208

Wynder EL, Hoffmann D (1994) Smoking and lung cancer: scientific challenges and opportunities. Cancer Res 54:5284–5295

Yang JL, Mahear VM, McCormick JJ (1987) Kinds of mutations formed when a shuttle vector containing adducts of (+/–)-7b,8a-dihydroxy-9a-epoxy-7,8,9,10-tetrahydrobenzo(a)pyrene. Proc Natl Acad Sci USA 84:3787–3791

Yang JL, Chen R-H, Maher VM, McCormick JJ (1991) Kinds and location of mutations induced by (+/–)-7b,8a-dihydroxy-9a,10a-epoxy-7,8,9,10-tetrahydrobenzo(*a*)pyrene in the coding region of the hypoxanthine(guanine)phosphoribosyltransferase gene in diploid human fibroblasts. Carcinogenesis 12:71–75

III. DNA Repair and Genetic Susceptibility

Relevance of DNA Repair to Carcinogenesis and Cancer Therapy

M. F. Rajewsky, J. Engelbergs, J. Thomale, and T. Schweer

Institute of Cell Biology (Cancer Research) [IFZ], University of Essen Medical School and West German Cancer Center Essen, Hufeland-Strasse 55, 45122 Essen, Germany

Abstract

DNA-reactive carcinogens and anticancer drugs induce many structurally distinct cytotoxic and potentially mutagenic DNA lesions. The capability of normal and malignant cells to recognize and repair different DNA lesions is an important variable influencing the risk of mutation and cancer as well as therapy resistance. Using monoclonal antibody-based immunoanalytical assays, very low amounts of defined carcinogen-DNA adducts can be quantified in bulk genomic DNA, individual genes, and in the nuclear DNA of single cells. The kinetics of DNA repair can thus be measured in a lesion-, gene-, and cell type-specific manner, and the DNA repair profiles of malignant cells can be monitored in individual patients. Even structurally very similar DNA lesions may be repaired with extremely different efficiency. The miscoding DNA alkylation products O^6-methylguanine (O^6-MeGua) and O^6-ethylguanine (O^6-EtGua), for example, differ only by one CH_2 group. These lesions are formed in DNA upon exposure to N-methyl-N-nitrosourea (MeNU) or N-ethyl-N-nitrosourea (EtNU), both of which induce mammary adenocarcinomas in female rats at high yield. Unrepaired O^6-alkylguanines cause transition mutations via mispairing during DNA replication. O^6-MeGua is repaired at a similar slow rate in transcribed (H-*ras*, *β-actin*) and inactive genes (*IgE heavy chain*; bulk DNA) of the target mammary epithelia (which express the repair protein O^6-alkylguanine-DNA alkyltransferase at a very low level). O^6-EtGua, however, via an alkyltransferase-independent mechanism, is excised ~ 20 times faster than O^6-MeGua from the transcribed genes selectively. Correspondingly, G:C → A:T transitions arising from unrepaired O^6-McGua at the second nucleotide of codon 12 (GGA) of the H-*ras* gene are frequently found in MeNU-induced mammary tumors, but are absent in their EtNU-induced counterparts.

Recent Results in Cancer Research, Vol. 154
© Springer-Verlag Berlin · Heidelberg 1998

Introduction

Carcinogenesis involves the stepwise evolution and selection of cells disobeying the physiological rules governing cell proliferation and differentiation, cell motility, and cell death (apoptosis) in a given tissue. The distinct pathways of differentiation and phenotypic properties of individual types of cells require that genes be switched on, up- or down-regulated, and turned off in specific combinations and sequence. Destabilization and disarrangement of these finely balanced, cell type-specific patterns of gene expression may be initiated and driven by diverse molecular alterations and mechanisms. Therefore, carcinogenesis is a multifactorial and multifaceted process conditioned by the genetic program and phenotype of the target cell, and a multitude of genes may potentially be involved. Of particular current interest, however, are those genes that encode "protective" proteins ensuring the integrity and stability of the genome (e.g., DNA repair proteins), proteins participating in cellular signal transduction pathways, and proteins associated with the control of cell proliferation and cell-cell and cell-matrix interactions.

There are "harder" and "softer" ways to upset regular gene expression. The former include the untimely gain, alteration, or loss of gene function as a result of structural modifications of DNA. Point mutations are frequent events following exposure to chemical or physical mutagens. Further important genetic alterations include deletions, insertions, inversions, DNA double-strand breaks, and chromosome rearrangements or losses (Friedberg et al. 1995). Examples of softer modulatory mechanisms are the epigenetic silencing of genes by 5-cytosine methylation at particular CpG dinucleotides (Costello et al. 1996; Baylin 1997; Kass et al. 1997; Lengauer et al. 1997; Ushijima et al. 1997; Woloschak et al. 1997; Zingg and Jones 1997), or alterations of gene expression levels via gene amplification receptor-mediated signaling pathways, transcription factors, and other molecules interfering with the nuclear transcription machinery.

Potentially mutagenic DNA lesions may either be exogenous, i.e., caused by DNA-reactive environmental chemicals (including many anticancer agents), solar UV light and ionizing radiation, or originate from endogenous cellular processes (Singer and Grunberger 1983; Dipple et al. 1990; Epstein 1990; Montesano et al. 1992; Dipple 1995; Friedberg et al. 1995; Loeb 1996). The latter include DNA replication (polymerase) errors that result in mismatched base pairs (Umar and Kunkel 1996; Kolodner 1997); the hydrolytic cleavage of N-glycosylic bonds generating misinstructive apurinic or apyrimidinic (AP) sites in DNA (Dogliotti et al. 1997); the deamination of 5-methylcytosine or cytosine in DNA to thymine or uracil, respectively (Gonzalgo and Jones 1997); various metabolic processes producing reactive oxygen species (ROS) which can cause a broad spectrum of DNA alterations, such as single-strand breaks, pyrimidine glycols, 8-hydroxyguanine, or glyoxal (Sies 1986; Demple and Harrison 1994; von Sonntag 1987; Loeb 1996; Croteau and Bohr 1997; Murata-Kamiya et al 1997); and alkylation of bases in DNA by, e.g., S-adenosylmethionine or alkylating compounds generated by bacterially catalyzed nitrosation of endogenous amides or amines (Lutz 1990; Sedgwick 1997).

DNA Repair

General Aspects

Mutagenesis by chemical or physical agents requires the persistence of structural lesions in genomic DNA for a period of time sufficient to give rise to heritable changes in nucleotide sequence. *The key protective mechanism counteracting the generation of mutations from premutational DNA lesions is timely and error-free DNA repair.* In principle, the cellular DNA repair machinery can process both potentially mutagenic and primarily cytotoxic DNA lesions. Besides decreasing the risk of mutation and cancer, DNA repair may thus enable cells to cope with an otherwise deleterious load of DNA damage (exception: mismatch repair, MMR, which may actually enhance cytotoxicity; Karran and Bignami 1994; Duckett et al. 1996; Fink et al. 1997). Most present-day anticancer drugs as well as radiation target DNA (along with other cellular macromolecules). In general, therefore, DNA repair synergizes with other adaptive mechanisms contributing to cancer therapy resistance (Fig. 1; Epstein 1990; Burt et al. 1991; Skovsgaard et al. 1994; Zeng-Rong et al. 1995; Chaney and Sancar 1996).

It is important to note that the efficiencies of specific pathways of DNA repair vary considerably between different types (and probably stages of differentiation) of mammalian cells – not to speak of their malignant counterparts (Goth and Rajewsky 1974; Harris 1989; Gerson et al. 1986; Müller et al. 1994; Preuss et al. 1995; Lee et al. 1996; Buschfort et al. 1997; White et al. 1997). Such variability would be predicted for the cells of malignant tumors, and between subpopulations of tumor cells, due to their genetic and phenotypic heterogeneity (Heppner and Miller 1998). What remains to be understood, however, is the physiological rationale underlying the differential DNA repair capacity of normal cells.

In contrast to the fundamental work on DNA repair in prokaryotes, research on genes, proteins and pathways operating in mammalian DNA repair had been sluggish for a long time (Friedberg et al. 1995; Wood 1996). Current rapid advances in this field have been fueled mainly by:
(1) the cloning of DNA repair genes of *Saccharomyces cerevisiae*, mostly found to be highly homologous to those identified earlier in bacteria and later on in mammalian cells;
(2) detailed genetic and biochemical analyses of heritable human disease syndromes involving defective DNA repair and increased susceptibility to cancer and/or other clinical phenotypes including neurological abnormalities (e.g., xeroderma pigmentosum, ataxia telangiectasia, Fanconi's anaemia, Lynch syndrome [HNPCC], Bloom's syndrome, Li-Fraumeni syndrome, and Cockayne syndrome; Hoeijmakers and Bootsma 1990;

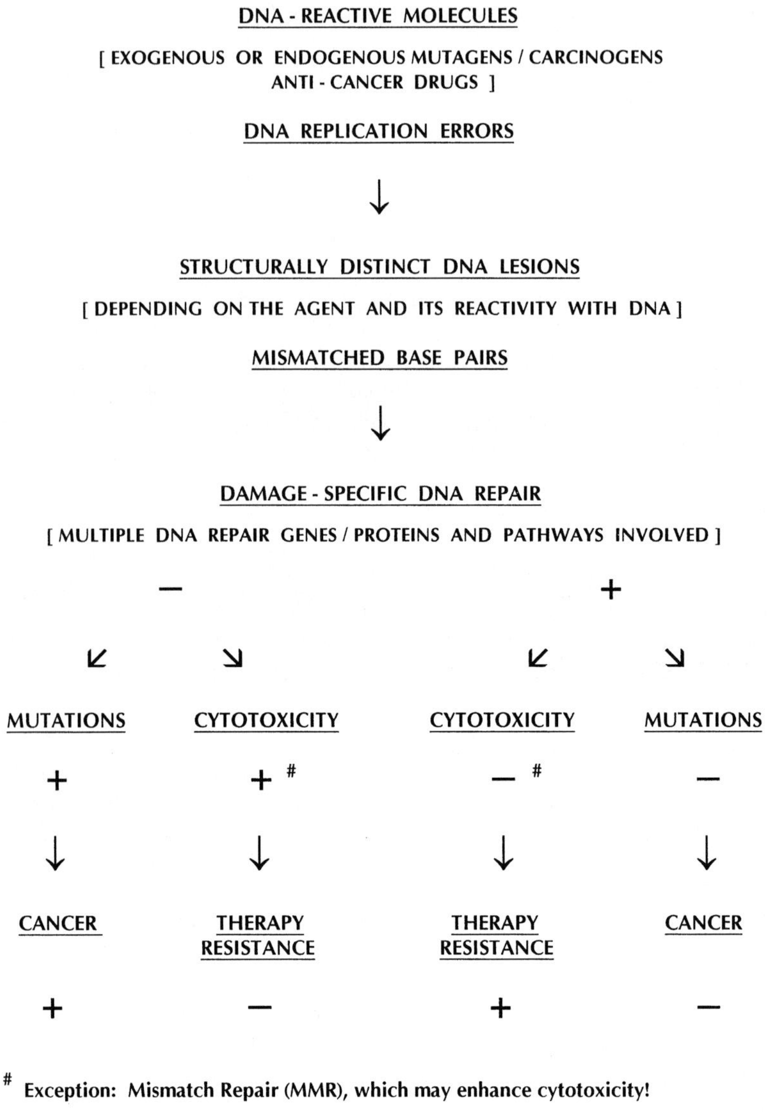

DNA - REACTIVE MOLECULES

**[EXOGENOUS OR ENDOGENOUS MUTAGENS / CARCINOGENS
ANTI - CANCER DRUGS]**

DNA REPLICATION ERRORS

$\downarrow$

STRUCTURALLY DISTINCT DNA LESIONS

[DEPENDING ON THE AGENT AND ITS REACTIVITY WITH DNA]

MISMATCHED BASE PAIRS

$\downarrow$

DAMAGE - SPECIFIC DNA REPAIR

[MULTIPLE DNA REPAIR GENES / PROTEINS AND PATHWAYS INVOLVED]

—   +

MUTATIONS	CYTOTOXICITY	CYTOTOXICITY	MUTATIONS
+	+[#]	—[#]	—
$\downarrow$	$\downarrow$	$\downarrow$	$\downarrow$
CANCER	THERAPY RESISTANCE	THERAPY RESISTANCE	CANCER
+	—	+	—

[#] **Exception: Mismatch Repair (MMR), which may enhance cytotoxicity!**

Fig. 1. DNA repair: Suppressor of mutation and cancer, accomplice of cancer therapy resistance

Ellis et al. 1995; Hanawalt 1996; Fishel and Wilson 1997; Kolodner 1997; Kraemer 1997);
(3) the revitalized notion that defective genes encoding DNA repair proteins and polymerases result in mutator phenotypes, i.e., in cells with reduced genomic stability and the propensity to rapidly accumulate mutations (Strauss 1977; Loeb 1996); and – of the same high relevance to carcinogenesis and cancer therapy –

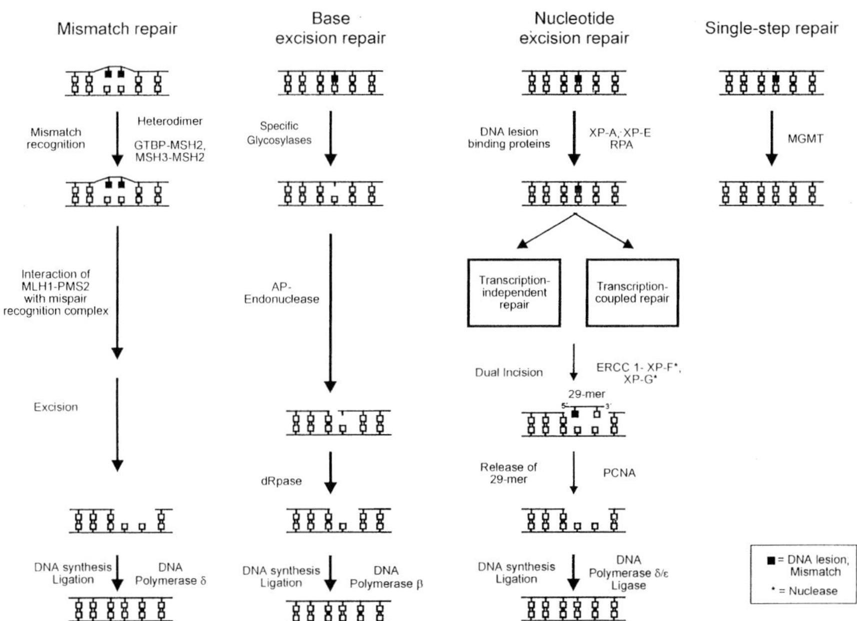

Fig. 2. DNA repair pathways in mammalian cells

(4) the unfolding interconnections between DNA repair and transcription on the one hand, and the genetic control of cell proliferation (cell cycle checkpoints) and apoptosis on the other (Bohr 1991; Bohr 1995; Hanawalt 1996; Kaufmann and Paules 1996; Sancar 1996; Wood 1996; Wahl et al 1997).

The number of genes and proteins identified as molecular players directly or more indirectly involved in DNA repair in mammalian cells has grown rapidly (Friedberg et al. 1995; Seeberg et al. 1995; Sancar 1996; Wood 1996; Hickson 1997; Kolodner 1997). What is being uncovered is an intricate multimodal system with multiple effector mechanisms, built-in redundancies and "backup" pathways, and endowed with the capacity for subtle distinction, in terms of recognition and processing, between specific types and sites of DNA damage. Comparable to the immune system with its surveillance function at the cellular level, this corrective network has evolved to preserve the integrity of the genome.

Figure 2 shows a simplified outline of major DNA repair pathways in mammalian cells. Two principal modes of the repair of DNA base damage are distinguished: *single-step repair* and *excision repair.* Not included in this scheme are: (1) the repair of DNA double-strand breaks (induced, e.g., by ionizing radiation, anticancer agents, or ROS generated in oxidative metabolism) by homologous recombination or by nonhomologous DNA end joining (Chu 1997); and (2) a potentially very important repair-associated process, *replicative bypass* (also referred to as *postreplication repair*), which has not yet been clarified sufficiently in terms of its molecular mechanisms (Naegeli 1994).

Single-step repair is performed by O^6-alkylguanine-DNA alkyltransferase (MGMT) through direct removal of an alkyl residue from the O^6-atom of guanine in the DNA of cells exposed to alkylating agents, and by photolyases in the direct reversion of UV-induced cyclobutane pyrimidine dimers (CPDs) in DNA in the presence of photoreactivating blue light (Lindahl et al. 1988; Pegg 1990; Friedberg et al. 1995; Singer and Hang 1997). Excision repair broadly encompasses the pathways of *base excision repair (BER)* (Seeberg et al. 1995; Wood 1996; Hickson 1997), *nucleotide excision repair (NER)* (Friedberg et al. 1995; Sancar 1996), and *mismatch repair (MMR)* (Karran 1996; Umar and Kunkel 1996; Kolodner 1997). Subpathways of NER are *transcription-coupled repair (TCR;* involving the general transcription factor TFIIH) in genes transcribed by RNA polymerase II, and *transcription-independent repair (TIR;* also referred to as *"global"* or *"overall"* NER) in transcriptionally silent genes (i.e., in most of genomic DNA; Link et al. 1991; Bohr 1995; Friedberg et al. 1995; Friedberg 1996; Hanawalt 1996). In addition to their involvement in the transcription machinery, certain NER proteins may also participate in subpathways involving genetic recombination (as probably required in the repair of DNA interstrand cross-links).

NER, BER and MMR are multistep pathways involving a large number of different proteins and protein complexes for the recognition and processing of DNA damage. NER is a highly versatile pathway acting upon a broad spectrum of structurally diverse DNA alterations ("bulky" DNA lesions) that cause substantial local distortions of the DNA helix (Gunz et al. 1996). The NER pathway involves the concerted action of about 30 proteins to excise a fragment of ~ 24–32 nucleotides after incision of the damaged strand on each side of the lesion, followed by DNA repair synthesis (by DNA polymerases δ and ε) using the intact strand as template, and closing of the gap by ligation. In contrast to BER, there appears to be little redundancy in the NER pathway. In BER, the removal of a single modified nucleotide from one DNA strand is performed by DNA glycosylases via hydrolytic cleavage of the N-glycosyl bond (Neddermann et al. 1996; Hickson 1997; Krokan et al. 1997). Some of these glycosylases exhibit pronounced lesion specificity, others recognize multiple, structurally different damaged bases, and certain glycosylases display considerable versatility regarding the range of reactions they catalyze. The apurinic/apyrimidinic (AP) site left behind after cleavage of the N-glycosyl bond is then hydrolyzed $5'$ by an AP endonuclease, and the $5'$deoxyribose phosphate is excised by a phosphodiesterase. The resulting single-nucleotide gap is filled by polymerase β and ligated. Alternatives to this common pathway of BER include, e.g., the excision of a short oligonucleotide patch containing the AP site and filling of the gap by polymerase δ or ε. Base alterations dealt with by the BER pathway may be caused by a large variety of agents and processes (e.g., spontaneous deamination, radiation, ROS, alkylating agents, DNA replication errors). Contrasting with the situation in NER, a common feature of the damaged or mismatched bases recognized by glycosylases in BER is that they do not significantly distort the DNA helix. While BER may well be the DNA repair mechanism used most frequently in mammalian cells, no disease has yet been clearly related to defects in this pathway, suggesting that some of its elements may be indispensable for viability.

Mainly based on analyses of repair rates of CPDs produced in the DNA of cells exposed to UV light, TCR has been found to operate faster than overall NER (TIR) – usually with a bias in favor of the transcribed strand. Depending on DNA sequence context and chromatin structure, however, extensive positional heterogeneity regarding the efficiency of CPD repair within defined genes has been documented by analyses at very high or even single-nucleotide resolution (Tu et al. 1997; Wellinger and Thoma 1997). Interestingly, pronounced intragenic heterogeneity has recently been observed along the *TP53* gene with respect to the distribution of sunlight-induced CPDs and benzo(a)pyrene-DNA adducts, dictated to a large extent by the absence or presence of 5-methylcytosines in target CpG dinucleotides (Denissenko et al. 1996; Tommasi et al. 1997). Obviously, both hotspots for the formation of premutational DNA lesions as well as "slow spots" regarding their repair may enhance the frequencies of critical mutations in proto-oncogenes or tumor suppressor genes.

The removal or persistence, respectively, of mutagenic DNA lesions in cancer-associated genes is critical to carcinogenesis. It is clear, therefore, that the relative capacity of target cells for corrective DNA repair is a key determinant for the probability of their malignant conversion. This is also true regarding the repair of cytotoxic DNA damage in tissues proficient for compensatory hyperplasia, where damage-induced cell loss leads to increased proliferative activity (Rajewsky 1972; Fong et al. 1997). Reparative cell proliferation enhances the probability of mutation fixation through DNA replication and is known to further promote the carcinogenic process through mechanisms as yet insufficiently understood.

Carcinogenesis: Human Cancer

The most impressive cases so far that link increased human cancer risk and the early onset of tumor development to defects in particular pathways of DNA repair, are: (1) the rare autosomal recessive disease xeroderma pigmentosum (XP), and (2) the HNPCC syndrome, a more common autosomal dominant cancer susceptibility disorder responsible for 1%–5% of all colorectal cancers. XP patients are defective in NER, exhibit very high sensitivity to sunlight, and their risk of developing skin cancer is ~2000 times that of the general population (Hoeijmakers and Bootsma 1990; Kraemer 1997). The age of onset of nonmelanoma skin cancer is reduced by ~50 years in these patients. Colorectal adenocarcinomas of HNPCC patients show genomic instability in the form of highly polymorphic mono- and dinucleotide microsatellites (microsatellite instability, MIN) (Karran 1996; Kolodner 1997). MIN reflects frameshift mutations resulting from uncorrected misalignments between template and daughter strands during DNA replication. The corresponding "replication error$^+$(RER$^+$) phenotype" has been observed in >90% of colorectal tumors of HNPCC families and in other cancers associated with the HNPCC syndrome. In nearly all cases analyzed so far, the underlying DNA repair defect was a germline mutation in one of four MMR genes (*hMSH2/hMSH6* and *hMLH1/hPMS2*). The proteins and sequential steps involved in human MMR, the substrate preferences of different MMR subpathways, and the possibility of dominant-negative mutations in MMR genes, are under investigation. Apparently, some MMR defects selectively result in an inability to repair single base mismatches and single nucleotide loops, while others affect the repair of both mono- and dinucleotide loops. It should be noted that DNA replication errors could, in principle, also accumulate as a result of polymerase alterations leading to decreased replication fidelity, or as a consequence of disproportionate deoxynucleotide triphosphate pools (Karran 1996).

Carcinogenesis: Animal Models and In Vitro-Studies

Numerous attempts have been made to demonstrate the cancer-suppressive function of DNA repair in established rodent models of chemical carcinogenesis complemented by cell culture experiments, and recently with the use of animals expressing a specific DNA repair transgene and repair gene knockout mice. Compared with human exposure to environmental carcinogens, experimental models have the obvious advantage that a single known carcinogen can be applied whose reaction products with DNA are well-defined and may be analyzed specifically in terms of their mutagenic potential and repair. For these reasons, alkylating N-nitroso carcinogens have been used in the majority of studies (Goth and Rajewsky 1974; Thomale et al. 1990; Engelbergs et al. 1998; Becker et al. 1997). However, UV light and some other mutagenic compounds, such as aralkylating agents (e.g., the polycyclic aromatic hydrocarbon 7,12-dimethylbenz[a]anthracene, DMBA), arylaminating agents (e.g., the aromatic amine N-acetoxy-2-acetylaminofluorene, N-AcOAAF), or heated food-derived, heterocyclic amines (e.g., 2-amino-1-methyl-6-phenylimidazo-[4,5-b]-pyridine, PhIP) have also been applied in recent analyses of cancer susceptibility in repair gene knockout mice (de Vries and van Steeg 1996).

Alkylating N-nitroso compounds either require enzymatic bioactivation (e.g., the N,N-dialkylnitrosamines) or decompose heterolytically (e.g., the N-alkyl-N-nitrosoureas) (Singer and Grunberger 1983; Eisenbrand et al. 1986; Colvin and Chabner 1990; Montesano et al. 1992). The resulting reactive electrophilic metabolites attack nucleophilic atoms in cellular macromolecules, and alkyl residues are thus covalently attached to O and N atoms in DNA. About 12 different alkylation products are formed in DNA at relative proportions that depend on the chemical nature of the respective N-nitroso compound (Singer et al. 1978; Beranek 1990). O^6-alkylguanines and O^4-alkylthymines are considered the most potent mutagenic DNA alkylation products (Singer and Grunberger 1983; Altshuler et al. 1996). Both lesions give rise to point mutations (G:C → A:T and T:A → C:G transitions, respectively) via mispairing during DNA replication. O^4-alkylthymines are formed in DNA at significantly lower yield than O^6-alkylguanines, in particular if the alkyl residue is a methyl group. O^6-methylguanine is predominantly repaired by the single-step "suicide repair protein" MGMT in a stoichiometric manner (Lindahl et al. 1988). This direct repair is effected through the transfer of the methyl residue from the O^6 atom of guanine to a cysteine in the active center of the MGMT molecule (which is thereby inactivated). The degree to which a given cell is able to clear its genomic DNA of O^6-methylguanine thus depends on its MGMT pool size and the rate of de novo MGMT synthesis. The expression of human MGMT appears to be controlled at the transcriptional level. Candidate regulatory mechanisms are 5-cytosine methylation and/or the interaction of a 45 kDa protein with a 59 base pair (bp) enhancer sequence located at the first exon-intron boundary of the MGMT gene (Chen et al. 1997). With increasing size of the alkyl group ($\geq$ethyl), the contribution of MGMT to the repair of O^6-alkylguanines decreases and excision repair steps in as a "backup" modality. In mammalian cells, both O^4-methyl- and O^4-ethylthymine are not repaired by MGMT, but are slowly removed from genomic DNA by excision mechanisms (O^4-methyl- $\gg O^4$-ethylthymine) (Altshuler et al. 1996; Singer and Hang 1997).

Using monoclonal antibody-based immunoanalysis, DNA alkylation products such as O^6-alkylguanines or O^4-alkylthymines can be quantified in the femtomole to attomole range (Thomale et al. 1996). The elimination kinetics of specific alkylation products from cellular DNA can thus be recorded as a reflection of their rate of repair. Specifically, available immunoanalytical methods include competitive radioimmunoassays following separation by HPLC of a given alkyl-2′-deoxynucleoside from DNA digests, immuno-slot-blot procedures, a combined immunoaffity-quantitative PCR assay to quantify specific DNA lesions in known gene sequences, immuno-electron microscopy, and an immunocytochemical assay to visualize and quantify specific alkylation products in the nuclear DNA of individual cells via digital imaging of electronically intensified fluorescence signals (Fig. 3; Seiler et al. 1993; Thomale et al. 1994 a, 1996).

Studies in rodent models of carcinogenesis induced by N-alkyl-N-nitrosoureas, and in vitro experiments using repair-competent vs repair-incompetent rodent cell variants, have shown a strong correlation between the persistence of unrepaired O^6-alkylguanines in the DNA of tissues with low MGMT activity and the development of malignant tumors (Goth and Rajewsky 1974; Thomale et al. 1990; Oda et al. 1997). Conversely, when rats were continuously exposed to the hepatocarcinogen N,N-diethylnitrosamine, unrepaired O^4-ethylthymines rapidly accumulated in the DNA of target cells with high MGMT activity (hepatocytes), thus substituting for the repaired O^6-ethylguanines as the predominant mutagenic DNA lesion (Swenberg et al. 1984).

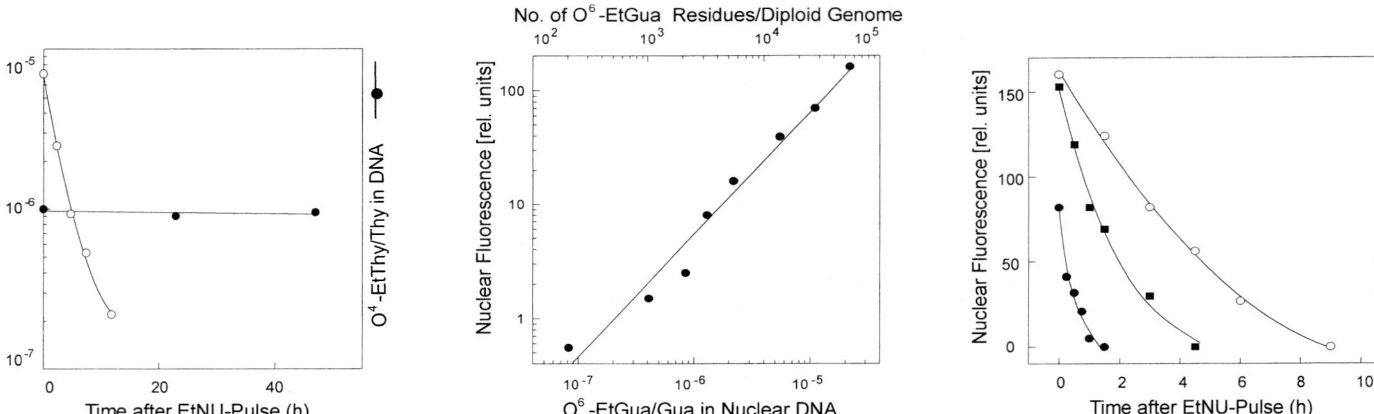

Fig. 3. Potentially mutagenic and cytotoxic DNA lesions and kinetics of their elimination from cellular DNA (repair): Quantification by monoclonal antibody-based immunoanalysis. *Left*: Elimination kinetics of O^6-ethylguanine (O^6-EtGua) and O^4-ethylthymine (O^4-EtThy) from genomic DNA of rat neural tumor cells after exposure to EtNU *in vitro* (competitive radioimmunoassay) (adapted from Huh and Rajewsky 1988). *Center*: Rat neural tumor cells after 20 min in vitro exposure to different concentrations of EtNU: Correlation of O^6-EtGua content of bulk genomic DNA (determined by competitive radioimmunoassay) with [O^6-EtGua]-specific nuclear immunofluorescence of individual cells (immunocytological analysis via digital imaging of intensified fluorescence signals; each point represents the average value for 100 cells). Adapted from Seiler et al. (1993). *Right*: Elimination kinetics of O^6-EtGua from the nuclear DNA of lymphocytes isolated from different patients with chronic lymphatic leukaemia, following 20 min *in vitro*-exposure to 100 μg of EtNU/ml (immunocytological analysis of individual cells; data points, average values for 100 cells each). *Filled circles*, patient resistant to therapy with alkylating drugs; *filled squares*, patient with intermediate sensitivity to alkylating drug therapy; *open circles*, patient sensitive to alkylating drug treatment. *Gua*, guanine; *Thy*, thymine. (Buschfort C, Müller MR, Thomale J, Seeber S, Rajewsky MF, unpublished data)

The evidence for the cancer-suppressive role of the repair of O^6-alkylguanine in target cell DNA has been corroborated impressively by recent studies showing: (1) almost complete protection from the induction of thymic lymphomas by single-dose exposure to N-methyl-N-nitrosourea (MeNU) in mice strongly expressing a human *MGMT* transgene in the thymus (Dumenco et al. 1993), and (2i) a reduced incidence of liver cancer following pulse-exposure to N,N-dimethyl- or -diethylnitrosamine in rats carrying the bacterial *MGMT* homologue *ada* as a transgene (Nakatsuru et al. 1993).

During the coming years, the relative contributions of different DNA repair pathways to the suppression of mutagenesis, carcinogenesis, and cytotoxicity, their individual substrate specificities, and their built-in redundancies and "backup" capacities will have to be investigated in depth under in vivo conditions. This can be achieved through functional analyses of DNA repair transgenes expressed in a cell type-specific manner, but most convincingly with the use of conventional and, in particular, cell type-specific, "conditional" gene targeting in mouse (and hopefully rat) models. Single and multiple gene knockouts, and their breeding into defined genetic backgrounds, will elucidate the interrelations of the DNA repair network with other critical regulatory systems, such as those controlling cell proliferation, senescence, and apoptosis. To date, mouse lines with a complete knockout of both alleles of a specific DNA repair gene have been generated for the *MGMT* gene, the *Aag* (alkyladenine DNA glycosylase) gene (BER), the *XPA*, and *XPC* and *CXB* genes (NER), the *PMS2, MLH1* and *MSH2* genes (MMR), the *PARP* (poly[ADP-ribose] polymerase) gene, and the *TP53* gene (Baker et al. 1995; Nakane et al. 1995; Sands et al. 1995; de Wind et al. 1995; Donehower 1996; Edelman et al. 1996; Prolla et al. 1996; de Vries and Steeg 1996; Engelward et al. 1997; Hang et al. 1997; van der Horst et al. 1997; Ménissier-de Murcia et al. 1997; Sakumi et al. 1997). Increased spontaneous and exogenously induced mutation rates and cancer risk are features common to these animals; however, detailed investigations, including the crossing of repair-defective mouse lines in different combinations, are being performed in various laboratories. Moreover, complete knockouts of a number of other DNA repair genes, such as the genes encoding DNA polymerase β (BER), the major AP endonuclease APE (BER), DNA ligase I (BER, NER), or the ERCC1 protein (NER) proved to be lethal during embryogenesis or early in postnatal life. In such cases, functional gene analyses will require conditional knockout methodology.

Differential Efficiency of DNA Repair Upon Subtle Variation of Target Lesion Structure in Transcriptionally Active vs Inactive Genes

As pointed out above, the efficiency of the repair of potentially mutagenic and carcinogenic DNA alterations is affected by the transcriptional status of target genes, DNA sequence context and chromatin structure. A further important determinant, however, lies in the molecular structure of the lesions

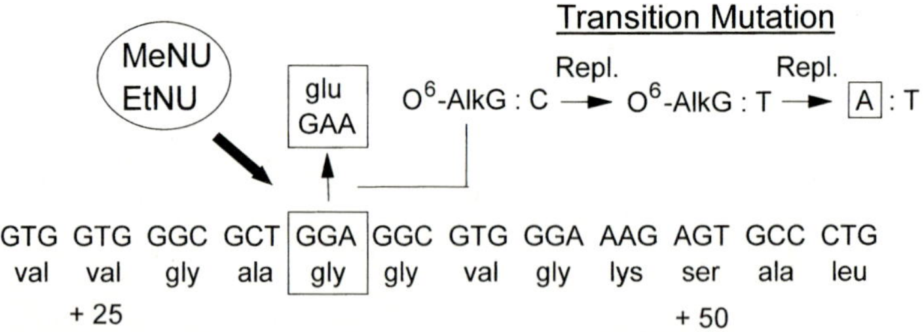

Fig. 4. N-ethyl-N-nitrosourea (EtNU) vs N-methyl-N-nitrosourea (MeNU)

to be recognized and processed. How small an alteration in substrate structure would be sufficient to significantly influence repair efficiency in transcriptionally active vs silent target genes? We have addressed this question by analyzing overall (global) and gene-specific repair of a mutagenic DNA lesion (O^6-alkylguanine), mutation frequencies in cancer-associated target genes (H-*ras*, K-*ras*), and tumor incidence in a model of mammary carcinogenesis induced in 50-day-old female Sprague-Dawley rats by a single application of MeNU vs N-ethyl-N-nitrosourea (EtNU) (Engelbergs et al. 1998). Both carcinogens induced mammary adenocarcinomas at high yield; the tumors were indistinguishable histologically and with respect to tumor progression. The structure of MeNU differs from that of EtNU only by one extra CH_2 group in the latter compound (Fig. 4); i.e., MeNU will induce O^6-methylguanine (O^6-MeGua) in DNA while EtNU induces O^6-ethylguanine (O^6-EtGua). Mispairing of an unrepaired O^6-alkylguanine with thymine during DNA replication results in a G:C $\rightarrow$ A:T transition mutation, which in MeNU-induced rat mammary tumors is very frequently observed at the second position of codon 12 (exon 1) of the H-*ras* gene (Fig. 5; Sukumar et al. 1983). This point mutation in the H-*ras* gene has, therefore, been considered a critical initiating gene alteration in the MeNU-induced malignant conversion of rat mammary epithelia (which exhibit a very low level of MGMT expression compared to other types of cells).

In our analyses of the repair of O^6-MeGua vs O^6-EtGua, we have compared bulk genomic DNA and the nontranscribed *IgE heavy chain* gene with the

Fig. 5. The rat H-*ras* proto-oncogene (exon 1): G:C $\rightarrow$ A:T transition mutation at the second base (guanine) of codon 12 following methylation of the O^6 atom of guanine by MeNU or EtNU and subsequent mispairing of unrepaired O^6-alkylguanine with thymine during DNA replication. *Repl.*, round of DNA replication

Table 1. Overall (global) and gene-specific repair of O^6-methylguanine vs O^6-ethylguanine in the DNA of rat mammary epithelia cells exposed to MeNU in vivo

	O^6-methylguanine $t_{50\%}$ [h]		O^6-ethylguanine $t_{50\%}$ [h]	
	– O^6-BeGua	+ O^6-BeGua	– O^6-BeGua	+ O^6-BeGua
Bulk genomic DNA	40	*	48	***
IgE heavy chain gene	48	*	50	**
H-*ras* gene	36	*	2.5	2.6
β-actin gene	42	*	2.4	2.4

$t_{50\%}$, Time (h) required for repair of 50% of input O^6-alkylguanines in DNA; O^6-BeGua: O^6-benzylguanine (MGMT inhibitor); * <10% of input O^6-methylguanine repaired during 48 h inhibition of MGMT by O^6-BeGua; ** 20% of input O^6-ethylguanine repaired during 48 h inhibition of MGMT by O^6-BeGua; *** 30% of input O^6-ethylguanine repaired during 48 h inhibition of MGMT by O^6-BeGua.

Table 2. G:C → A:T transition mutations at the second nucleotide of codon 12 (GGA) of the H-*ras* and K-*ras* genes in rat mammary adenocarcinomas induced by EtNU vs MeNU

	EtNU		MeNU	
	A [a]	B [a]	A [a]	B [a]
H-*ras* gene	0/12 *	0/7	6/8	6/10
K-*ras* gene	0/12	0/3	0/15	n.d.

Mutations were found neither at any other position of H-*ras* exon 1 in EtNU-induced tumors, nor in exon 1 of K-*ras* in 12 EtNU- and 15 MeNU-induced tumors analyzed. Likewise, no mutations were detected at codon 61 (CAA), exon 2, of H-*ras* and K-*ras* in a total of 23 MeNU-induced tumors and 31 tumors induced by EtNU; 1 EtNU-induced tumor exhibited a transversion (CAA → CTA) at codon 61 of H-*ras*.
[a] O^6-alkylguanine-DNA alkyltransferase activity of mammary epithelia at the time of carcinogen exposure. A, Normal (low) MGMT activity; B, MGMT activity supplemented by the bacterial MGMT homolog ada (the alkyltransferase activity of mammary epithelia in *ada* transgenic rats was ~6.5-fold that of wild-type animals).
[b] Number of tumors with mutant gene/number of tumors analyzed.

transcriptionally active H-*ras* and *β-actin* genes. In mammary epithelia exposed to MeNU on postnatal day 50 in vivo, O^6-MeGua was eliminated from the transcribed H-*ras* and *β*-actin genes at the same slow rate as from bulk DNA and the silent *IgE heavy chain* gene (Table 1). This comparatively high persistence of O^6-MeGua in DNA correlated with a high frequency of G:C → A:T transitions at codon 12 of H-*ras* in the MeNU-induced tumors (Table 2). The repair of O^6-EtGua was similarly slow in bulk DNA and the *IgE heavy chain* gene (Table 1). In sharp contrast to O^6-MeGua, however, O^6-EtGua was removed about 20 times faster from both strands of the transcriptionally active H-*ras* and *β-actin* genes by an *MGMT*-independent excision repair process (Table 1). Correspondingly, no H-*ras* codon 12 mutations were observed in the EtNU-induced tumors (Table 2), and surplus MGMT activity of the mammary epithelia – via a bacterial *ada* transgene – did not significantly counteract mammary tumorigenesis in EtNU-exposed rats in contrast to the MeNU-treated animals.

Neither the MeNU- nor the EtNU-induced mammary carcinomas exhibited mutations at codons 13 and 61 of H-*ras* or at codons 12, 13 and 61 of K-*ras*.

A small molecular change (methyl to ethyl) in the alkyl residue bound to the O^6 atom of guanine in a transcribed gene (H-ras) thus dramatically influences the rate of repair of a potentially mutagenic DNA lesion, thereby modifying the risk of mutation of a critical gene. The apparent disregard of O^6-MeGua by the fast repair system of active genes is intriguing (might this barrier perhaps be installed to avoid interference with molecular recognition of the methyl group in [5-methylC]pG?). The selective fast repair of O^6-EtGua obviously prevents the activation of H-*ras* through mutation at codon 12 when rat mammary carcinogenesis is initiated by EtNU in place of MeNU, leaving open the question which genetic alteration(s) is (are) involved in the initiation of EtNU-induced mammary cancer in the rat.

DNA Repair and Cancer Therapy Resistance

Cancer therapy resistance is multifactorial and involves the pronounced capacity of malignant cells to adapt to altered microenvironmental conditions (including exposure to cytocidal agents). The ranking of DNA repair as part of the repertoire of synergistic mechanisms used by cancer cells to evade cytotoxic therapy has not yet been firmly established, in spite of active past and currrent investigation (excellently reviewed by Chaney and Sancar 1996). However, DNA repair is a particularly important protective mechanism in cancer cells when the type and extent of DNA damage caused by a given anticancer agent is primarily responsible for triggering apoptotic pathways or other forms of cell death.

Perhaps most impressively, resistance of cancer cells to the widely used chloroethylnitrosoureas (e.g., N,N'-bis[2-chloroethyl]-N-nitrosourea, BCNU; N-[2-chloroethyl]-N'-cyclohexyl-N-nitrosourea, CCNU) has been found to be strongly correlated with the expression of MGMT (Chaney and Sancar 1996). In the formation of cytotoxic interstrand cross-links, chloroethylnitrosoureas initially chloroethylate the O^6 atom of guanine in target cell DNA. The levels of MGMT expression in different types of human tumors have been found to be highly variable (Preuss et al. 1995; Lee et al. 1996; White et al. 1997). The efficiency of DNA repair pathways other than single-step repair by MGMT in human malignancies has so far not been investigated in any detail. Clearly, however, the development of specific inhibitors of distinct pathways of DNA repair (dictated by the form of DNA damage, i.e., by the chemistry of the therapeutic agent) and their tumor-selective (!) application is an important objective. The only efficient inhibitor of a specific DNA repair pathway available, and currently in clinical testing, is the MGMT inhibitor O^6-benzylguanine (Crone et al. 1994; Pegg 1990).

The selection of effective anticancer drugs based on the avoidance of therapy resistance due to DNA repair requires the establishment of methods (i) for testing human primary malignant cells with respect to their capacity to repair specific DNA lesions prior to therapy, and (ii) for the "intratherapeutic" monitoring of target cells for changes in their DNA repair properties which may translate into resistance to the therapeutic agent initially applied. Standardized in vitro assays of this kind have thus far only been focused on the pre- and intratherapeutic testing of leukaemic cells from individual patients in connection with alkylating drug therapy (O^6-alkylguanines as model DNA lesions to be repaired; Fig. 3) (Müller et al. 1994; Thomale et al. 1994b; Buschfort et al. 1997).

Contrary to strategies attempting inhibition of DNA repair to avoid therapy resistance, it may also be possible to exploit enhanced DNA repair to achieve more effective cancer therapy; e.g., via selective protection of haematopoietic stem cells in the bone marrow. Due to their high sensitivity to cytotoxic drugs, these cells constitute the main limiting factor in cancer chemotherapy. Normal bone marrow cells express MGMT at an exceedingly low level (Gerson et al. 1986). However, the *MGMT* gene can be retrovirally transduced and expressed in haematopoietic progenitor cells (e.g., human $CD34^+$ cells) (Moritz et al. 1995; Maze et al. 1996; Rafferty et al. 1996). Using an (O^6-benzylguanine)-insensitive mutant *MGMT* gene for transduction, malignant tumors can thus be sensitized to chloroethylnitrosoureas via inhibition of their endogenous MGMT by O^6-benzylguanine, while haematopoietic cells continuing to express the mutant *MGMT* gene remain protected (Reese et al. 1996; Davis et al. 1997).

Acknowledgements. The authors are indebted to their colleagues, past and present, who have contributed to work carried out in this laboratory and referred to here. We apologize to all those whose original publications and reviews pertaining to the broad topic of this article could not be directly referenced due to space constraints. The secretarial assistance of Ms. Ute Häusler is gratefully acknowledged. Our research is supported by the Dr. Mildred Scheel Stiftung für Krebsforschung, the Deutsche Forschungsgemeinschaft, and the National Foundation for Cancer Research (USA) through Krebsforschung International e.V. (Germany).

References

Altshuler KB, Hodes CS, Essigmann JM (1996) Intrachromosomal probes for mutagenesis by alkylated DNA bases replicated in mammalian cells: a comparison of the mutagenicities of O^4-methylthymine and O^6-methylguanine in cells with different DNA repair backgrounds. Chem Res Toxicol 9:980–987

Baker SM, Bronner CE, Zhang L, Plug AW, Robatzek M, Warren G, Elliott M, Yu J, Ashley T, Arnheim N, Flavell RA, Liskay RM (1995) Male mice defective in the DNA mismatch repair gene *PMS2* exhibit abnormal chromosome synapsis in meiosis. Cell 82:309–319

Baylin SB (1997) Tying it all together: epigenetics, genetics, cell cycle, and cancer. Science 277:1948–1949

Becker K, Gregel CM, Kaina B (1997) The DNA repair protein O^6-methylguanine-DNA methyltransferase protects against skin tumor formation induced by antineoplastic chloroethylnitrosourea. Cancer Res 57:3335–3338

Beranek DT (1990) Distribution of methyl and ethyl adducts following alkylation with monofunctional alkylating agents. Mutat Res 231:11–30

Bohr VA (1991) Gene specific DNA repair. Carcinogenesis 12:1983–1992

Bohr VA (1995) DNA repair fine structure and its relation to genomic instability. Carcinogenesis 16:2885–2892

Burt RK, Poirier MC, Link CJ Jr, Bohr VA (1991) Antineoplastic drug resistance and DNA repair. Ann Oncol 2:325–334

Buschfort C, Müller MR, Seeber S, Rajewsky MF, Thomale J (1997) DNA excision repair profiles of normal and leukemic human lymphocytes: functional analysis at the single-cell level. Cancer Res 57:651–658

Chaney SG, Sancar A (1996) DNA repair: enzymatic mechanisms and relevance to drug response. J Natl Cancer Inst 88:1346–1360

Chen FY, Harris LC, Remack JS, Brent TP (1997) Cytoplasmic sequestration of an O^6-methylguanine-DNA methyltransferase enhancer binding protein in DNA repair-deficient human cells. Proc Natl Acad Sci USA 94:4348–4353

Chu G (1997) Double strand break repair. J Biol Chem 171:24097–24100

Colvin M, Chabner BA (1990) Alkylating agents. In: Chabner BA, Collins JM (eds) Cancer chemotherapy: principles and practice. Lippincott, Philadelphia, pp 276–314

Costello JF, Berger MS, Huang H-JS, Cavenee WK (1996) Silencing of *p16/CDKN2* expression in human gliomas by methylation and chromatin condensation. Cancer Res 56: 2405–2410

Crone TM, Goodtzova K, Edara S, Pegg AE (1994) Mutations in human O^6-alkylguanine-DNA alkyltransferase imparting resistance to O^6-benzylguanine. Cancer Res 54:6221–6227

Croteau DL, Bohr VA (1997) Repair of oxidative damage to nuclear and mitochondrial DNA in mammalian cells. J Biol Chem 272:25409–25412

Davis BM, Reese JS, Ko ON, Lee K, Schupp JE, Gerson SL (1997) Selection for G156A O^6-methylguanine DNA methyltransferase gene–transduced hematopoietic progenitors and protection from lethality in mice treated with O^6-benzylguanine and 1,3-bis(2-chloroethyl)-1-nitrosourea. Cancer Res 57:5093–5099

De Vries A, van Steeg H (1996) *Xpa* knockout mice. Semin Cancer Biol 7:229–240

De Wind N, Dekker M, Berns A, Radman M, te Riele H (1995) Inactivation of the mouse *Msh2* gene results in postreplicational mismatch repair deficiency, methylation tolerance, hyperrecombination, and predisposition to tumorigenesis. Cell 82:321–330

Demple B, Harrison L (1994) Repair of oxidative damage to DNA: enzymology and biology. Annu Rev Biochem 63:915–948

Denissenko MF, Pao A, Tang M-S, Pfeifer GP (1996) Preferential formation of benzo(a)pyrene adducts at lung cancer mutational hotspots in P53. Science 274:430–432

Dipple A (1995) DNA adducts of chemical carcinogens. Carcinogenesis 16:437–441

Dipple A, Chau Cheng S, Bigger AH (1990) Polycyclic aromatic hydrocarbon carcinogens. In: Pariza M (ed) Mutagens and carcinogens in the diet. Wiley-Liss, New York, pp 109–127

Dogliotti E, Fortini P, Pascucci B (1997) Mutagenesis of abasic sites. In Hickson ID (ed) Base excision repair of DNA damage. Landes Bioscience, Austin, pp 81–101

Donehower LA (1996) The p53-deficient mouse: a model for basic and applied cancer studies. Semin Cancer Biol 7:269–278

Duckett DR, Drummond JT, Murchie AIH, Reardon JT, Sancar A, Lilley DMJ, Modrich P (1996) Human MutSα recognizes damaged DNA base pairs containing O^6-methylguanine, O^4-methylthymine, or the cisplatin d(GpG) adduct. Proc Natl Acad Sci USA 93:6443–6447

Dumenco LL, Allay E, Norton K, Gerson SL (1993) The prevention of thymic lymphomas in transgenic mice by human O^6-alkylguanine-DNA alkytransferase. Science 259:219–222

Edelman W, Cohen P, Kane M, Lan K, Morrow B, Bennet S, Umar A, Kunkel T, Cattoretti G, Chaganti R, Pollard J, Kolodner R, Kucherlapati R (1996) Meiotic pachytene arrest in MLH1-deficient mice. Cell 85:1125–1134

Eisenbrand G, Müller N, Denkel E, Sterzel W (1986) DNA adducts and DNA damage by antineoplastic and carcinogenic N-nitroso compounds. J Cancer Res Clin Oncol 112:196–204

Ellis NA, Groden J, Ye T-Z, Straughen J, Lennon DJ, Ciocci S, Proytcheva M, German J (1995) The Bloom's syndrome gene product is homologous to RecQ helicases. Cell 83:655–666

Engelbergs J, Thomale J, Galhoff A, Rajewsky MF (1998) Fast repair of O^6-ethylguanine, but not O^6-methylguanine, in transcribed genes prevents mutation of H-*ras* in rat mammary tumorigenesis induced by ethylnitrosourea in place of methylnitrosourea. Proc Natl Acad Sci USA 95:1635–1640

Engelward BP, Weeda G, Wyatt MD, Broekhof JL, De Wit J, Donker I, Allan JM, Gold B, Hoeijmakers JHL, Samson LD (1997) Base excision repair deficient mice lacking the Aag alkyladenine DNA glycosylase. Proc Natl Acad Sci USA 94:13087–13092

Epstein RJ (1990) Drug-induced DNA damage and tumor chemosensitivity. J Clin Oncol 8:2062–2084

Fink D, Zheng H, Nebel S, Norris PS, Aebi S, Lin T-Z, Nehmé A, Christen RD, Haas M, MacLeod CL, Howell SB (1997) In vitro and in vivo resistance to cisplatin in cells that have lost DNA mismatch repair. Cancer Res 57:1841–1845

Fishel R, Wilson T (1997) MutS homologs in mammalian cells. Curr Opin Genet Dev 7:105–113

Fong LYY, Lau K-M, Huebner K, Magee PN (1997) Induction of esophageal tumors in zinc-deficient rats by single low doses of N-nitrosomethylbenzylamine (NMBA): analysis of cell proliferation, and mutations in H-*ras* and *p53* genes. Carcinogenesis 18:1477–1484

Friedberg EC (1996) Relationships between DNA repair and transcription. Annu Rev Biochem 65:15–42

Friedberg EC, Walker GC, Siede W (1995) DNA Repair and mutagenesis. ASM, Washington DC

Gerson SL, Trey JE, Miller K, Berger NA (1986) Comparison of O^6-alkylguanine-DNA alkyltransferase activity based on cellular DNA content in human, rat and mouse tissues. Carcinogenesis 7:745–749

Gonzalgo ML, Jones PA (1997) Mutagenic and epigenetic effects of DNA methylation. Mutat Res 386:107–118

Goth R, Rajewsky MF (1974) Persistence of O^6-ethylguanine in rat-brain DNA: correlation with nervous system-specific carcinogenesis by ethylnitrosourea. Proc Natl Acad Sci USA 71:639–643

Gunz D, Hess MT, Naegeli H (1996) Recognition of DNA adducts by human nucleotide excision repair. J Biol Chem 271:25089–25098

Hanawalt PC (1996) Role of transcription-coupled DNA repair in susceptibility to environmental carcinogenesis. Environ Health Perspect 104 Suppl 3:547–551

Hang B, Singer B, Margison GP, Elder RH (1997) Targeted deletion of alkylpurine-DNA-N-glycosylase in mice eliminates repair of $1,N^6$-ethenoadenine and hypoxanthine but not of $3,N^4$-ethenocytosine or 8-oxoguanine. Proc Natl Acad Sci USA 94:12869–12874

Harris CC (1989) Interindividual variation among humans in carcinogen metabolism, DNA adduct formation and DNA repair. Carcinogenesis 10:1536–1566

Heppner GH, Miller FR (1998) The cellular basis of tumor progression. Int Rev Cytol 177:1–56

Hickson ID (ed) (1997) Base excision repair of DNA damage. Landes Bioscience, Austin

Hoeijmakers JHJ, Bootsma D (1990) Molecular genetics of eukaryotic DNA excision repair. Cancer Cells 2:311–320

Huh N-H, Rajewsky MF (1988) Enzymatic elimination of O^6-ethylguanine from the DNA of ethylnitrosourea–exposed normal and malignant rat brain cells grown under cell culture versus in vivo conditions. Int J Cancer 41:76–766.

Karran P (1996) Microsatellite instability and DNA mismatch repair in human cancer. Semin Cancer Biol 7:15–24

Karran P, Bignami M (1994) DNA damage tolerance, mismatch repair and genome instability. Bioessays 16:833–839

Kass SU, Pruss D, Wolffe AP (1997) How does DNA methylation repress transcription? Trends Genet 13:444–449

Kaufmann WK, Paules RS (1996) DNA damage and cell cycle checkpoints. FASEB J 10:238–247

Kolodner RD (1997) DNA mismatch repair and cancer susceptibility. In: Fortner JG, Sharp PA (eds) Accomplishments in cancer research 1996. Lippincott - Raven, Philadelphia, pp 56–69

Kraemer KH (1997) Sunlight and skin cancer: another link revealed. Proc Natl Acad Sci USA 94:11–14

Krokan HE, Standal R, Slupphaug G (1997) DNA glycosylases in the base excision repair of DNA. Biochem J 325:1–16

Lee SM, Reid H, Elder RH, Thatcher N, Margison GP (1996) Inter- and intracellular heterogeneity of O^6-alkylguanine-DNA alkyltransferase expression in human brain tumors: possible significance in nitrosourea therapy. Carcinogenesis 17:637–641

Lengauer C, Kinzler KW, Vogelstein B (1997) DNA methylation and genetic instability in colorectal cancer cells. Proc Natl Acad Sci USA 94:2545–2550

Lindahl T, Sedgwick B, Sekiguchi M, Nakabeppu Y (1988) Regulation and expression of the adaptive response to alkylating agents. Annu Rev Biochem 57:133–157

Link CJ Jr, Burt RK, Bohr VA (1991) Gene-specific repair of DNA damage induced by UV irradiation and cancer chemotherapeutics. Cancer Cells 3:427–436

Loeb LA (1996) Many mutations in cancers. Cancer Sur 28:329–342

Lutz WK (1990) Endogenous genotoxic agents and processes as a basis of spontaneous carcinogenesis. Mutat Res 238:287–295

Maze R, Carney JP, Kelley MR, Glassner BJ, Williams DA, Samson L (1996) Increasing DNA repair methyltransferase levels via bone marrow stem cell transduction rescues mice from the toxic effects of 1,3-bis(chloroethyl)-1-nitrosourea, a chemotherapeutic alkylating agent. Proc Natl Acad Sci USA 93:206–210

Ménissier-de Murcia J, Niedergang CP, Trucco C, Ricoul M, Dutrillaux B, Mark M, Oliver FJ, Masson M, Dierich A, LeMeur M, Walztinger C, Chambon P, de Murcia G (1997) Requirement of poly(ADP-ribose) polymerase in recovery from DNA damage in mice and in cells. Proc Natl Acad Sci USA 94:7303–7307

Montesano R, Hall J, Wild CP (1992) Alkylating agents relating to carcinogenesis in man. In: D'Amato R, Slaga TJ, Farland WH, Henry C (eds) Relevance of animal studies to the evaluation of human cancer risk. Wiley-Liss, New York, pp 175–196

Moritz T, Mackay W, Glassner BJ, Williams D, Samson L (1995) Retrovirus-mediated expression of a DNA repair protein in bone marrow protects hematopoietic cells from nitrosourea-induced toxicity in vitro and in vivo. Cancer Res 55:2608–2614

Müller MR, Seiler F, Thomale J, Buschfort C, Rajewsky MF, Seeber S (1994) Capacity of individual chronic lymphatic leukemia lymphocytes and leukemic blast cells for repair of O^6-ethylguanine in DNA: Relation to chemosensitivity in vitro and treatment outcome. Cancer Res 54:4524–4531

Murata-Kamiya N, Kamiya H, Kaji H, Kasai H (1997) Glyoxal, a major product of DNA oxidation, induces mutations at G:C sites on a shuttle vector plasmid replicated in mammalian cells. Nucleic Acids Res 25:1897–1902

Naegeli HP (1994) Roadblocks and detours during DNA replication: mechanisms of mutagenesis in mammalian cells. Bioessays 16:557–564

Nakane H, Takeuchi H, Yuba S, Saijo M, Nakatsu Y, Murai H, Nakatsuru Y, Ishikawa T, Hirota S, Kitamura Y, Kato Y, Tsunoda Y, Miyauchi H, Horio T, Tokunaga T, Matsunaga T, Nikaido O, Nishimune Y, Okada Y, Tanaka K (1995) High incidence of ultraviolet-B- or chemical-carcinogen-induced skin tumours in mice lacking the xeroderma pigmentosum group A gene. Nature 377:165–168

Nakatsuru Y, Matsukuma S, Nemoto N, Sugano H, Sekiguchi M, Ishikawa T (1993) O^6-methylguanine-DNA methyltransferase protects against nitrosamine-induced hepatocarcinogenesis. Proc Natl Acad Sci USA 90:6468–6472

Neddermann P, Gallinari P, Lettieri T, Schmid D, Truong O, Hsuan JJ, Wiebauer K, Jiricny J (1996) Cloning and expression of human G/T mismatch-specific thymine-DNA glycosylase. J Biol Chem 271:12767–12774

Oda H, Zhang S, Tsurutani N, Shimizu S, Nakatsuru Y, Aizawa S, Ishikawa T (1997) Loss of p53 is an early event in induction of brain tumors in mice by transplacental carcinogen exposure. Cancer Res 57:646–650

Pegg AE (1990) Mammalian O^6-alkylguanine-DNA alkyltransferase: regulation and importance in response to alkylating carcinogens and therapeutic agents. Cancer Res 50:6119–6129

Preuss I, Eberhagen I, Haas S, Eibl RH, Kaufmann M, von Minckwitz G, Kaina B (1995) O^6-methylguanine-DNA methyltransferase activity in breast and brain tumors. Int J Cancer 61:321–326

Prolla TA, Abuin A, Bradley A (1996) DNA mismatch repair deficient mice in cancer research. Semin Cancer Biol 7:241–247

Rafferty JA, Hickson I, Chinnasamy N, Lashford LS, Margison GP, Dexter TM, Fairbairn LJ (1996) Chemoprotection of normal tissues by transfer of drug resistance genes. Cancer Metastasis Rev 15:365–383

Rajewsky MF (1972) Proliferative parameters of mammalian cell systems and their role in tumor growth and carcinogenesis. Z Krebsforsch 79:12–30

Reese JS, Ko ON, Lee K, Liu L, Allay JA, Phillips WP, Gerson SL (1996) Retroviral transduction of a mutant *MGMT* into human $CD34^+$ cells confers resistance to O^6-benzylguanine plus BCNU. Proc Natl Acad Sci USA 93:14088–14093

Sakumi K, Shiraishi A, Shimizu S, Tsuzuki T, Ishikawa T, Sekiguchi M (1997) Methylnitrosourea-induced tumorigenesis in MGMT gene knockout mice. Cancer Res 57:2415–2418

Sancar A (1996) DNA excision repair. Annu Rev Biochem 65:43–81

Sands AT, Abuin A, Sanchez A, Conti CJ, Bradley A (1995) High susceptibility to ultraviolet-induced carcinogensis in mice lacking XPC. Nature 377:162–165

Sedgwick B (1997) Nitrosated peptides and polyamines as endogenous mutagens in O^6-alkyguanine-DNA alkyltransferase deficient cells. Carcinogenesis 18:1561–1567

Seeberg E, Eide L, Bjoras M (1995) The base excision repair pathway. Trends Biochem Sci 20:391–397

Seiler F, Kirstein U, Eberle G, Hochleitner K, Rajewsky MF (1993) Quantification of specific DNA O-alkylation products in individual cells by monoclonal antibodies and digital imaging of intensified nuclear fluorescence. Carcinogenesis 14:1907–1913

Sies H (1986) Biochemistry of oxidative stress. Angew Chem [Int Ed] 25:1058–1071

Singer B, Grunberger D (1983) Molecular biology of mutagens and carcinogens. Plenum, New York

Singer B, Hang B (1997) What structural features determine repair enzyme specificity and mechanism in chemically modified DNA? Chem Res Toxicol 10:713–732

Singer B, Bodell WJ, Cleaver JE, Thomas GH, Rajewsky MF, Thon W (1978) Oxygens in DNA are main targets for ethylnitrosourea in normal and xeroderma pigmentosum fibroblasts and fetal rat brain cells. Nature 276:85–88

Skovsgaard T, Nielsen D, Maare C, Wassermann K (1994) Cellular resistance to cancer chemotherapy. Int Rev Cytol 156:77–157

Strauss BS (1977) Silent and multiple mutations in *p53* and the question of the hypermutability of tumors. Carcinogenesis 18:1445–1452

Sukumar S, Notario V, Martin-Zanka D, Barbacid M (1983) Induction of mammary carcinomas in rats by nitrosomethylurea involves malignant activation of H-ras-1 locus by single point mutations. Nature 306:658–661

Swenberg JA, Dyroff MC, Bedell MA, Popp JA, Huh N-H, Kirstein U, Rajewsky MF (1984) O^4-ethyldeoxythymidine, but not O^6-ethyldeoxyguanosine, accumulates in hepatocyte DNA of rats exposed continuously to diethylnitrosamine. Proc Natl Acad Sci USA 81:1692–1695

Thomale J, Huh N-H, Nehls P, Eberle G, Rajewsky MF (1990) Repair of O^6-ethylguanine in DNA protects rat 208F cells from tumorigenic conversion by N-ethyl-N-nitrosourea. Proc Natl Acad Sci USA 87:9883–9887

Thomale J, Hochleitner K, Rajewsky MF (1994a) Differential formation and repair of the mutagenic DNA alkylation product O^6-ethylguanine in transcribed and non-transcribed genes of the rat. J Biol Chem 269:1681–1686

Thomale J, Seiler F, Müller MR, Seeber S, Rajewsky MF (1994b) Repair of O^6-alkylguanines in the nuclear DNA of human lymphocytes and leukaemic cells: analysis at the single-cell level. Br J Cancer 69:698–705

Thomale J, Engelbergs J, Seiler F, Rajewsky MF (1996) Monoclonal antibody-based quantification and repair analysis of specific alkylation products in DNA. In: Pfeifer GP (ed) Technologies for detection of DNA damage and mutations. Plenum, New York, pp 87–101

Tu Y, Bates S, Pfeifer GP (1997) Sequence-specific and domain-specific DNA repair in xeroderma pigmentosum and Cockayne syndrome cells. J Biol Chem 272:20747–20755

Umar A, Kunkel TA (1996) DNA-replication fidelity, mismatch repair and genome instability in cancer cells. Eur J Biochem 238:297–307

Ushijima T, Morimura K, Hosoya Y, Okonogi H, Tatematsu M, Sugimura T, Nagao M (1997) Establishment of methylation-sensitive-representational difference analysis and isolation of hypo- and hypermethylated genomic fragments in mouse liver tumors. Proc Natl Acad Sci USA 94:2284–2289

Van der Horst GTJ, van Steeg H, Berg RJW, Morreau H, Beems RB, van Kreij CF, de Gruiji FR, Bootsma D, Hoeijmakers JHJ (1997) Defective transcription-coupled repair in Cockayne syndrome B mice is associated with skin cancer predisposition. Cell 89:425–435

Von Sonntag C (1987) The chemical basis of radiation biology. Taylor and Francis, London

Wahl GM, Linke SP, Paulson TG, Huang L-C (1997) Maintaining genetic stability through TP53 mediated checkpoint control. Cancer Surv 29:183–219

Wellinger RE, Thoma F (1997) Nucleosome structure and positioning modulate nucleotide excision repair in the non-transcribed strand of an active gene. EMBO J 16:5046–5056

White A, Kibitel J, Garcia Y, Belanich M, Yarosh D, Wideroff J, Levin L, Held D, Fuchs A, Citron M (1997) O^6-alkylguanine-DNA alkyltransferase in normal colon tissue and colon cancer. Oncol Res 9:149–153

Woloschak M, Yu A, Post KD (1997) Frequent inactivation of the *p16* gene in human pituitary tumors by gene methylation. Mol Carcinog 19:221–224

Wood RD (1996) DNA repair in eukaryotes. Annu Rev Biochem 65:135–167

Zeng-Rong N, Paterson J, Alpert L, Tsao M-S, Viallet J, Aloui-Jamali MA (1995) Elevated DNA repair capacity is associated with intrinsic resistance of lung cancer to chemotherapy. Cancer Res 55:4760–4764

Zingg J-M, Jones PA (1997) Genetic and epigenetic aspects of DNA methylation on genome expression, evolution, mutation and carcinogenesis. Carcinogenesis 18:869–882

Molecular Basis of DNA Repair Mechanisms and Syndromes

G. Weeda, J. de Boer, I. Donker, J. de Wit, S. B. Winkler,
G. T. J. van der Horst, W. Vermeulen, D. Bootsma, and J. H. J. Hoeijmakers

Department of Cell Biology and Genetics, Medical Genetic Centre,
Erasmus University, P.O. Box 1738, 3000 DR Rotterdam, The Netherlands

Introduction

Numerous chemical agents and various types of radiation (e.g. UV-light, X-rays) induce a wide range of lesions in DNA. Such damage can lead to changes in the nucleotide sequence varying from point mutations to gross chromosomal aberrations which can alter the expression or functioning of genes implicated in regulation of cell proliferation and differentiation, thereby forwarding the cell in the multistep process of carcinogenesis. To prevent these and other deleterious consequences of DNA injury, all living organisms are equipped with a complex network of DNA repair systems. One of the best studied repair processes is the nucleotide excision repair (NER) pathway which removes a wide diversity of DNA lesions including cyclobutane pyrimidine dimers and (6-4) photoproducts as well as chemical adducts and cross-links. In most – if not all – organisms two NER subpathways operate. One deals with the rapid and efficient removal of lesions that block transcription and thus need to be eliminated urgently (transcription-coupled repair, TCR). The other accomplishes the slower and less efficient global genome repair (GGR) of bulk DNA, including the nontranscribed strand of active genes.

Mutants and Diseases

Since the isolation of NER deficiency mutants in *E. coli*, a large number of eukaryotic mutants has been discovered. These were isolated in many species including yeast, *Drosophila*, rodent cell lines and humans. The collection of *Saccharomyces cerevisiae* NER mutants includes at least 14 different complementation groups, comprising the RAD3 epistasis group representing as many genes involved in NER (Friedberg et al. 1995). Similarly, a large number of mammalian NER mutants has been generated in the laboratory using rodent cell lines. Cell fusion experiments has identified a minimum of 11 complementation groups. By introducing human DNA into these rodent mutant cells the NER defect could be complemented. These genes were desig-

Recent Results in Cancer Research, Vol. 154
© Springer-Verlag Berlin · Heidelberg 1998

nated *ERCC* (for excision repair cross complementing) followed by the number of the rodent complementation group corrected by the human gene.

In humans the source of NER mutants is an interesting and still expanding group of rare genetic diseases characterized by hypersensitivity of the skin of patients to sunlight (UV) (Hoeijmakers 1993). The prototype DNA repair disorder is xeroderma pigmentosum (XP). Strongly reduced DNA-repair synthesis (the gap-filling step), demonstrating the NER defect, has been observed in situ in cultured cells from patients with XP by autoradiographically monitoring the incorporation of radioactive nucleotides. Complementation tests via cell fusion have demonstrated genetic heterogeneity within XP and provided evidence of at least seven excision-deficient complementation groups (XP-A to -G) implying the existence of as many distinct genes (Bootsma et al. 1997). Several of them have been shown to be similar to genes cloned by transfection of rodent cells. An NER defect was also found in two other rare inborn disorders: Cockayne syndrome (CS) (Nance and Berry 1990) and PIBIDS (Itin and Pittelkow 1990), the photosensitive form of brittle hair disease trichothiodystrophy (TTD). CS is represented by two complementation groups (CS-A and CS-B), whereas the NER defect of PIBIDS patients has been assigned to three complementation groups (XPB, XPD and TTD-A). In exceptional cases individuals display a combination of XP and CS or XP and TTD. These have been assigned to XP complementation groups B, D and G, indicating the molecular and connected clinical intricacy of mammalian NER. XP patients show, in addition to sun sensitivity, other cutaneous manifestations including pigmentation abnormalities and an over 2000-fold elevated frequency of skin cancer, often accompanied by progressive neurological degeneration. A different and much more severe type of neurologic dysfunction, namely, demyelination of neurons, is seen in CS. PIBIDS manifests essentially all of the CS symptoms and in addition two hallmarks of TTD: ichthyosis and brittle hair. The latter is due to a reduced content of cysteine-rich matrix proteins. In contrast to XP, CS and PIBIDS individuals do not appear to be particularly cancer-prone. Thus, a remarkable clinical heterogeneity is found to be associated with NER impairment.

Nucleotide Excission Repair Proteins and Excision of Damaged DNA

The XPA protein is thought to play an important role in damage recognition as it specifically binds to damaged DNA (Jones and Wood 1993), and interacts with RPA as well as with other DNA repair proteins including the structure-specific endonucleases XPG and the ERCC1 complex (consisting of XPF and ERCC1) and the basal transcription factor IIH (TFIIH). The multiprotein-containing complex TFIIH was first described as an essential factor required for the transcription of RNA polymerase II (RNAPII) genes (Gerard et al. 1991). This complex contains the DNA helicases XPB and XPD (Schaeffer et al. 1993, 1994). Microinjection and in vitro repair experiments with purified TFIIH as well as antibody depletions revealed that probably the entire complex is an integral part of the NER reaction. The bidirectional helicase activity of the complex has implicated TFIIH in a helix-opening step during both transcription initiation and NER. The complex consists of at least nine components, which have been cloned and characterized: XPB (p89, $3' \rightarrow 5'$ helicase), XPD (p80, $5' \rightarrow 3'$ helicase), p62, p52 (WD repeat), p44 (two Zn^{2+} fingers), p34 (Zn^{2+} finger) (Marinoni et la. 1997) and in addition the CAK subcomplex, harbouring CDK7 which was identified as the catalytic subunit of the kinase activity of TFIIH that is able to phosphorylate the COOH-terminal domain of the large subunit of RNA polymerase II. Interestingly, CDK7 also constitutes a separate trimeric kinase complex possibly involved in cell-cycle regulation together with the cyclin H and Mat1 subunits of TFIIH (Adamczewski et al. 1996). In order to investigate the function of TFIIH in NER, we developed a simplified purification scheme by generating stably transfected human and CHO cell lines containing functional tagged XPB. The affinity-purified TFIIH contains all the known components, as judged from immunoblots and corrects the repair defect of XPB, XPD and TTDA-deficient extracts in vitro (Winkler et al. 1998). Starting from repair-competent whole cell extracts fractionated under native conditions, we identified interactions of TFIIH with p53 and the human homologue of the yeast SUG1, a protein associated with the 26S proteasome and the RNA polymerase II holoenzyme. Interestingly, the interaction with hSUG1 was weakened by a XPB mutation, providing clues to some of the clinical manifestations of CS and TTD (Weeda et al. 1997a). Furthermore this suggests a link between TFIIH functioning and protein remodelling systems involving the proteosome machinery. In addition, we did not find any evidence of copurification of other significant quantities of NER and basal transcription activities. Obviously, these results do not rule out fragile or transient interactions.

During NER, TFIIH is thought to convert a recognized damaged site into a substrate for XPG (3' incision) and the XPF/ERCC1 (5' incision) structure-specific nucleases by locally opening DNA around a lesion allowing dual incision at some distance from the lesion (Fig. 1) (O'Donovan et al. 1997; Sijbergs et al. 1996). The gap is subsequently filled in by DNA polymerase δ and/or ε with the help of RPA, PCNA and RFC, and the newly synthesized DNA is ligated to the existing strand by DNA ligase I (Aboussekhra et al. 1995).

The above scheme of the NER reaction is still tentative and some pieces of the model are still missing. The XPE DNA-damage-binding protein (Chu and Chang 1988), (consisting of a heterodimer of 125 and 41 kDa) may have an accessory function in NER. A newly recognized and poorly defined activity, initiation factor (IF7) (Aboussekhra et al. 1995) is essential in the reconstituted in vitro NER reaction, but its composition is not known.

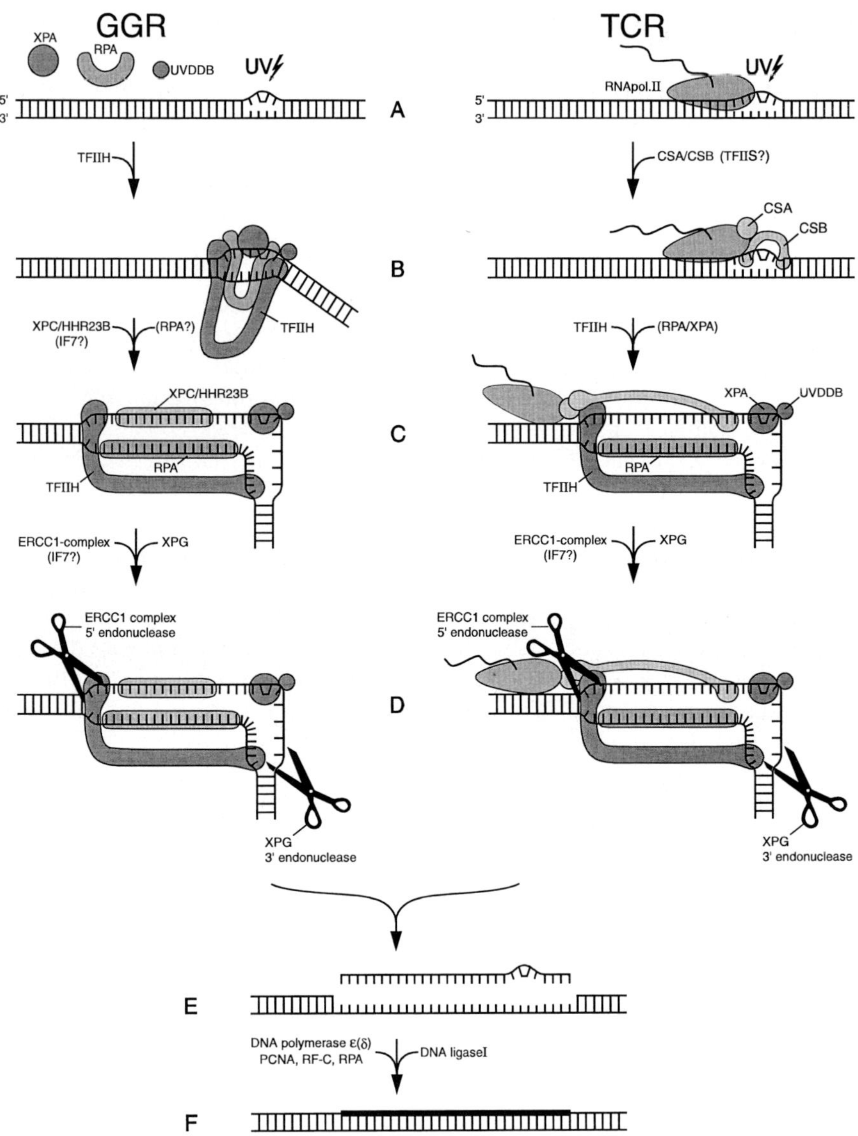

Fig. 1 A–F. Models of the two NER pathways, global genome repair (GGR) and transcription-coupled rapair (TCR) are shown. For an explanation of the mechanisms, see text

Transcription-Coupled Repair and Global Genome Repair

Although, in principle, NER acts on the entire genome, a profound heterogeneity exists in the efficiency with which at least some types of lesions are removed in different parts of the genome. Two subpathways of NER exist, a fast and efficient repair of lesions in the transcribed strand of RNAPII-driven genes and the slower repair of untranscribed DNA (Hanawalt et al. 1994). Interestingly, it turned out that this TCR pathway enhances only the repair of the transcribed strand of active genes, while the nontranscribed strand is repaired at a slower rate (Mellon et al. 1997). Damage recognition in the TCR pathway is probably performed by the elongating RNAPII complex itself. Since it is known that RNAPII stalls on UV-induced lesions (Donahue et al. 1994), this stalled RNAPII complex may serve as a substrate for the NER machinery. Both complementation groups of CS (CS-A and CS-B) exhibit deficient TCR but normal GGR. *CSB* encodes a putative ATPase belonging to the superfamily SWI/SNF helicases (Gorbalenya and Koonin 1993). CSA belongs to a protein family containing WD repeats (Henning et al. 1995). The WD repeats in CSA could serve to stabilize transient interactions between CSB and the stalled transcription complex. In addition, these domains, perhaps together with unidentified regions in CSB, may be involved in the transient interaction with the repair machinery, and thus stimulate repair of the lesion. Finally, the recently documented presence of CSB in an RNAPII complex is consistent with the idea that CS is in part due to impaired transcription (van Gool et al. 1997).

Most of the XP complementation groups are deficient in both TCR and GGR, except XP-C which has a proficient TCR mechanism and is unable to remove UV-induced pyrimidine dimers and (6-4) photoproducts from untranscribed sequences including the nontranscribed strand of active genes (Venema et al. 1991). Despite its specific role in GGR, the exact function of the XPC protein, which forms a heterodimer with the abundantly present HHR23B polypeptide (Matsutani et al. 1994), in NER is still unclear.

Nucleotide Excision Repair and Transcription Deficiency Syndromes

A specific correlation is apparent between TFIIH and the three NER-deficient complementation groups exhibiting the TTD features, XP-B, XP-D and TTD-A (van Vuuren et al. 1994; Vermeulen et al. 1994). The unexpected dual role of these proteins provided a rationale for the complex clinical features specifically associated with inherited defects in TFIIH that were difficult to explain solely on the basis of a NER defect, such as the combined XP/CS and TTD symptoms. This combined "repair/transcription" syndrome concept dissects the pleiotropic clinical features into those derived from a NER defect and those explained by a subtle transcription impairment. Some mutations in TFIIH may lead to only an affected NER function and thus explain the classical XP patients. Alternatively, other mutations may inactivate NER and

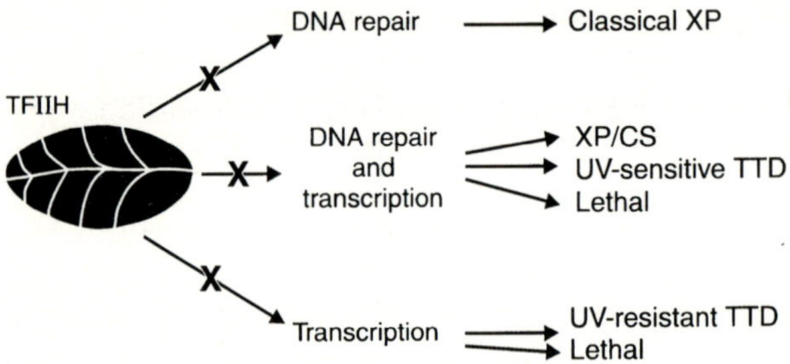

Fig. 2. Mutations in TFIIH components affect NER or basal transcription, or both processes. This results in the indicated inherited diseases, which can be categorized as repair, repair/transcription and transcription syndromes

concomitantly partly disrupt the transcription function giving rise to the combined XP/CS and photosensitive TTD patients (Fig. 2). Furthermore, this model provides an explanation for the category of TTD (and CS) patients in whom only the transcription function is slightly altered, without NER defects: such nonphotosensitive individuals harbour mutations that only cripple the transcription function of TFIIH. Recently, it was shown that TFIIH isolated from a lymphoblastoid cell of an XP-B (XP/CS) patient had reduced $3' \rightarrow 5'$ XPB-dependent helicase, DNA repair and basal transcription activity compared to wild-type cells (Huang et al. 1996). These data provide evidence for the proposed concept of repair/transcription syndromes.

Mouse Models for Human DNA Repair/Transcription Syndromes

To gain more insight into the complex genotype-phenotype relationship in these syndromes and the role of these proteins in preventing mutagenesis and carcinogenesis, we utilized gene targeting in ES-cells for the generation of repair-deficient mouse mutants.

The *ERCC1* gene specifically corrects rodent group 1 (mutant sensitive for UV and DNA cross-linking agents) and appears not to be involved in any of the known XP and CS complementation groups. For *ERCC1* homozygous knockout and a more subtle point mutant proved viable, although in both cases the frequency of –/– offspring was below Mendelian expectation. The homozygous mutant mice exhibit severe growth defects and have a reduced lifespan, the extent of which is dependent on the genetic background (Weeda et al. 1997 b). Pathological findings included absence of subcutaneous fat, striking polyploidy and chromatin abnormalities in liver and kidney as well as ferritin deposition in the spleen. These mice probably die as a consequence of liver failure. An important clue to the cause of the very severe *ERCC1*-mutant phenotypes is the finding that *ERCC1*-mutant cells undergo premature senescence, unlike cells from mice with a defect only in NER, such as $XPA^{-/-}$ mice (de Vries et al. 1995; Nakane et al. 1995). Importantly the latter mice, – like *ERCC1*$^{-/-}$ mice – are totally deficient in NER, yet fail to display many of the severe ERCC1 characteristics. This suggests that the ERCC1 features are not due to accumulation of NER lesions but may be caused by endogenously generated DNA interstrand cross-links which are normally repaired by ERCC1-dependent recombination repair. This probably underlies both the early onset of cell cycle arrest and polyploidy in the liver and kidney and highlights the role of ERCC1 and interstrand cross-links.

The *CSB* gene was shown to correct the repair defect in CS-B cells. It is involved in the repair of actively transcribed genes. Surprisingly, *CSB*-deficient mice showed only mild Cockayne syndrome features: minor developmental and neurological abnormalities. Repair studies with embryonic fibroblasts from *CSB*$^{-/-}$ mice revealed an increased UV sensitivity, normal global genome repair, defective transcription-coupled repair and impaired RNA synthesis recovery. However, contrary to the situation in CS, *CSB*-deficient mice showed increased cancer incidence following either UV-B or DMBA treatments (van der Horst et al. 1977). *XPC/CSB* double knockouts were severely runted, with disturbed gait and died early after birth.

To investigate the dual role of XPB, we have generated several mouse mutants that mimic a causative mutation found in the XP/CS patient XP11BE of XP group B. This mutation is a C → A transversion in the splice-acceptor site 4 bp upstream of the normal 3′ splice site of the very last exon (Weeda et al. 1990). Mimicking this mutation by inserting 4 bp in the last exon close to the splice site resulted in embryonic lethality in the mouse. In addition, we generated mice harbouring an extra splice acceptor site 4 bp in front of the normal 3′ splice sequence, more precisely reflecting the mutation in the human patient. In this case the most 5′ splice site is preferentially used in both embryonic stem cells and in mouse tissues, resulting in a COOH-terminal truncated XPB protein and a viable phenotype. These results establish the essential function of the XPB protein in mammals and in cellular viability and show that the COOH-terminal of XPB is essential for NER (Weeda et al., unpublished observations).

Recently, we generated a null allele for *XPD* in mice which proved to be embryonic lethal, which is consistent with its essential role in basal transcription (de Boer et al. 1998). In addition, we decided to mimic the causative XPD mutation of the photosensitive TTD1BEL patient in the mouse germline. Mice homozygous for the *XPD*^{TTD1BEL} mutation display many of the clinical symptoms of TTD, such as growth retardation, reduced lifespan, ichthyosis, reduced female fertility and UV sensitivity. Interestingly, homozygous mutant *XPD*^{TTD1BEL} mice have reduced hair specific cysteine-rich matrix proteins which normally cross-link the hair keratin filament. As a result the hair of *XPD*^{TTD1BEL} mice is brittle, mimicking the hallmarks of the human disorder. Finally, as in the case of *CSB* mice, *XPD*^{TTD1BEL} mice, in contrast to TTD patients, show increased susceptibility to skin cancer.

It is expected that the above mouse mutants will improve our understanding of the contribution of repair to mutagenesis, carcinogenesis, aging and neurodegeneration.

Acknowledgements. Research is supported by the Dutch Cancer Society, Netherlands Scientific Organisation (NWO) and Human Frontiers. The research of G.W. is supported by a fellowship of the Royal Netherlands Academy of Arts and Sciences.

References

Aboussekhra A, Biggerstaff M, Shivji MKK, Vilpo JA, Moncollin V, Podust VN, Protic M, Hubscher U, Egly J-M, Wood RD (1995) Mammalian excision repair reconstituted with purified components. Cell 80:859–868

Adamczewski JPA, Rossignol M, Tassan J-P, Nigg EA, Moncollin V, Egly J-M (1996) MAT1, cdk7 and cyclin H form a kinase complex which is UV light-sensitive upon association with TFIIH. EMBO J 15:1877–1884

Bootsma D, Kraemer KH, Cleaver JE, Hoeijmakers JHJ (1997) Nucleotide excision repair syndromes: xeroderma pigmentosum, Cockayne syndrome and trichothiodystrophy. In: Vogelstein B, Kinzler K (eds) The genetic basis of human cancer. McGraw-Hill, New York

Chu G, Chang E (1988) Xeroderma pigmentosum group E lacks a nuclear factor that binds to damaged DNA. Science 242:564–567

De Boer J, Donker I, de Wit J, Hoeijmakers JHJ, Weeda G (1998) Disruption of the mouse *XPD* DNA repair/basal transcription gene results in preimplantation lethality. Cancer Res 1998 (in press)

De Vries A, van Oostrom CThM, Hofhuis FMA, Dortant PM, Berg RJW, de Gruijl FR, Wester PW, van Kreijl CF, Capel PJA, van Steeg H, Verbeek SJ (1995) Increased susceptibility to ultraviolet-B and carcinogens of mice lacking the DNA excision repair gene *XPA*. Nature 377:169–173

Donahue BA, Yin S, Taylor J-S, Reines D, Hanawalt PC (1994) Transcript cleavage by RNA polymerase II arrested by a cylobutane pyrimidine dimer in the DNA template. Proc Natl Acad Sci USA 91:8502–8506

Friedberg EC, Walker GC, Siede W (1995) DNA repair and mutagenesis. ASM, Washington, DC

Gerard M, Fischer L, Moncollin V, Chipoulet M, Chambon P, Egly J-M (1991) Purification and interaction properties of the human RNA polymerase B (II) general transcription factor BTF2. J Biol Chem 266:20940–20945

Gorbalenya AE, Koonin EC (1993) Helicase: amino acid sequence comparison and structure-function relationships. Curr Biol 3:419–429

Hanawalt PC, Donahue BA, Sweder KS (1994) Collision or collusion? Curr Biol 4:518–521

Henning KA, Li L, Iyer N, McDaniel LD, Reagan MS, Legerski R, Schultz RA, Stefanini M, Lehmann AR, Mayne L, Friedberg EC (1995) The Cockayne syndrome group A gene encodes a WD repeat protein that interacts with CSB protein and a subunit of RNA polymerase II TFIIH. Cell 82:555–564

Hoeijmakers JHJ (1993) Nucleotide excision repair II: From yeast to mammals. Trends Genet 9:211–217

Huang JR, Moncollin V, Vermeulen W, Seroz T, van Vuuren H, Hoeijmakers JHJ, Egly J-M (1996) A $3' \rightarrow 5'$ XPB helicase defect in repair/transcription factor TFIIH of xeroderma pigmentosum group B affects both DNA repair and transcription. J Biol Chem 271: 15898–15904

Itin PH, Pittelkow MR (1990) Trichothiodystrophy: review of sulphur-deficient brittle hair syndromes and association with ectodermal dysplasias. J Am Acad Dermatol 22: 705–717

Jones CJ, Wood RD (1993) Preferential binding of xeroderma pigmentosum group A complementing protein to damaged DNA. Biochemistry 32:12096–12104

Marinoni J-C, Roy R, Vermeulen W, Miniou P, Lutz Y, Weeda G, Seroz T, Gomez DM, Hoeijmakers JHJ, Egly J-M (1997) Cloning and characterization of p52, the fifth subunit of the core of the transcription/DNA repair factor TFIIH. EMBO J 16:1093–1102

Masutani C, Sugasawa K, Yanagisawa J, Sonoyama T, Ui M, Enemoto T, Takio K, Tanaka K, van der Spek PJ, Bootsma D, Hoeijmakers JHJ, Hanaoka F (1994) Purification and cloning of a nucleotide excision repair complex involving the xeroderma pigmentosum group C protein and a human homologue of yeast RAD23. EMBO J 13:1831–1843

Mellon, I, Spivak G, Hanawalt PC (1997) Selective removal of transcription-blocking DNA damage from the transcribed strand of the mammalian *DHFR* gene. Cell 51:241–249

Nakane H, Takeuchi S, Yuba S, Saijo M, Nakatsu Y, Murai H, Nakatsuru Y, Ishikawa T, Hirota S, Kitamura Y, Kato Y, Tsunoda Y, Miyauchi H, Horio T, Tokunaga T, Matsunaga T, Nikaido O, Nishimune Y, Okada Y, Tanaka K (1995) High incidence of ultraviolet-B- or chemical-carcinogen-induced skin tumours in mice lacking the xeroderma pigmentosum group A gene. Nature 377:165–168

Nance NA, Berry SA (1992) Cockayne syndrome. Review of 140 cases. Am J Med Genet 42:68–84

O'Donovan A, Davies AA, Moggs J, West SC, Wood RD (1994) XPG endonuclease makes the 3′ incision in human DNA nucleotide excision repair. Nature 371:432 435

Schaeffer L, Roy R, Humbert S, Moncollin V, Vermeulen W, Hoeijmakers JHJ, Chambon P, Egly J-M (1993) DNA repair helicase: a component of BTF2(TFIIH) transcription factor. Science 260:58–63

Schaeffer L, Moncollin V, Roy R, Staub A, Mezzina M, Sarasin A, Weeda G, Hoeijmakers JHJ, Egly J-M (1994) The ERCC2/DNA repair protein is associated with the class II BTF2/TFIIH transcription factor EMBO J 13:2388–2392

Sijbers AM, de Laat WL, Ariza RR, Biggerstaff M, Wei YF, Moggs JG, Carter KC, Shell BK, Evans, de Jong MC, Rademakers S, de Rooij J, Jaspers NGJ, Hoeijmakers JHJ, Wood RD (1996) Xeroderma pigmentosum group F caused by a defect in a structure-specific DNA repair endonuclease. Cell 86:811–822

Van der Horst GTJ, van Steeg H, Berg RJW, van Gool AJ, de Wit J, Weeda G, Morreau H, Beems RB, van Kreijl CF, de Gruijl FR, Bootsma D, Hoeijmakers JHJ (1997) Defective transcription-coupled repair in Cockayne syndrome B mice is associated with skin cancer predisposition. Cell 89:425–435

Van Gool AJ, Citterio E, Rademakers S, van Os R, Vermeulen W, Constantinou A, Egly J-M, Bootsma D, Hoeijmakers JHJ (1997) The Cockayne syndrome B protein, involved in transcription-coupled DNA repair resides in an RNA polymerase II-containing complex. EMBO J 16:5955–5956

Van Vuuren AJ, Vermeulen W, Ma L, Weeda G, Appeldoorn E, Jaspers NGJ, van der Eb AJ, Bootsma D, Hoeijmakers JHJ, Humbert S, Schaeffer L, Egly J-M (1994) Correction of xeroderma pigmentosum repair defect by basal transcription factor BTF2 (TFIIH). EMBO J 13:1645–1653

Venema J, van Hoffen A, Karcagi V, Natarajan AT, van Zeeland AA, Mullenders LHF (1991) Xeroderma pigmentosum complementation group C cells remove pyrimidine selectively from the transcribed strand of active genes. Mol Cell Biol 11:4128–4134

Vermeulen W, van Vuuren AJ, Chipoulet M, Schaeffer L, Appeldoorn E, Weeda G, Jaspers NGJ, Priestley A, Arlett CF, Lehmann AR, Stefanini M, Mezzina M, Sarasin A, Bootsma D, Egly J-M, Hoeijmakers JHJ (1994) Three unusual repair deficiencies associated with transcription factor BTF2(TFIIH): evidence for the existence of a transcription syndrome. Cold Spring Harbor Symp Quant Biol 59:317–329

Weeda G, van Ham RCA, Vermeulen W, Bootsma D, van der Eb AJ, Hoeijmakers JHJ (1990) A presumed DNA helicase encoded by *ERCC-3* is involved in the human repair disorders xeroderma pigmentosum and Cockayne's syndrome. Cell 62:777–791

Weeda G, Rossignol M, Fraser RA, Winkler GS, Vermeulen W, van't Veer LJ, Ma L, Hoeijmakers JHJ, Egly J-M (1997a) The XPB subunit of repair/transcription factor TFIIH directly interacts with SUG1, a subunit of the 26S proteasome and putative transcription factor. Nucleic Acids Res 25:2274–2283

Weeda G, Donker I, de Wit J, Morreau H, Janssens R, Vissers CJ, Nigg A, van Steeg H, Bootsma D, Hoeijmakers JHJ (1997b) Disruption of the mouse *ERCC1* results in a novel repair syndrome with growth failure, nuclear abnormalities and senescence. Curr Biol 7:427–439

Winkler SB, Vermeulen W, Coin F, Egly J-M, Hoeijmakers JHJ, Weeda G (1998) Affinity purification of human DNA repair/transcription factor TFIIH using epitope tagged XPB protein. J Biol Chem (in press)

The Ataxia Telangiectasia Gene in Familial and Sporadic Cancer

M. A. R. Yuille and L. J. A. Coignet

Institute for Cancer Research, Academic Department of Haematology
and Cytogenetics, Haddow Laboratories, 15 Cotswold Road, Sutton,
Surrey SM2 5NG, UK

Abstract

The ataxia telangiectasia (A-T) gene, *ATM*, predisposes affected homozygotes to a wide range of malignancies. It has been suggested that this is a consequence of the genomic instability associated with the syndrome. The elevated risk of malignancy is not, however, observed among A-T heterozygotes (except, apparently, regarding breast cancer). In this report we describe results from the study of the rare sporadic disease, T cell prolymphocytic leukaemia (T-PLL). In all individuals tested, we observed that at least one *ATM* allele was disrupted by rearrangement, that in many cases both alleles were disrupted and that there were additional mutations, predominantly missense, that clustered toward the 3′ end of the gene corresponding to the protein's phosphatidylinositol 3-kinase (PIK)-related domain. We conclude that the *ATM* gene can act as a tumour suppressor in the development of sporadic T-PLL. Our finding of a surfeit of mutations within *ATM* may reflect the involvement of the gene at more than one step in tumorigenesis. In particular, we suggest that the clustering of missense mutations may pertain to the late-onset character of both sporadic and A-T-related T-PLL, since the closest homologue of Atm protein is the yeast TEL1 protein that maintains telomere length. *ATM* inactivation may not be the initiating event in T-PLL tumorigenesis: prior mutation of another gene – perhaps *TCL1* activation – may be obligate. This would explain the recessive character of T-PLL risk in A-T.

Introduction

The theme of this volume is the role of the environment in cancer. This chapter is concerned, in particular, with defective DNA repair as a mediator of increased cancer risk. However, we shall be arguing that defective DNA repair due to inactivation of both copies of the ataxia telangiectasia (A-T) gene is not the major cause of an elevated risk of a haematological malignancy in A-T. Moreover, rather than suggest that the external environment is of signif-

Recent Results in Cancer Research, Vol. 154
© Springer-Verlag Berlin · Heidelberg 1998

icance to a sporadic leukaemia involving the A-T gene, we shall instead speculate that the "internal environment" may play a role in this malignancy.

The A-T Gene

The first clinical description of ataxia telangiectasia (A-T) appeared in 1926 (Syllaba and Henner 1926). The second better known one by Madame Denise Louis-Bar, appeared in 1941. She described a 9-year-old Belgian boy with progressive cerebellar ataxia and telangiectasiae of the skin and conjunctivae. In 1957, a simple recessive mendelian inheritance was proposed and the disease was named ataxia telangiectasia (Boder and Sidgwick 1958). As well as neurological abnormalities and progeric changes, the condition was associated with abnormal development (including athymia), radiosensitivity, cell cycle abnormalities, cancer predisposition and immunological abnormalities (including hypogammaglobulinemia, selective deficiency of serum IgA and IgE, abnormalities of IgG subclasses, depressed blastogenic response, faulty development or complete absence of the thymus, failure to produce virus-specific histocompatibility-restricted cytotoxic T lymphocytes and an overall poor response to skin test allergens). More features of this disease were described as antibiotics were discovered that helped patients shake off their frequent infections. One of these, seen in older patients, was a rapidly progressive leukaemia with a mature T cell immunophenotype and a preceding relatively stable T cell lymphocytosis, both with characteristic cytogenetic abnormalities (Taylor et al. 1996). It is this mature T cell leukaemia and a similar sporadic disease that will mostly concern us here.

The A-T trait was mapped (Gatti et al. 1988) to chromosome 11q23 in 1988, leading to the cloning in 1995 by Savitsky et al. (1995a) of the 66 exon gene – called *ATM* for A-T-mutation – encoding a large 350 kDa protein. Its -COOH terminal is homologous to a group of phosphatidyl-3 kinases and the closest homologue is the *TEL 1* gene of *S. cerevisiae* that controls telomere length and chromosome integrity. Upstream of this is a region of homology to three genes in yeast and *D. melanogaster (MEC1, rad3* and *mei-41)* that all share a property: arrest at G2 in the cell cycle after DNA damage (Savitsky et al. 1995b). Recently the 146 kb of genomic *ATM* sequence was published by workers from Jena here in Germany (Platzer et al. 1997). Most A-T mutations so far described – and there are over 100 apparently randomly distributed throughout the gene (see the *ATM* mutation database at http://www.vmmc.org/vmrc/atm.htm) – result in truncation of the ATM protein (Fig. 1). These data have opened up new vistas for research into A-T, into the cellular function of the protein and into sporadic diseases in which the gene is implicated. We shall focus on the relationship between *ATM* and cancer.

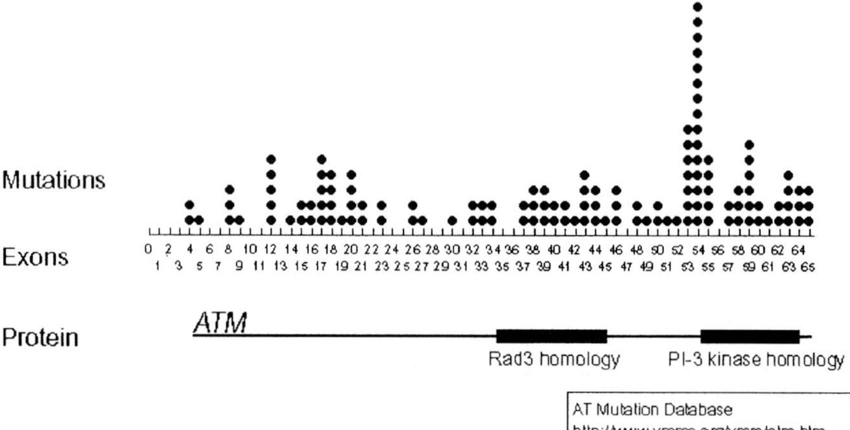

Fig. 1. The distribution of reported A-T mutations is shown. *Circles* above the *numbered line* representing the exons of *ATM* identify the exon location of mutations. Each *circle* represents a report and hence the same mutation is in some instances shown more than once. Homology domains in the protein are identified at *bottom*

A-T and Cancer

Complete autopsy reports (Hecht and Hecht 1990) on over 100 A-T patients revealed that the two leading causes of death were pulmonary disease and cancer, with cancers present in 47% of autopsies. Many of the neoplasms recorded in A-T patients have been collated at the Immunodeficiency Cancer Registry and these are summarised in Table 1. This reveals that mutation of both *ATM* alleles predisposes A-T individuals at a young age to a wide range of neoplasms. These are rarely observed in corresponding normal individuals, or, indeed, in A-T heterozygotes. Among female A-T heterozygotes there is an elevated risk of breast cancer, ranging from an odds ratio of 2.9 (CI 1.1–7.6) for onset before 60 years to an odds ratio of 6.4 (CI 1.4–28.8) for onset 60-plus (Athma et al. 1996). Note that only one A-T homozygote breast cancer case was reported to the Immunodeficiency Cancer Registry. Linkage studies in breast cancer families have excluded the A-T locus (Wooster et al. 1993). For all other cancers, the situation is less clear: in A-T families, the relative risk of all other cancers has been calculated (Easton 1994) at 1.9 (CI 1.5–2.5), but this data is inhomogeneous, with European studies showing no evidence of any excess risk.

Many of the Registry A-T patients had multiple neoplasms, most commonly non-Hodgkin's lymphoma (NHL). In a study of UK A-T patients (Taylor et al. 1996), 17 haematological malignancies were observed of which eight were NHL. Of these, five were T-NHL and three were B-NHL. Since T-NHL is rarer than B-NHL in the general population it would appear that while all NHL is elevated in A-T, the risk of T-NHL is even greater. Among

Table 1. Neoplasms in A-T patients

Type of Neoplasm	N	%
Non-Hodgkin's lymphoma	49	41
Solid tumours Brain (3); breast(1); GI (11); laryngeal (1); liver (2); ovarian (5); parotid (1); skin (4); uterine (3)	32	27
Leukaemia ALL (20); acute leukaemia (4); subacute lymphocytic leukaemia (1); chronic lympho- blastic leukaemia (2) Hodgkin's disease	26 12	22 10
Total	119	100

the five acute leukaemias reported, four were T-ALL and one was of mixed lineage. The mean life expectancy of A-T patients is about 17 years but the mature T cell leukaemia we shall consider here has an average age of onset of over 30 years. It is thus an infrequent cause of death among A-T patients as a whole. This prevalence of T cell malignancy is of special interest in light of the frequent athymia of A-T patients.

Theories on the Role of *ATM* in Tumorigenesis

It appears that one mutated copy of the *ATM* gene in the germline predisposes to breast cancer and two mutated copies predispose to a variety of solid tumours and lymphoproliferative diseases. This is rather a puzzling picture. Other cancer predisposition syndromes – be it the well-known conditions such as familial retinoblastoma or Li-Fraumeni syndrome or the various mutator genes implicated in cancer families – show a simple dominant mode of inheritance. An idea (Hecht and Hecht 1990) that began to address this problem is that there might be more than one way that *ATM* is linked to cancer, with one copy predisposing to solid tumours and two mutated copies predisposing to solid and haematological tumours. Knudson (1971) who proposed the two-hit hypothesis defining dominant tumour suppressors, has suggested that, as far as breast cancer is concerned, *ATM* may be classified as a dominant cancer gene (Knudson 1997). This however avoids the issue of cancer predisposition in A-T patients.

However, the favoured view of the role of *ATM* in tumorigenesis has been based on the early observation (Hecht et al. 1966) of chromosomal instability in A-T cells. The observation has been replicated by many other groups and has led implicitly and also, more recently, explicitly (Bebb et al. 1997) to the proposition that *ATM* is a mutator gene: loss of *ATM* function is said to result in a chromosomal instability that is characterised by frequent chromosomal aberrations. Some of these may affect the function of genes involved in tumorigenesis. Hence the frequency of cancer is elevated. This model is not however entirely satisfactory:

1. With the mutator genes *MSH2* and *MLH1* that have been described in hereditary nonpolyposis colon cancer (HNPCC), the total number of DNA errors per genome is very great: inactivation of these genes yields a phenotype that includes somatic microsatellite instability in noncoding DNA. Only a small number of microsatellites need to be examined for a somatic mutation to be detected. Hence the total number of errors arising is very large. But in A-T, no microsatellite instability has been reported: the syndrome is characterised by cells that fairly frequently have complex karyotypes with perhaps 20 breakpoints. This makes breakages less frequent than errors of replication in HNPCC and thus may well reduce the relative risk of mutating a cancer gene.

2. The common chromosomal aberrations seen in A-T cells can be regarded as especially labile genomic regions according to the mutator hypothesis. But they could also be indicators of precancerous states. Where such aberrations have been cloned (as at 14q32.1), the latter explanation has been favoured.

3. There is good evidence of cell cycle defects in A-T (see below) and hence the mutator hypothesis at least requires modification.

4. The different patterns of malignancy between A-T homozygotes and heterozygotes are explicable by considering tissue-specific effects of constitutive *ATM* expression in regulation of the cell cycle. But these patterns are much harder to explain based on the mutator hypothesis.

5. The mutator hypothesis does not readily explain different patterns of chromosome breakage in different A-T tissues. Lymphocytes and fibroblasts have different patterns of breakage while bone marrow samples show no chromosomal abnormalities (Hecht et al. 1973; Al Saadi et al. 1980; Cohen et al. 1975). The chromosomal breakages seen in A-T T cells are highly nonrandom since they commonly involve the T cell receptor loci on chromosomes 7 and 14. A-T B cell translocations commonly involve immunoglobulin loci on chromosomes 2, 22 and 14. Such nonrandomness is at variance with a general mutator hypothesis. The other main cytogenetic abnormality suggesting chromosomal instability is the prevalence in both lymphocytes and fibroblasts of telomeric fusions (Kojis et al. 1989). Telomeric fusions are also found in A-T T cell clonal lymphocytoses (Metcalfe et al. 1996) (suggesting that the mutations that give rise to the lymphocytosis do not rescue telomere integrity). However, the disease of which these clones are a precursor – a mature T cell leukaemia (see below) – do not have telomeric fusions. Hence rescue of telomeric integrity is a step in progression toward T-PLL. Thus progression involves suppression of at least one aspect of *ATM* inactivation. The mutator hypothesis can only explain this with difficulty. There is probably much significance in telomeric fusions of A-T because of the high degree of homology between the 3′ end of the *ATM* cDNA and the yeast *TEL1* gene. Mutation of this gene reduces telomere length, and, just like *ATM* inactivation (Meyn

1993), elevates aneuploidy and recombination rates (Greenwell et al. 1995). Note that an elevated frequency of legitimate recombination may contribute to specific steps in tumorigenesis (e.g. where one allele only is normally methylated).

6. The mutator hypothesis may require an additional postulate (Bridges and Harnden 1981): that A-T involves faulty recombinase activity. Cloning of chromosomal breakpoints in A-T T cells has usually identified consensus sequences implicating recombinase-mediated events (Mengle-Gaw et al. 1987, 1988; Russo et al. 1989; Baer et al 1987; Davey et al. 1988). But in vitro assays suggest that A-T cell extracts are associated with a distinct pattern of DNA misrepair (Thacker 1994) that has no obvious relationship to recombinase activity. Thus the postulate is not supported.

7. The observation of chromosomal abnormalities in A-T cells need not implicate *ATM* inactivation as the sole, immediate cause of those abnormalities. Rather the absence of *ATM* may select for the chromosomal abnormality. For example, in A-T stable T cells with inv(14)(q11;q32) or t(14;14)(q11;q32) are elevated 50-fold over their frequency in normal individuals (Aurias et al. 1980). For the record, smaller transient lymphocytoses with inv(7) and t(7;14) clones have also been reported in normal and in A-T (Aurias 1981)

The mutator hypothesis is thus an incomplete description of the role of *ATM* in tumorigenesis. A key test of the mutator hypothesis is whether the gene is occasionally mutated in sporadic cancers. The microsatellite instability phenotype is certainly observed sporadically at varying frequencies. But it has not been observed – nor would the mutator hypothesis predict that it would – in all cases of a sporadic malignancy. Let us now turn to these malignancies.

Sporadic Cancers and *ATM*

Based on the frequency of breast cancer among A-T heterozygotes, some 10% of sporadic breast cancers were predicted (Easton 1994) to involve *ATM* and with the cloning of gene this has now been investigated. Early onset breast cancers and those with loss of heterozygosity at 11q23 showed no truncating or point mutations (FitzGerald et al. 1997; Vorechovsky et al. 1996a). Breast cancer in families also manifesting haematological malignancies showed no nucleotide changes (Vorechovsky et al. 1996b). This of course immediately raises the question as to whether these are the appropriate risk groups to examine.

However, positive results have been obtained for some of the malignancies seen in A-T homozygotes. We have reported, so far, on two sporadic malignancies: B-NHL and T-prolymphocytic leukaemia (T-PLL) (Yuille et al. 1996a, 1998; Vorechovsky et al. 1997) and these reports have been confirmed by others for T-PLL (Stilgenbauer et al. 1997).

The reason for examining NHL is obvious: it is common among A-T patients. T-PLL is far less frequent in A-T but nonetheless the risk is substantially elevated compared with the normal population. It is a rare sporadic leukaemia of cells with a mature T cell phenotype that is highly aggressive (mean survival: 7 months) (Matutes et al. 1991), and our clinical colleagues at the Royal Marsden Hospital and their collaborators have shown (Pawson et al. 1997) that the disease responds well to a monoclonal antibody, CAMPATH-1H, directed at the cell surface antigen CD52. Antigen-CD52 antibodies activate resting rat T cells via a Ca^{2+}-dependent signal transduction pathway (Rowan et al. 1995). It is worth investigating whether CAMPATH binds to CD52 to cause apoptosis (rather than complement-mediated lysis) via this pathway, since: (1) T-PLL is exquisitely sensitive to CAMPATH-1H; (2) B cell tumour lines undergo Ca^{2+}-dependent apoptosis when the pathway is inhibited (Bonnefoyberard et al. 1994); (3) the pathway includes genes that are homologues of the ataxia telangiectasia gene (Brown et al. 1994).

Our colleagues at the Marsden noted, some years ago, (Brito-Babapulle and Catovsky 1991), the striking cytogenetic and immunophenotypic similarity between T-PLL first described by workers including Profs. David Galton and Daniel Catovsky – who has been collecting for two decades the samples we have now studied (Catovsky et al. 1973; Galton et al. 1974); and the mature T cell leukaemia found in older A-T patients. This indirect evidence implicates the *ATM* gene in T-PLL, as summarised in Table 2. The differences between the two diseases are: (1) The risk of disease is greater for A-T homozygotes than for the general population. (2) A lower age of onset is indicated in A-T homozygotes than in the population. (3) We observed in the sporadic disease breakpoints at chromosome 11q23 – where *ATM* maps – but this has not been reported in A-T-related mature T cell leukaemia. This latter observation encouraged us to consider *ATM* as a candidate gene in T-PLL. We had previously examined other genes in this chromosome band impli-

Table 2. Mature T cell leukaemia in A-T patients and sporadic T-PLL

Property	A-T mature T-cell leukaemia	T-PLL
Age of onset	34 years (8 patients)	66 years (85 patients)
CD1a–	4/4	100%
CD3+	5/5	100%
CD4+	2/5	63%
CD8+	4/7	10%
CD4+/CD8+	2/5	26%
TdT–	2/2	100%
11q23 breakpoint	0/8	10%
14q32 breakpoint	5/8	76%
Xq28 breakpoint	2/8	5%
Trisomy 8q	2/8	67%

A-T, ataxia telangiectasia; T-PLL, T cell prolymphocytic leukaemia.

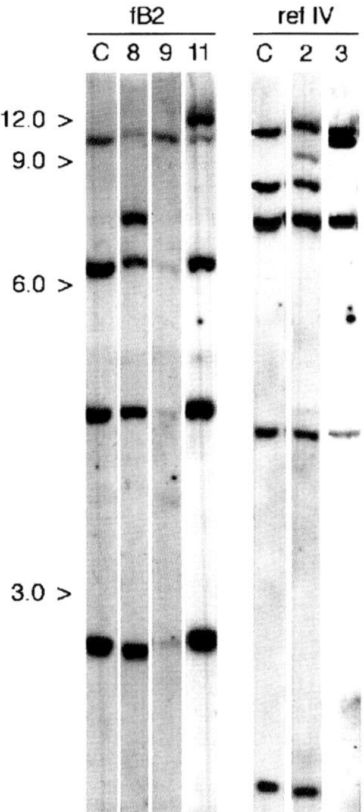

Fig. 2. Southern blots were prepared with restricted DNA from a panel of 20 T-PLL samples (identified by *sample number* above each lane) and a healthy volunteer *(C* above lane) and probed with cDNA probes fB2 (spanning exons 27–31) and reflV (spanning exons 56–65). Representative rearrangements are shown for samples 2, 3, 8, 9 and 11. The multiple bands seen with cDNA probes often make difficult the detailed interpretation of the rearrangements. Samples 2 and 3 were also examined by Fibre FISH (see text)

cated in lymphoproliferative disorders – *PLZF* and *MLL* among others – but had no indication of their involvement (Yuille et al. 1996b). The search for a gene on 11q23 started before *ATM* was cloned and so relied on nearby sequence-tagged sites as probes on Southern blots. Rearrangements were detected in two cases: one with D11S384 (which maps immediately centromeric of *ATM)*, and another with a probe for the transcription cofactor *BOB-1* (which we showed maps immediately telomeric of *ATM)*. This approach, however, was overtaken by the positional cloning of the *ATM* gene (Savitsky et al. 1995a). Using cDNA probes we then identified rearrangements in one in four of 20 T-PLL samples (Fig. 2). The use of cDNA probes involves numerous problems of interpretation and when we observed cases with highly complex patterns of rearrangement, we decided it was necessary to use a technique that could give a complete overview of the 150 kb *ATM* gene.

We examined a smaller panel of seven T-PLL samples by fibre FISH (Yuille et al. 1996a, 1998). In this technique, DNA fibres are released from tumour cells on glass slides and the fibres stretched out by gravity prior to hybridisation using, in our case, four fluorochrome-labeled cosmids spanning the *ATM* locus. We discovered that all the cases had at least one lesion disrupting the locus (Fig. 3). It was difficult to escape the conclusion that the gene is usually a target for mutation in T-PLL. It is rather rare to identify a gene mutated in all cases of a sporadic disease and it implies, of course, that

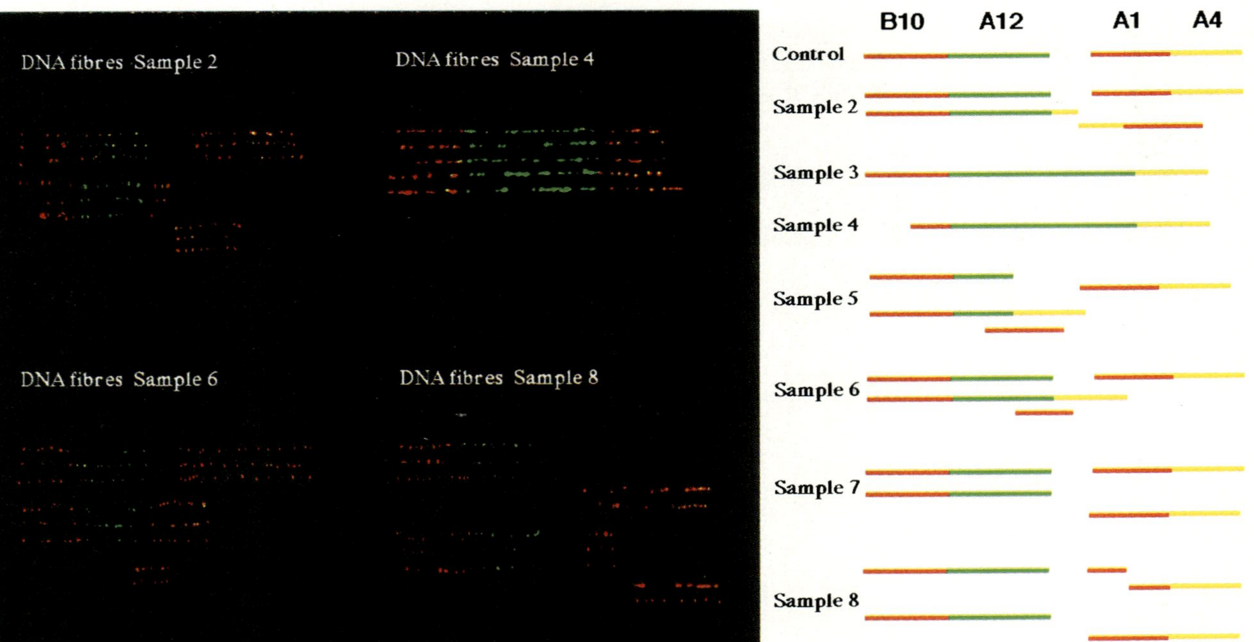

Fig. 3. At *left* are shown DNA fibres from T-PLL samples 2, 4, 6 and 8 hybridised with cosmids B10, A12, A1 and A4 that span most of the *ATM* gene and that had been labeled with *red, green, red* and *yellow* fluorochromes, respectively. At *right* is a cartoon showing the rearrangements in these and three other T-PLL samples, based on an interpretation of the staining pattern and lengths of stained regions of their DNA fibres

the gene is crucial to the pathogenesis of the disease. By definition, this is not the case for a mutator gene. In four of the seven cases neither allele was intact. Close inspection of the DNA fibres indicated that in some cases more than one event had occurred. For example, in case 2 (Fig. 3, left) we deduced that an intragenic inversion had occurred followed by a translocation-type event. In case 4 (Fig. 3, left), one allele appeared to be lost entirely and on the other there was an apparent deletion at the centromeric end of the gene, a probable duplication event had occurred more distally and a transposition was inferred distal of that. Thus one allele had undergone at least three separate events involving a minimum of five breakages. Consideration of the limited resolution of the technique leaves open the possibility that the apparently intact alleles contained cryptic abnormalities. We were concerned that these multiple events might not be restricted to the *ATM* region; but no abnormalities were found when we examined a region of the genome not implicated in T-PLL using another cosmid contig from the *ETV-6* gene on chromosome 12. Therefore these multiple lesions appeared to be specific to the *ATM* gene in T-PLL.

Three of the cases had one intact *ATM* allele, but was that allele expressed? To test this, we also performed, in collaboration with Prof S. P. Jackson (Cambridge UK), a western blot with anti-ATM antibody (Lakin et al. 1996) (corresponding to consecutive exons in cosmids A1 and A4, as shown in Fig. 3, right) and found that two of these three lacked an *ATM* band. Thus in six of seven cases there was good evidence that both *ATM* alleles were inactivated.

Could the final case with one intact *ATM* allele have acquired (or even inherited) a missense mutation that led to inactivation without loss of protein? We performed exon-scanning using single-strand conformation polymorphism (SSCP) mutation detection, in collaboration with Dr. Igor Vorechovsky (Karolinska Institute, Sweden), with PCR primers spanning each of the coding exons of the gene (exons 3–65) and identified in this final case a homozygous nucleotide change in exon 44 in the *rad3* domain. This change was acquired, since it was absent from a germline sample (evidence from other cases indicated that all nucleotide changes were acquired). The change had not been reported as a polymorphism (nor has any other change we detected subsequently, see below). We concluded that *ATM* was mutated on both alleles in all the cases of T-PLL examined. Therefore the sporadic disease, T-PLL, is as commonly mutated at *ATM* as is the A-T-related mature T cell leukaemia: the two diseases are nearly indistinguishable both by phenotype and at the molecular level. Moreover, such frequent *ATM* inactivation in T-PLL is not predicted by the mutator hypothesis on the mode of action of ATM in causing cancer susceptibility. Rather, it points to *ATM* acting as a type of tumour suppressor, consistent with its known effects in relieving cell cycle checkpoints (Meyn 1995).

In the panel of seven cases examined by fibre FISH we also found two other missense mutation, both at exons in the 3′ end of the cDNA in the so-called kinase domain of *ATM*. A fourth case had a deletion that removed a splice site and was predicted to lead to truncation. All four nucleotide changes showed loss of the wild-type allele: there was a reduction to homozygosity. Note, however, that the two cases with one remaining intact allele and with no detectable *ATM* protein had no nucleotide change. This may be due to the limited sensitivity of SSCP, to an event proximal or distal to exons 3 and 65 or to an epigenetic event (e.g. examination of the mutational spectrum of A-T mutations [see the *ATM* mutation database at http://www.vmmc.org/vmrc/atm.htm] indicates that C→T transitions are the most common type of point mutation, consistent with mutation by deamination of methyl cytosine and thus implying that *ATM* is methylated).

Both *ATM* alleles were mutated in the seven cases examined. But why did a single allele so often contain more than one breakpoint? Why were nucleotide changes present when the allele was also disrupted by one or more breakages? Why was there a reduction to homozygosity when the DNA fibres showed the presence of two distinct alleles? In other words, why was there an apparent surfeit of mutations?

One possibility was that the nucleotide changes we had observed were actually rare in T-PLL. To test this, we examined, in collaboration with Dr. I. Vorechovsky (Karolinska Institute, Sweden), a panel of 37 T-PLL cases (Vorechovsky et al. 1997). Nearly half (46%, 17 samples) showed nucleotide changes (Table 3). In all except three, the wild-type allele was absent. Five cases showed truncating mutations (in exons 15, 30, 40, 55 and 65). Three were mutations reported as A-T mutations and two cases had the same point mutation. Two cases had more than one mutation (a frameshift plus a downstream missense mutation). But the major observation was the clustering of 15 out of 23 nucleotide changes (30% of all T-PLL cases) in the 3′ end of the gene: in the domain most closely homologous to *TEL1* in yeast. Thus, not only are point mutations present in a third of all T-PLL cases, but their distribution suggests impairment of a specific function of the gene. (Note that among the 35 B-NHLs tested, three had point mutations, one of which was in the *TEL1* domain. This indicates the need to test a large panel of NHL cases.)

The clustering of mutations implies a defect in the function of the *TEL1* domain. If this domain controls telomere integrity in humans as in yeast, then we may imagine that a function of *ATM* is to switch between progression of the cell cycle (when telomere integrity is confirmed) and delay or death (when it is not). The choice between delay and death could be determined by the actual length of telomeres. These shorten with age, leading telomere fusions and correlating with aneuploidy and senescence (death) (Norrback and Roos 1997). In A-T, this is more pronounced (Metcalfe et al. 1996). Moreover, late onset is observed in both sporadic T-PLL (at 66 years) and A-T-related T-PLL [at 34 years (Taylor et al. 1996), twice the mean survival of A-T homozygote]. Thus T-PLL may be a disease of old age because it requires age-compromised telomeres as a starting condition. In other words, T-PLL may be favoured by a change in the "internal environment", i.e. by ageing.

Table 3. *ATM* nucleotide changes in sporadic T-PLL and B-NHL

Sample	*ATM* exon	Nucleotide change	Wild-type allele (%)	Protein change
T-PLL				
5b3	15	2119delTCTGA	0	Frameshift
1c8	30	4174insC	0	Frameshift
5b3	30	4220T → C	20	I1407T
1b8	36	5044G → C	0	D1682H
1b2	40	5729T → A	15	L1910H
5	40	5763-22del31	0	Splice site loss
6	44	6116A → G	0	E2139G
1d4	47	6490G → A	0	E2164K
1c8	51	7187C → G	0	T2396S
1c10	51	7271T → G	0	V2424G
1a9	52	7325A → C	0	Q2442P
1d5	54	7636del9	0	S2546del, R2547del, I2548del
6c4	55	7880insT	25	Frameshift
1a8	57	8084G → C	0	G2695A
1b4	58	8165T → G	0	L2722R
1b7	58	8174A → T	10	D2725V
5a6	58	8194T → C	0	F2732L
t1a5	60	8430delAAA	50	K2810del
1a1	61	8613delACA	50	R2871S, H2872del
6b1	61	8668C → G	40	L2890V
3	61	8668C → G	0	L2890V
BJ01	65	9139C → T	0	R3047X
4	65	9022C → T	0	R3008C
B-NHL				
NHL20	23	3118A → G	0	M1040V
NHL34	31	4387T → C	10	F1463S
G519	60	8494C → T	45	R2832C

ATM, ataxia telangiectasia gene; T-PLL, T cell prolymphocytic leukaemia, B-NHL, B non-Hodgkin's lymphoma.

Impairment of the *ATM TEL1* domain's function cannot constitute the sole role of the gene in T-PLL tumorigenesis since our fibre FISH results indicate that complete *ATM* inactivation due to rearrangement is also common. So, if *ATM* is involved at two distinct steps in T-PLL tumorigenesis, the first might require impairment and the second loss of all *ATM* function. Logically, this imposes an order on events: the point mutation would arise first and the re-arrangements second.

However, there is also a need to explain the recessive character of T-PLL in A-T families: no case of T-PLL has been reported among A-T heterozygotes, yet there is a substantial risk of T-PLL in A-T homozygotes. Why does the presence of a single mutated *ATM* allele in an A-T heterozygote not lead to any detectable risk of T-PLL? Other cancer predisposition syndromes, such as familial retinoblastoma or Li-Fraumeni disease, show a dominant

Sporadic T-PLL

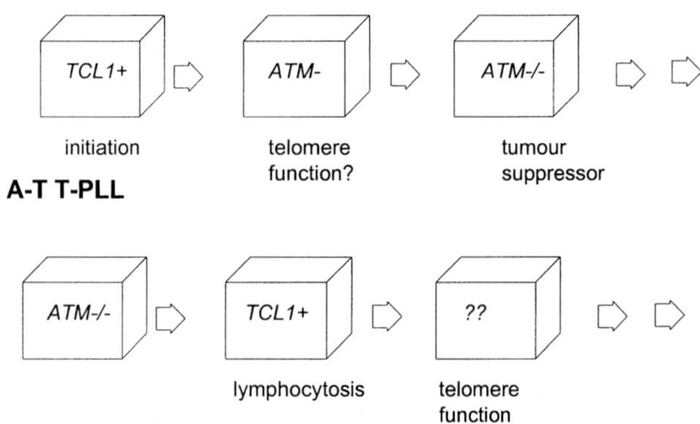

Fig. 4. In sporadic cases, a mature T cell undergoes a rearrangement giving, first, *TCL1* expression and then a point mutation in the *ATM TEL1* domain. This combination bypasses limits set on growth (arising from age-related loss of telomere integrity). Subsequent complete *ATM* inactivation then bypasses restriction points in the cell cycle, resulting in a large, clonal lymphocytosis. In A-T patients, ectopic *TCL1* expression in a mature T cell directly permits this large clonal lymphocytosis

pattern of inheritance and are the basis for Knudson's two-hit hypothesis (Knudson 1971). The answer is surely related to the consequence to a heterozygote of acquiring a hit at the second *ATM* allele: this hit fails to confer a growth advantage or it confers a disadvantage relative to all its sister cells. A disadvantage seems more likely in light of the observations that A-T cells are prone to aneuploidy and spontaneous apoptosis (Duchaud et al. 1996). Now, if this disadvantage were overcome by some prior mutation of another gene, then the development of T-PLL would be dependent on the risk of that prior mutation. If this risk were low then the risk of T-PLL to the A-T heterozygote might not be detectably different than the risk of T-PLL in the general population. What might this other gene be? An excellent candidate is *TCL1*. This maps to 14q32.1 and breakpoints at this band are the most common cytogenetic abnormality in sporadic and A-T-related T-PLL (Brito-Babapulle et al. 1987). In A-T, T cell clones with 14q32.1 breakpoints are frequently observed as significant nonpathological proliferations and are known in some cases to have preceded the emergence of T-PLL in those patients (Taylor et al. 1996). Thus these large stable clones carry a mutation that gives a growth advantage to the T cell bearing it. Such large stable clones are not observed in the general population. Thus it seems likely that expression of *TCL1* in T cells suppresses the general growth disadvantage of loss of *ATM* function and specifically may block the path toward apoptosis that putatively arises from loss of *ATM TEL1* domain function. This then permits us to propose a model for the development of sporadic and A-T-related T-PLL (Fig. 4): (1) Sporadic T-PLL is initiated by *TCL1* activation (in some cases we observe no breakpoint at 14q32.1, but rather at Xq28 which results in expression of an alternate transcript of the *MTCP1* gene called *MTCP1* B1 – the corresponding protein has 41% amino acid identity to *TCL1* (Stern et al. 1993; Madani et al. 1996). (2) A missense mutation arises in the *ATM TEL1* domain on one allele. The second, wild-type allele is lost or acquires the same mutation by somatic homologous recombination. This subverts the maintenance of the integrity of telomere function which, in the context of *TCL1/MTCP1* B1 expression, constitutes a growth advantage. This step may be restricted to those T-PLL cases that acquire TEL1 domain missense mutations (about a third of all cases); other cases bypass this step. (3) Further mutations arise at *ATM* resulting in complete *ATM* inactivation and thus relief of cell cycle checkpoints. This permits progression to a stable clonal lymphocytosis (as seen in A-T patients). The inactivation implicates domains additional to *TEL1* in cell cycle control.

It is difficult to see why a locus should involve multiple disruptions in order that its function be disrupted. It is unlike the situation in *BCL2* in which more than one breakpoint is occasionally seen in association with gene activation (Seite et al. 1993), or the situation at the *DMD* dystrophin locus in which the severity of the muscular dystrophy can depend on multiple mutational events in a 5 mb region (Bartlett et al. 1989; Laing et al. 1992). For the moment, the multiple disruptions at *ATM* must remain as intriguing observations, although they are reminiscent of the chromosomal fragmentation seen in the developing *ATM-/-* knockout mouse spermatocyte (Xu et al. 1996). Another possible explanation for multiple disruption of an allele is that there might be a nearby gene also involved in tumorigenesis.

In summary, we have observed an intriguing difference in the pattern of mutation of the *ATM* gene in A-T as compared to T-PLL. A-T seems to require complete inactivation of the gene and this is achieved primarily by truncating mutations. This suggests that most missense mutations leave intact functions of *ATM* which if lost in the germline do not give a recognisable A-T phenotype. While loss of *ATM* function substantially elevates the risk of T-PLL, the pattern of mutation in sporadic cases suggests that the gene is involved at two distinct steps in tumorigenesis: a step requiring impairment of the *TEL1* domain and a subsequent step requiring loss of all functions. The first step is achieved by missense mutation while the second step often involves unusual complex rearrangements. The rarity of A-T heterozygotes among sporadic T-PLL cases and the absence of T-PLL in A-T heterozygotes points to the recessive nature of the predisposition to T-PLL and thus implicates another gene, quite possibly *TCL1*, in initiation of T-PLL tumorigenesis. The finding of occasional *ATM* mutations in B-NHL demonstrates that the cancer epidemiology of A-T patients does not predict the relative frequency of involvement of *ATM* in sporadic malignancy: in A-T, T-PLL is rare but NHL common, while the reverse is true for *ATM* mutations in the sporadic counterparts of these diseases. Similarly while A-T heterozygotes have elevated risk of breast cancer, no *ATM* mutations have yet been reported in the sporadic form. That said, T-PLL demonstrates that *ATM* should be considered a candidate gene in a wide range of malignancies, perhaps

Table 4. Sporadic solid tumours with frequent loss of heterozygosity at 11q22-23

Site	Reference
Breast	Kerangueven et al. (1997)
Bladder	Shaw et al. (1995)
Colorectal	Keldysh et al. (1993)
Lung	Iizuka et al. (1995)
	Rasio et al. (1995)
Nasopharyngeal	Hui et al. (1996)
Ovarian	Foulkes et al. (1993)
	Davis et al. (1996)
	Gabra et al. (1996)
Stomach	Baffa et al. (1996)
Melanoma	Tomlinson et al. (1993)

especially those that show loss of heterozygosity in the *ATM* region (Table 4).

Acknowledgements. We wish to thank Prof. D. Catovsky and Dr. M. J. S. Dyer for their support and encouragement; all our collaborators especially Dr. Igor Vorechovsky (Karolinska Institute, Sweden) and Prof S. P. Jackson (Wellcome-CRC Institute, Cambridge); our colleagues (S. M. Abraham, V. Brito-Babapulle, E. Matutes, R. Hamoudi, F. Yaqub); and the Leukaemia Research Fund (M.Y.) and the Kay Kendall Leukaemia Trust (M.Y. and L.C.).

References

Al Saadi A, Palutke M, Krishna-Kuma G (1980) Evolution of chromosomal abnormalities in sequential cytogenetic studies of ataxia telangiectasia. Hum Genet 55:23–29

Athma P, Rappoport R, Swift M (1996) Molecular genotyping shows that Ataxia-Telangiectasia heterozygotyes are predisposed to breast cancer. Cancer Genet Cytogenet 92:130–134

Aurias A (1981) Analyse cytogénétique de 21 cas d'ataxie telangiëctasie. J Genet Hum 29:235–247

Aurias A, Dutrillaux B, Buriot D, Lejeune J (1980) High frequencies of inversions and translocations of chromosome 7 and 14 in ataxia telangiectasia. Mutat Res 69:369–374

Baer R, Heppel A, Taylor AMR, Rabbitts PH, Boulier B, Rabbitts TH (1987) The breakpoint of an inversion of chromosome 14 in a T-cell leukemia: sequences downstream of the immunoglobulin heavy chain locus are implicated in tumorigenesis. Proc Natl Acad Sci US 84:9069–9073

Baffa R, Negrini M, Mandes B, Rugge M, Ranzani G, Hirohashi S, Croce C (1996) Loss of heterozygosity for chromosome 11 in adenocarcinoma of the stomach. Cancer Res 56:268–272

Bartlett RJ, Walker AP, Laing NG, Koh J, Secore SL, Speer MC, Pericak-Vance MA, Hung W-Y, Yamaoka LH, Siddique T, Kandt R, Roses AD (1989) Inherited deletion at Duchenne dystrophy locus in normal male. Lancet 1:496–497

Bebb G, Glickman B, Gelmon K, Gatti R (1997) "AT risk" for breast cancer. Lancet 349:1784–1785

Boder E, Sidgwick RP (1958) Ataxia-Telangiectasia. Pediatrics 21:526

Bonnefoyberard N, Genestier L, Flacher M, Revillard JP (1994) The phosphoprotein phosphatase calcineurin controls calcium-dependent apoptosis in B-cell lines. Eur J Immunol 24:325–329

Bridges BA, Harnden DG (1981) Untangling ataxia telangiectasia. Nature 289:222–223

Brito-Babapulle V, Catovsky D (1991) Inversions and tandem translocations involving chromosome 14q11 and 14q32 in T-cell prolymphocytic leukemia and T-cell leukemias in patients with ataxia-telangiectasia. Cancer Genet Cytogenet 55:1–9

Brito-Babapulle V, Pomfret M, Matutes E, Catovsky D (1987) Cytogenetic studies on prolymphocytic leukaemia II T-cell prolymphocytic leukaemia. Blood 70:926–931

Brown EJ, Albers MW, Shin TB, Ichikawa K, Keith CT, Lane WS, Shreiber SL (1994) A mammalian protein targeted by G1-arresting rapamycin-receptor complex. Nature 369:756–758

Catovsky D, Galetto J, Okos A, Galton DAG, Wiltshaw E, Stathopoulos G (1973) Prolymphocytic leukaemia of B and T cell type. Lancet 2: 232–234

Cohen MM, Shamam M, Dagan J, Shmueli E, Korn J (1975) Cytogenetic investigations in families with ataxia telangiectasia. Cytogenet Cell Genet 15:338–356

Davey MP, Bertness V, Nakahara K, Johnson JP, McBride OW, Waldmann TA, Kirsch I (1988) K Juxtaposition of the T-cell receptor α-chain locus (14q11) and a region (14q32) of potential importance in leukemogenesis by a 14,14 translocation in a patient with T-cell chronic lymphocytic leukemia and ataxia telangiectasia. Proc Natl Acad Sci USA 85:9287–9291

Davis M, Hitchcock A, Foulkes W, Campbell I (1996) Refinement of two chromosome 11q regions of loss of heterozygosity in ovarian cancer. Cancer Res 56:741–744

Duchaud E, Ridet A, Stoppa-Lyonnet D, Janin N, Moustacchi E, Rosselli F (1996) Deregulated apoptosis in ataxia telangiectasia: association with clinical stigmata and radiosensitivity. Cancer Res 56:1400–1404

Easton DF (1994) Cancer risks in A-T heterozygotes. Int J Radiat Biol 66:S177–S182

FitzGerald MG, Bean JM, Hegde SR, Unsal H, MacDonald DJ, Harkin DP, Finkelstein DM, Isselbacher KJ, Haber DA (1997) Heterozygous ATM mutations do not contribute to early onset of breast cancer. Nature [Genet] 15:307–310

Foulkes W, Campbell I, Stamp G, Trowsdale J (1993) Loss of heterozygosity and amplification on chromosome 11q in human ovarian cancer. Br J Cancer 67:268–273

Gabra H, Watson V, Taylor K, Mackay J, Leonard R, Steel M, Porteous D, Smyth J (1996) Definition and refinement of a region of loss of heterozygosity at 11q233-q243 in epithelial ovarian cancer associated with poor prognosis. Cancer Res 56:950–954

Galton DAG, Goldman JM, Wiltshaw F, Catovsky D, Kenry K, Goldenberg GJ (1974) Prolymphocytic leukaemia. Br J Haematol 27:7–23

Gatti RA, Berkel I, Boder E, Braedt G, Charmley P, Concannon P, Ersoy F, Foroud T, Jaspers NGJ, Lange K, Lathrop GM, Leppert M, Nakamura Y, O'Connell P, Paterson M, Salser W, Sanal O, Silver J, Sparkes RS, Susi E, Weeks DE, Wei S, White R, Yoder F (1988) Localization of an ataxia-telangiectasia gene to chromosome 11q22-23. Nature 336:577–578

Greenwell PW, Kronmal SL, Porter SE, Gassenhuber J, Obermaier B, Petes TD (1995) TEL1, a gene involved in controlling telomere length in S cerevisiae, is homologous to the human ataxia telangiectasia gene. Cell 82:823–829

Hecht F, Hecht BK (1990) Cancer in ataxia-telangiectasia patients. Cancer Genet Cytogenet 46:9–19

Hecht F, Koler RD, Rigas DA, Dahnke GS, Case MP, Tisdale Y, Miller RW (1966) Leukaemia and lymphocytes in ataxia-telangiectasia. Lancet 2:1193

Hecht F, McCaw BK, Koler RD (1973) Ataxia telangiectasia: clonal growth of translocation lymphocytes. N Engl J Med 289:286–291

Hui A, Lo KW, Leung SF, Choi PHK, Fong Y, Lee JCK, Huang DP (1996) Loss of heterozygosity on the long arm of chromosome 11 in nasopharyngeal carcinoma. Oncogene 56:3225–3229

Iizuka M, Sugiyama Y, Shiraishi M, Jones C, Sikya T (1995) Allelic losses in human chromosome 11 in lung cancers. Genes Chromosomes Cancer 13:40–46

Keldysh P, Dragani T, Fleischman E, Konstantinova L, Perevoschikov A, Pierotti M, Della Porta G, Kopnin B (1993) 11q deletions in human colorectal carcinomas: cytogenetics and restriction fragment length polymorphism analysis. Genes Chromosomes Cancer 6:45–50

Kerangueven F, Eisinger F, Noguchi T, Allione F, Wargniez V, Eng C, Padberg G, Theillet C, Jacquemier J, Longy Mm, Sobol H, Birnbaum D (1997) Loss of heterozygosity in human breast carcinomas in the ataxia telangiectasia, Cowden disease and *BRCA1* gene regions. Oncogene 14:339–347

Knudson AG (1971) Mutation and cancer: statistical study of retinoblastoma. Proc Natl Acad Sci USA 68:820–823

Knudson AG (1997) Hereditary cancer: theme and variations. J Clin Oncol 15:3280–3287

Kojis TL, Schreck RR, Gatti RA, Sparkes RS (1989) Tissue specificity of chromosomal rearrangements in ataxia telangiectasia. Hum Genet 83:347–352

Laing NG, Layton MG, Johnsen RD, Chandler DC, Mears ME, Goldblatt J, Kakulas BA (1992) Two distinct mutations in a single dystrophin gene – chance occurrence or premutation? Am J Med Genet 42:688–692

Lakin ND, Weber P, Stankovic T, Rottinhaus ST, Taylor AMR, Jackson SP (1996) Analysis of the *ATM* protein in wild-type and ataxia telangiectasia cells. Oncogene 13:2707–2716

Louis-Bar D (1941) Sur un syndrome progressif comprenant des télangiéctasies capillaires cutanées et conjonctivales symétriques, à disposition naevoïde et de troubles cérébelleux. Confirm Neurol (Basel) 4:32

Madani A, Choukroun V, Soulier J, Cacheux V, Claisse JF, Valensi F, Daliphard S, Cazin B, Levy V, Leblond V, Daniel M-T, Sigaux F, Stern M-H (1996) Expression of p13*(MTCP1)* is restricted to mature T-cell proliferations with t(X;14) translocations. Blood 87:1923–1927

Matutes E, Brito-Babapulle V, Swansbury J, Ellis J, Morilla R, Dearden C, Sempere A, Catovsky D (1991) Clinical and laboratory features of 78 cases of T-prolymphocytic leukemia. Blood 78:3269–3274

Mengle-Gaw L, Willard HF, Smith CIE, Hammarstrom L, Fischer P, Sherrington P, Lucas G, Thompson PW, Baer R, Rabbitts TH (1987) Human T-cell tumours containing chromosome 14 inversion or translocation with breakpoints proximal to immunoglobulin joining regions at 14q32. EMBO J 6:2273–2280

Mengle-Gaw L, Albertson DG, Sherrington PD, Rabbitts TH (1988) Analysis of a T-cell tumor-specific breakpoint cluster at human chromsome 14q32. Proc Natl Acad Sci USA 85:9171–9175

Metcalfe JA, Parkhill J, Campbell L, Stacey M, Biggs P, Byrd PJ, Taylor AMR (1996) Accelerated telomere shortening ataxia-telangiectasia. Nature [Genet] 13:350–353

Meyn MS (1993) High spontaneous intrachromosomal recombination rates in ataxia telangiectasia. Science 260:1327–1330

Meyn MS (1995) Ataxia telangiectasia and cellular responses to DNA damage. Cancer Res 55:5991–6001

Norrback K-F, Roos G (1997) Telomeres and telomerase in normal and malignant haemopoietic cells. Eur J Cancer 33:774–780

Pawson R, Dyer MJS, Barge R, Matutes E, Thornton PD, Emmett E, Kluin-Nelemans JC, Fibbe WE, Willemze R, Catovsky D (1997) Treatment of T-cell prolymphocytic leukaemia with human CDw52 antibody. J Clin Oncol 15:2667–2672

Platzer M, Rotman G, Bauer D, Uziel T, Savitsky K, BarShira A, Gilad S, Shiloh Y, Rosenthal A (1997) Ataxia-telangiectasia locus: sequence analysis of 184 kb of human genomic DNA containing the entire *ATM* gene. Genome Res 7:592–605

Rasio D, Negrini M, Manenti G, Dragani T, Croce C (1995) Loss of heterozygosity at chromosome 11q in lung adenocarcinoma: identification of three independent regions. Cancer Res 55:3988–3991

Rowan WC, Hale G, Tite JP, Brett SJ (1995) Cross-linking of the CAMPATH-1 antigen (CD52) triggers activation of normal human T lymphocytes. Int Immunol 7:69–77

Russo G, Isobe M, Gatti R, Finan J, Batuman O, Huebner K, Nowell PC, Croce CM (1989) Molecular analysis of a t(14,14) translocation in leukemic T-cells of an ataxia telangiectasia patient. Proc Natl Acad Sci USA 86:602–606

Savitsky K, Bar-Shira A, Gilad S, Rotman G, Ziv Y, Vanagaite L, Tagle DA, Smith S, Uziel T, Sfez S, Ashkenazi M, Pecker I, Frydman M, Harnik R, Patanjali SR, Simmons A, Clines GA, Sartiel A, Gatti RA, Chessa L, Sanal O, Lavin MF, Jaspers NJ, Taylor AR, Arlett CF, Miki T, Weissman SM, Lovett M, Collins FS, Shiloh YA (1995a) A single ataxia-telangiectasia gene with a product similar to PI-3 kinase. Science 268:1749–1752

Savitsky K, Sfez S, Tagle DA, Ziv Y, Sartiel A, Collins FS, Shiloh Y, Rotman G (1995b) The complete sequence of the coding region of the *ATM* gene reveals similarity to cell cycle regulators in different species Hum Mol Genet 4:2025–2032

Seite P, Hillion J, D'Agay MF, Berger R, Larsen CJ (1993) *BCL2* complex rearrangement in follicular lymphoma – translocation MBR J(H) and deletion in the VCR region of the same *BCL2* allele. Oncogene 8:3073–3080

Shaw M, Knowles M (1995) Deletion mapping of chromosome 11 in carcinoma of the bladder. Genes Chromosomes Cancer 29:222–233

Stern M-H, Soulier J, Rosenzwajg M, Nakahara K, Canki-Klain N, Aurias A, Sigaux F, Stern IR (1993) *MTCP1*: a novel gene on the human chromosome Xq28 translocated to the T cell receptor a/δ locus in mature T cell proliferations. Oncogene 8:2475–2483

Stilgenbauer S, Schaffner C, Litterst A, Liebisch P, Gilad S, Bar-Shira A, James MR, Lichter P, Dohner H (1997) Biallelic mutations in the *ATM* gene in T-prolymphocytic leukemia. Nature [Medicine] 3:1155–1159

Syllaba L, Henner K (1926) Contribution à l'independence de l'athétose double idiopathique et congénitale: atteinte familiale, syndrome dystrophique, signe du reseau vasculaire conjonctival, intégrite psychique. Rev Neurol (Paris) 5:541–562

Taylor AMR, Metcalfe JA, Thick J, Mak Y-F (1996) Leukemia and lymphoma in ataxia telangiectasia. Blood 87:423–428

Thacker J (1994) Cellular radio sensitivity in ataxia-telangiectasia. Int J Radiat Biol 66:S87–S96

Tomlinson I, Gammack A, Stickland J, Mann G, Mackie R, Kefford R, McGee JO'D (1993) Loss of heterozygosity in malignant melanoma at loci on chromosomes 11q and 17 implicated in the pathogenesis of other cancers. Genes Chromosomes Cancer 7:169–172

Vorechovsky I, Rasio D, Luo L, Monaco C, Hammarstrom L, Webster ADB, Zaloudik J, Barbanti-Brodano G, James M, Russo G, Croce CM, Negrini M (1996a) The *ATM* gene and susceptibility to breast cancer: analysis of 38 breast tumours reveals no evidence for mutation. Cancer Res 56:2726–2732

Vorechovsky I, Luo LP, Lindblom A, Negrini M, Webster ADB, Croce CM, Hammarström L (1996b) *ATM* mutations in cancer families. Cancer Res 56:4130–4133

Vorechovsky I, Luo L, Dyer MJS, Catovsky D, Amlot PL, Yaxley JC, Foroni L, Hammarström L, Webster ADB, Yuille MAR (1997) Clustering of missense mutations in the ataxia-telangiectasia gene in a sporadic T-cell leukaemia. Nature [Genet] 17:96–99

Wooster R, Ford D, Mangion J, Ponder BAJ, Peto J, Easton DF, Stratton MR (1993) Absence of linkage to the ataxia telangiectasia locus in familial breast cancer. Hum Genet 92:91–94

Xu Y, Ashley T, Brainerd EE, Bronson RT, Meyn MS, Baltimore D (1996) Targeted disruption of *ATM* leads to growth retardation, chromosomal fragmentation during meiosis, immune defects and thymic lymphoma. Genes Dev 10:2411–2422

Yuille MAR, Abraham SM, Coignet LJA, Lakin ND, Yaqub F, Matutes E, Brito-Babapulle V, Jackson SP, Dyer MJS, Catovsky D (1996a) Abnormalities of the ataxia telangiectasia gene (*ATM*) in T-prolymphocytic leukemia. Blood 8:477a

Yuille MAR, Galiegue-Zouitina S, Hiorns L, Jadayel D, De Schouwer PJJC, Catovsky D, Dyer MJS, Kerckaert J-P (1996b) Heterogeneity of breakpoints at the transcriptional co-activator gene, *BOB-1*, in lymphoproliferative disease. Leukemia 10:1492–1496

Yuille MAR, Coignet LA, Abraham SM, Yaqub F, Luo L, Matutes E, Brito-Babapulle V, Vorechovsky I, Dyer MJS, Catovsky D (1998) *ATM* is usually rearranged in T-cell prolymphocytic leukemia. Oncogene (in press)

IV. Induced Chromosome Damage and Cancer

Cancer Predictive Value of Cytogenetic Markers Used in Occupational Health Surveillance Programs

L. Hagmar[1], S. Bonassi[2], U. Strömberg[1], Z. Mikoczy[1], C. Lando[2], I.-L. Hansteen[3], A.H. Montagud[4], L. Knudsen[5], H. Norppa[6], C. Reuterwall[7], H. Tinnerberg[1] et al.[*]

[1] Department of Occupational and Environmental Medicine, Lund University, 221 85 Lund, Sweden
[2] Department of Environmental Epidemiology, Istituto Nazionale per la Ricerca sul Cancro, Viale Benedetto XV, 1016132 Genoa, Italy
[3] Department of Occupational Medicine, Telemark Central Hospital, 3710 Skien, Norway
[4] Centro Nacional de Condiciones de Trabajo, Instituto Nacional de Seguridad e Higiene en el Trabajo, Dulcet 2-10, 08034 Barcelona, Spain
[5] National Institute of Occupational Health, Lersø Parkallé 105, 2100 Copenhagen Ø, Denmark
[6] Finnish Institute of Occupational Health, Topeliuksekatu 41 a A, 00250 Helsinki, Finland
[7] National Institute of Work Life, 171 84 Solna, Sweden

Abstract

It has not previously been clear whether cytogenetic biomarkers in healthy subjects will predict cancer. Earlier analyses of a Nordic and an Italian cohort indicated predictivity for chromosomal aberrations (CAS) but not for sister chromatid exchanges (SCES). A pooled analysis of the updated cohorts, forming a joint study base of 5271 subjects, will now be performed, allowing a more solid evaluation. The importance of potential effect modifiers, such as gender, age at testing, and time since testing, will be evaluated using Poisson regression models. Two other potential effect modifiers, occupational exposures and smoking, will be assessed in a case-referent study within the study base.

[*] Anton Brøgger, Norwegian Radium Hospital, Oslo, Norway, Alessandra Forni, Istituto di Medicina del Lavoro Clinica del Lavoro "L. Devoto", Milano, Italy; Inger-Lise Hansteen,; Benkt Högstedt, Department of Occupational Medicine, Central Hospital, Halmstad, Sweden; Bo Lambert, Department of Environmental Medicine, Centre for Nutrition and Toxicology, Karolinska Institute, Stockholm, Sweden; Felix Mitelman, Department of Clinical Genetics, Lund University, Sweden; Ingrid Nordenson, National Institute of Work Life, Umeå, Sweden; Sisko Salomaa, Finnish Center for Radiation and Nuclear Safety, Helsinki, Finland; Staffan Skerfving, Department of Occupational and Environmental Medicine, Lund University, Sweden.

Recent Results in Cancer Research, Vol. 154
© Springer-Verlag Berlin · Heidelberg 1998

Background

Cytogenetic biomarkers such as chromosomal aberrations (CAs), sister chromatid exchanges (SCEs), and micronuclei (MN) in peripheral blood lymphocytes have been used for decades in surveying workers exposed to mutagens or carcinogens. It has been proposed that these cytogenetic endpoints may serve as biomarkers not only of exposure, but also of an early mutagen effect indicating increased cancer risk (Aitio et al. 1988; International Commission for Proctection against Environmental Mutagens and Carcinogens 1988). This hypothesis had, however, been left unproven until the Nordic Study Group on the Health Risk of Chromosome Damage in the late 1980s established a cohort of 3182 subjects from Sweden, Finland, Norway and Denmark who had been examined for at least one of the cytogenetic tests (Nordic Study Group on the Health Risk of Chromosome Damage 1990a). A predictive value of CA frequency for total cancer incidence was observed (Nordic Study Group on the Health Risk of Chromosome Damage 1990b; Hagmar et al. 1994), whereas no such associations were observed for SCEs or MN. These estimates were based on a relatively limited number of observations which hampered a firm conclusion. It was therefore of interest that an Italian cohort study, designed in a similar way as the Nordic one, also showed an association between CA frequency and cancer risk (Bonassi et al. 1995).

Economic support from the European Union Biomed-2 program has enabled a collaborative effort, creating a joint Nordic and Italian data base of cytogenetically examined subjects and allowing pooled analyses. The main objectives of this collaboration were to evaluate the type of association between cytogenetic biomarkers and cancer risk in a large study base and to assess whether gender, age at cytogenetic testing, time since testing, smoking habits, and exposure to mutagens/carcinogens may modify the cancer-predictive value of the biomarkers.

We will here report on the basic design of this 3-year project, and give some descriptive data on the joint study base. Furthermore, we will outline some methodological aspects regarding cohort analysis of the joint data base and a case-referent study within the study base.

Establishment of a Joint Data Base

Altogether 5271 subjects, examined between 1965 and 1988 for at least one cytogenetic biomarker, constituted the study base (Table 1). Looking separately at the various endpoints, 3540 subjects had been examined for CAS, 2702 for SCES and 1496 for MN. The CA tests in the the study base were performed between 1965 and 1987. The corresponding time interval for the SCE tests was 1970–1987, and for the MN tests 1980–1987. The cohorts of cytogentically examined subjects from Sweden, Norway, Finland, or Denmark which were included in the joint data base were identical with those described before (Nordic Study Group on the Health Risk of Chromsome

Table 1. Number of subjects tested for chromosomal aberrations (CAs), sister chromatid exchanges (SCEs), or micronuclei (MN), with respect to tumor diagnosis[a] during follow-up

Cytogenetic endpoint	Country	Number of subjects in cohort	
		With a tumor diagnosis	All
CAs			
	Sweden	33	749
	Finland	26	557
	Norway	30	471
	Denmark	2	191
	Italy	64	1573
SCEs			
	Sweden	23	850
	Finland	27	669
	Norway	20	289
	Denmark	3	202
	Italy	4	692
MN			
	Sweden	18	686
	Italy	9	810

[a] Number of incident cancer cases for Sweden, Finland, Norway, and Denmark and number of deaths in cancer for Italy.

Damage 1990 a, b; Hagmar et al. 1994), The included Italian cohort was, however, only partly identical with the one previously reported on (Bonassi et al. 1995), due to the required application of the same inclusion criteria for all cohorts: (a) cytogenetic tests should have been performed because of potentially harmful environmental/occupational exposures or because the subjects had served as unexposed control subjects (thus excluding subjects tested due to medical reasons), (b) the subjects should have been at least 15 years of age at cytogenetic testing, (c) and should not have had a cancer diagnosis before testing, and (d) the personal identification code and (e) the date for cytogenetic testing should be known. These data, which were included in the joint data base, could thus be used to assess the potentially modifying effect on cancer risk of gender, age at testing, and time since test. The available data on smoking habits and occupational exposure were to scarce too allow an evaluation of the modifying effect of these factors without additional information.

Classification of Cytogenetic Endpoints

Ten Nordic and ten Italian cytogenetic laboratories contributed with data. In order to standardize for interlaboratory variation, the results for the various cytogenetic endpoints were trichotomized within each laboratory as follows:

Table 2. Agreement between trichotomization for chromosomal aberrations (CAs) and sister chromatid exchanges (SCEs) in 1553 subjects examined for both endpoints (κ-value = 0.03)

SCEs frequency	CAs frequency		
	Low	Medium	High
Low	219	144	150
Medium	218	138	146
High	188	157	193

"low" (1–33 percentile), "medium" (34–66 percentile), or "high" (67–100 percentile), as described in detail earlier (Hagmar et al. 1994; Bonassi et al. 1995).

At least 100 metaphases were scored with respect to CAs (gaps not included) for each individual. The culture time was 48 or 72 h. The CA data based on 48-h culture time were trichotomized separately from those with a 72-h culture time. The scoring of mean SCEs, after replication of a DNA template containing BrdU, was based on the analysis of 20–50 cells/individual in the Nordic cohorts and 20–100 cells/individual in the Italian cohort. The MN estimate was, in both the Swedish and Italian data bases, based on at least 1000 interphase cells; 78% of the Italian MN tests were performed using the cytokinesis block technique, and thus binuclear cells were analysed. The remaining Italian tests and all Swedish tests were performed using the traditional technique and scoring of mononuclear cells. The trichotomization of the MN results was made with respect to the technique used.

Agreement Between Cytogenetic Endpoints

Altogether 1553 subjects were examined for both CAs and SCEs, but there was poor agreement between the trichotomizations for these two endpoints (Table 2, κ-value = 0.03). The corresponding figure for those 773 subjects examined for both CA and MN was similarly low (Table 3, κ-value = 0.07). Considering this astonishing lack of agreement, one should not expect a similar cancer predictive value from the three cytogenetic endpoints.

Cohort Analysis of Mortality and Cancer Incidence

After linkage to national registers, the data base was supplemented with information on vital status. The follow-up period was defined as the time from the date of cytogenetic testing until the date of death, tumor diagnosis (Nordic cohort only), emigration, 85th birthday, or end of the calendar-year of follow-up, whichever occurred first.

Table 3. Agreement between trichotomization for chromosomal aberrations (CAs) and micronuclei (MN) in 773 subjects examined for both endpoints (κ-value = 0.07)

MN frequency	CAs frequency		
	Low	Medium	High
Low	192	107	57
Medium	92	66	57
High	83	65	54

Information on incident malignant tumors, from the start of the follow-up period until the end of 1993 (Sweden, Denmark), 1994 (Norway), or 1995 (Finland), were obtained from the National Cancer Registries. In the Italian cohort, the specific causes of death until April 30, 1996 were obtained from the Municipality of Residence.

During the follow-up period 91 Nordic subjects examined for CAs were diagnosed with cancer and 64 Italian subjects examined for CAs died from a malignant tumor (Table 1). The relative distributions of tumor diagnoses differs somewhat between the Nordic cohorts and the Italian cohort. About 40% of the tumor deaths in the Italian cohort were caused by neoplasms in the lower respiratory tract, but these tumors contributed only to 12% of the observed cancer cases in the Nordic cohorts. By contrast, only one prostate cancer death (2%) was found in the Italian cohort, whereas 15% of the incident cases in the Nordic cohorts were due to prostate cancer. This can partly be explained by a varying survival with respect to cancer diagnosis. It underlines, however, the difficulties in assessing the predictive value of CAs for specific tumor diagnoses in the joint data base. Such analyses will be more meaningful after a prolonged follow-up period.

Seventy-three subjects from the Nordic cohorts examined for SCEs were diagnosed with cancer, but only four Italian SCE-examined subjects had died from a malignant tumor (Table 1). The corresponding figures for MN were 18 in the Swedish cohort and nine in the Italian cohort.

Expected cancer incidence for the Nordic cohorts will be calculated by calendar year-, gender-, and 5-year age-group specific incidences for each country. Correspondingly, the expected cancer mortality in the Italian cohorts can be calculated by calendar year-, gender-, and 5-year age-group specific death rates for the Italian population. Stratified calculations of standardized cancer incidence ratios (SIRs) and standardized mortality ratios (SMRs), with respect to the trichotomized results of the cytogenetic biomarkers, will thereafter be performed.

Table 4. Distribution of the potential effect modifying factors, gender, age at test, and length of follow-up time in the Nordic and Italian cohorts, with respect to frequency of chromosomal aberrations (CAs) andsister choromatid exchanges (SCEs)

Cytogenetic endpoint	Cohort	Frequency of CAs	Females (%)	Age at test (years) Percentiles			Follow-up time (years) Percentiles		
				10th	50th	90th	10th	50th	90th
CAs	Nordic	Low	23.3	23	33	55	6.8	11.2	16.5
		Medium	21.5	23	36	55	6.8	12.6	16.9
		High	28.0	25	38	57	12.2	12.2	17.8
	Italian	Low	21.3	25	38	54	3.5	10.9	22.1
		Medium	26.1	25	39	55	3.8	11.7	19.7
		High	28.0	26	41	57	3.8	11.9	20.0
SCEs	Nordic	Low	32.9	23	35	55	6.9	10.2	15.6
		Medium	35.6	23	35	58	6.8	10.8	16.1
		High	32.0	25	38	56	6.9	12.6	16.2
	Italian	Low	27.6	24	36	53	2.2	5.2	10.9
		Medium	27.8	26	37	54	2.4	4.5	11.5
		High	32.7	26	38	55	2.2	3.8	12.2

Low, 1–33 percentiles; medium, 34–66 percentiles; high, 67–100 percentiles.

Poisson Regression Models

The distributions of gender, age at testing, and length of follow-up, with respect to the frequency of the cytogenetic endpoints, are displayed in Table 4. One aim of the present study is to assess the importance of potential effect modifiers on the predictive values of the cytogenetic endpoints regarding cancer risk. The potential modifying effect of gender, age at testing, time since testing, and country (only for cancer incidence) will be assessed by means of Poisson regression (Clayton and Hill 1993). As the the presently available data on smoking habits and occupational exposure are not sufficient, the importance of these factors will therefore be assessed in a case-referent study within the joint study base.

Cohort-Based Case-Referent Study

The aim of this study is to investigate if the predictivity of CA frequency regarding cancer risk is modified by certain exposures (occupational exposures, smoking habits, radiotherapy and cytostatic drugs). For each subject with cancer in the study base, four referents will be selected, independent of their CA frequency and exposure status. The referents will be matched with respect to country, gender, birth year, and year of cytogenetic testing.

Available exposure data for cases and referents will be retrieved from medical records and protocols from the original cytogenetic studies. Moreover, skilled industrial hygienists from each participating country will contact the companies in which the cases and referents were employed at the time of cytogenetic testing in order to ascertain supplementary exposure data. A lifelong occupational history will be obtained by means of a postal questionnaire to cases/referents (or next-of-kin if they are deceased), followed by a structured telephone interview performed by the occupational hygienists. Based on available exposure data, each subject will be classified in a semiquantitative way for a number of exposures included in an exposure matrix. This exposure matrix has basically been constructed with respect to the mutagen/carcinogen exposures described in the original cytogenetic studies, forming the present study base. The assessment according to the exposure matrix will be performed for each calendar year during the subjects occupational history, until end of follow-up. Data on smoking habits, radiotherapy and treatment with cytostatic drugs will also be obtained through the telephone interview, and if necessary checked with medical records. Logistic regression models will be used for the data analysis. The case-referent study must be approved by ethics committees in each participating country before it can be implemented.

Discussion

A validation of candidate biomarkers of excess cancer risk to be used in occupational health surveys hopefully will result in the enhanced quality of health surveillance programs, and increased preventive measures at the workplace. Cytogenetic biomarkers, which have been used for decades and to a large extent in occupational health surveys, are presently the only endpoints allowing a reasonable epidemiologic evaluation of cancer predictivity in healthy subjects. The prerequisites for prospective cohort studies needed for such a validation are that the identity of the subjects examined for cytogenetic endpoints can be retrieved and that an adequate follow-up for cancer can be performed. These conditions were at hand in the Nordic countries and in Italy, but do not seem to be present in other countries. The data base presented here are therefore unique, and their further analysis will allow a more detailed understanding of the predictive value of cytogenetic biomarkers, possibly also providing some mechanistic knowledge relevant to cancer development.

Acknowledgements. We are indebted to Aage Andersen, Harri Paakkulainen, Eero Pukkala, and Hans Storm for epidemiologic assistance. This study was supported by grants from the European Union Biomed-2 program, the Swedish Medical Research Council, the Swedish Cancer Society, the Swedish Council for Work Life Research, the Academy of Finland, Associazione Italiana per la Ricerca sul Cancro (AIRC), the Italian Ministry of the University and of the Scientific and Technological Research, and the Italian Ministry of Health.

References

Aitio A, Becking G et al (1988) Indicators for assessing exposure and biological effects of genotoxic chemicals. Consensus and technical reports. Commission of the European Communities. International Programme on Chemical Safety (UNEP-ILO-WHO), World Health Organization Regional Office for Europe, Institute of Occupational Health, Finland

Bonassi S, Abbondandolo A et al (1995) Are chromosome aberrations in circulating lymphocytes predictive of a future cancer onset in humans? Preliminary results of an Italian cohort study. Cancer Genet Cytogenct 79:133–135

Clayton D, Hills M (1993) Statistical models in epidemiology. Oxford University Press, Oxford

Hagmar L, Brøgger A et al (1994) Cancer risk in humans predicted by increased levels of chromosome aberrations in lymphocytes: Nordic Study Group on the Health Risk of Chromosome Damage. Cancer Res 54:2919–2922

International Commission for Protection against Environmental Mutagens and Carcinogens (1988) Considerations for population monitoring using cytogenetic techniques. Mutat Res 204:379–406

Nordic Study Group on the Health Risk of Chromosome Damage (1990a) A Nordic data base on somatic chromosome damage in humans. Mutat Res 241:325–337

Nordic Study Group on the Health Risk of Chromosome Damage (1990b) An inter-Nordic prospective study on cytogenetic endpoints and cancer risk. Cancer Genet Cytogenet 45:85–92

Instability at Chromosomal Fragile Sites

T. W. Glover

Deparmtents of Pediatrics and Human Genetics, 4708 Medical Sciences II,
University of Michigan, Ann Arbor, MI 48109-0618, USA

Abstract

Chromosomal fragile sites are loci that are especially prone to forming gaps
or breaks on metaphase chromosomes when cells are cultured under conditions that inhibit DNA replication or repair. The relationship of "rare" folate
sensitive fragile sites with (CCG)n expansion and, in some cases, genetic disease is well established. Although they comprise the vast majority of fragile
sites, much less is known at the molecular level about the "common" fragile
sites. These fragile sites may be seen on all chromosomes as a constant feature. In addition to forming fragile sites on metaphase chromosomes, they
have been shown to display a number of characteristics of unstable and
highly recombinogenic DNA in vitro, including chromosome rearrangements,
sister chromatid exchanges and, more recently, intrachromosomal gene amplification. Only one such fragile site, FRA3B at 3p14.2, has been extensively
investigated at the molecular level. It extends over a broad region of possibly
500 kb, and no trinucleotide or other simple repeat motifs have been identified in the region. FRA3B has recently been shown to lie within the *FHIT*
gene locus. This region and the *FHIT* gene are unstable in a number of tumors and tumor cell lines. It thus appears that common fragile sites are also
associated with unstable regions of DNA in vivo, at least in some tumor cells,
and may cause this instability. Current challenges include determining the
mechanism of fragile site expression and instability, and both the environmental and genetic factors that influence this process. Candidate factors include those genes involved in DNA repair and cell cycle and common carcinogens such as those in cigarette smoke.

Background

Chromosomal fragile sites are chromosome regions that are especially sensitive to forming chromosome gaps or breaks on metaphase chromosomes
(reviewed in Sutherland and Hecht 1985). They are site-specific in that they

Recent Results in Cancer Research, Vol. 154
© Springer-Verlag Berlin · Heidelberg 1998

occur at cytogenetically identifiable points in the genome and do not generally appear on metaphase chromosomes unless the cells are cultured under conditions that inhibit DNA synthesis or repair. Today, we know of over 100 fragile sites, which are generally grouped into two classes based on their relative frequency of occurrence and means of induction. These are the "rare" fragile sites, such as FRAXA in the fragile X mental retardation (*FMR1*) gene, and "common" (or "constitutive") fragile sites, such as FRA3B at 3p14.2, which are found in many if not all chromosomes. Appearance of the rare fragile sites is a manifestation of mutation and genetic variation while common fragile sites apparently represent a constant feature of chromosome structure, but which may be unstable in somatic cells under certain conditions.

Rare Fragile Sites

Growth of cells under conditions of folate or thymidylate stress has led to the identification of 17 rare folate-sensitive fragile sites, a class which includes FRAXA. Other rare fragile sites are induced by 5-bromodeoxyuridine (BrdU) or distamycin A (Sutherland and Hecht 1985). Seven of the rare fragile sites have been cloned and six, including the fragile X site, FRAXA, are associated with CCG trinucleotide repeats (Warren 1996). These fragile site loci therefore represent a subclass of the trinucleotide repeat expansion mutations involved in a number of human diseases. However, only the CCG repeat expansion disorders are known to be associated with chromosomal fragile sites. Expanded CAG, CTG or GAA repeats apparently do not give rise to fragile sites (Jalal et al. 1993). The associated fragile site contributed immensely to the positional cloning of the *FMR1* gene and the discovery that an expanded CCG repeat in the 5′ untranslated region of the *FMR1* gene leads to inactivation of the gene and associated chromosomal instability (Verkerk et al. 1991; Kremer et al. 1991; Oberle et al. 1991). The trinucleotide repeat expansion explains the unusual inheritance and genetic anticipation seen in the fragile X syndrome (Fu et al. 1991), and accounts for the appearance of the associated fragile site on metaphase chromosomes from affected individuals and some carrier females.

In addition to FRAXA, expanded CCG repeats have also been found at the FRAXE and FRAXF loci in Xq27–28, FRA16A in 16p13, and FRA11B in 11q23 (Knight et al. 1993; Parrish et al. 1994; Nancarrow et al. 1994). FRAXE is associated with mild mental retardation in males with expanded repeats. FRA11B, found in the *CBL2* gene, is believed to lead to terminal deletions of distal chromosome 11 in some cases of Jacobsen syndrome. FRA16A lies adjacent to a CpG island but is not associated with disease in heterozygotes. A related, but different, rare fragile site was recently cloned and characterized by Yu et al. (1997). This fragile site, FRA16B, is associated with an expanded 33 bp AT-rich microsatellite repeat. The finding that this sequence contains long AT tracts was predicted based on the fact that it and a few other rare fragile sites are induced by AT-binding drugs such as distamycin A and netropsin.

In all of these cases, the instability observed at the nucleotide level as expanded repeats is translated through an apparent change in chromatin structure to a higher order instability observed at the level of the metaphase chromosome. These changes can give rise to genetic disease by modifying the expression of neighboring genes, as is the case with FRAXA and FRAXF, or by mediating chromosome deletions, as is seen in some cases of Jacobsen syndrome. In all cases, the changes give rise to fragile sites on metaphase chromosomes by mechanisms that likely involve formation of complex intramolecular structures that act as a block to DNA synthesis.

Common Fragile Sites

In the early investigations of the cytogenetics of the fragile X syndrome, the occurrence of site-specific chromosomal gaps and breaks was noted on chromosomes of all individuals, hence the term "common fragile sites" (Glover et al. 1994). Certain sites such as 3p14.2, 16q23, Xp22.3 and others repeatedly display gaps and breaks which appear on the cytological level just like the fragile X site. While common fragile sites are seen when cells are grown under those conditions of folate or thymidylate stress that also induce the rare (CCG)n-associated fragile sites, they are more efficiently seen when cells are treated with aphidicolin, an inhibitor of DNA polymerases α and γ (Glover et al. 1984). However, the rare fragile sites are not induced by aphidicolin, suggesting related, but different, mechanisms for instability.

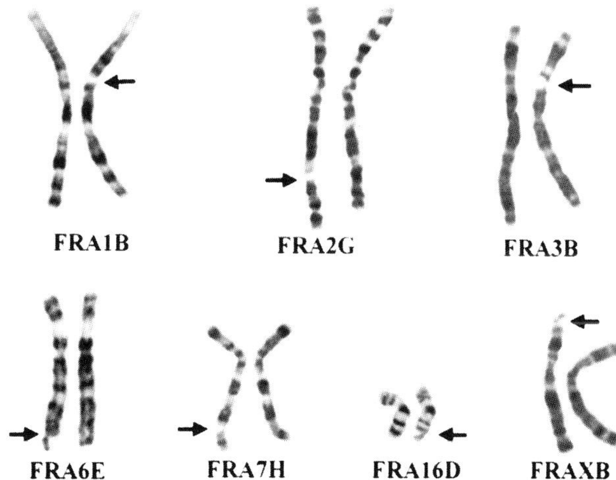

Fig. 1. Examples of common fragile sites induced by aphidicolin in normal human lymphocytes (from Glover 1988)

At present, 84 common fragile sites are listed in the Genome Database (GDB). The exact number of common fragile sites that exist is a matter of interpretation based on criteria for inclusion and statistical analyses of data. The greater the stress placed on DNA replication or G2 repair, the more breaks and gaps are observed until replication ceases altogether. The most frequently observed common fragile sites occur at 3p14.2 (FRA3B), 16q23 (FRA16D, 6q26 (FRA6E), 7q32 (FRA7H), Xp22.3 (FRAXB) and five to ten other sites (Glover et al. 1984) (Fig. 1).

Most common fragile sites occur in G-light bands, leading to suggestions that they may be associated with active gene regions (Yunis and Soreng 1984; Hecht 1988). Variation among normal individuals in the proportion of treated cells expressing common fragile sites has been reported (Austin et al. 1992), and a study of expression in twins (Tedeschi et al. 1992) has suggested that the level of expression is under stringent genetic control. However, there are also very likely environmental influences on fragile site expression, such as cigarette smoking (Ban et al. 1995; Stein et al., submitted) (discussed below).

Common Fragile Sites and Cancer

Instability In Vitro

Common fragile sites have been of interest because they represent an unknown component of chromosome structure, and because of their instability and high recombination *in vitro*. However, even though these sites comprise the vast majority of fragile sites, little is known about their structure or biological significance. Based on their behavior *in vitro* and their locations, numerous suggestions have been made that fragile sites may play a mechanistic role in chromosome breakage and rearrangements involved in cancer (Austin et al. 1992; LeBeau and Rowley 1984; Hecht and Glover 1984; Hecht and Sutherland 1984). This association is based on the coincident location of a number of fragile sites and the location of breakpoints of common and characteristic chromosome aberrations in cancer. However, these studies have been based largely on statistical correlation of breakpoints and fragile sites with little direct evidence either to support or refute this suggestion. They make the assumption that instability at fragile sites can lead to chromosome breakage *in vivo*, as they do *in vitro*, and that these breaks result in chromosome rearrangements or deletions.

In addition to forming gaps or breaks on metaphase chromosomes, common fragile sites have been shown to display a number of characteristics of unstable and highly recombinogenic DNA *in vitro*. All of these characteristics are consistent with the hypothesis that DNA strand breaks are associated with fragile site induction. Following induction, these sites are "hotspots" for increased sister chromatid exchange on metaphase chromosomes (Glover and Stein 1987) and show a high rate of translocation and deletions in somatic cell hybrid systems (Glover and Stein 1988; Wang et al. 1993). Rassool et al. (1916) showed that FRA3B (and likely other common fragile sites) is a preferred site of recombination, or integration, with pSV2neo-plasmid DNA transfected into cells pretreated for fragile site induction. Perhaps related to this characteristic are the findings of Wilke et al. (1996), that FRA3B was the site of integration of HPV16 in a primary cervical carcinoma, and other reports of the coincidence of viral integration sites in tumors or tumor cell lines and fragile sites as studied by FISH (De Braekeleer et al. 1992; Popescu and DiPaolo 1989; Smith et al. 1992).

Fragile sites have also recently been implicated in intrachromosomal gene amplification events in cultured CHO cells. Kuo et al. (1994) found a fragile site in CHO cells to be consistent with the site of three independently established P-glycoprotein gene amplification events, and that pretreatment of cells with aphidicolin greatly increased such amplification events. These results suggested that fragile sites might also play a pivotal role in some gene amplification by initiating a breakage-fusion bridge cycle. More recently, Coquelle et al. (1997 and this volume) have expanded on the findings that show a relationship between fragile sites and gene amplification. They showed that actinomycin D, a known clastogen with CG binding preference, and related compounds that induce fragile sites in CHO cells also induce amplification of flanking genes and regions. The investigators hypothesize that DNA strand breaks preferentially at fragile sites initiate a breakage-bridge-fusion cycle, triggering and setting limits to amplification of large DNA segments. Additional studies of the connection between fragile sites and gene amplification are necessary to understand this process and are important in fully understanding the significance of fragile site expression in cancer cells, where gene amplification plays a major role in tumor progression.

Molecular Analysis of FRA3B

Only one common fragile site, FRA3B, has so far been extensively studied on the molecular level. FRA3B was targeted for study because it is the most frequently seen fragile site on human metaphase chromosomes and can be induced in the majority of treated cells. It maps to a region of 3p known to be associated with deletions in a number of solid tumors, including small cell lung cancer (SCCL) (Hibi et al. 1992), hereditary and sporadic renal cell cancer (RCC) (Cohen et al. 1979; Yamakawa et al. 1991), and cervical cancer (Wistuba et al. 1997). In addition, FRA3B was found to lie very near the t(3;8) translocation breakpoint segregating in a family described with familial renal cell carcinoma (Glover et al. 1988).

Sequences at FRA3B have been identified by a number of related approaches. Wilke et al. (1994, 1996) used a positional cloning approach and FISH to localize the fragile site to a large region of >100 kb that is ~160 kb telomeric to the renal cell carcinoma t(3;8) breakpoint. Sequence analysis of 9 kb at the "center" of the defined region revealed a site of integration of

HPV 16 in a human cervical carcinoma, suggesting that fragile sites may be hotspots for integration of viral DNA in vivo, as they are for transfected DNA in vitro (Rassool et al. 1991). Pardee et al. (1995, 1996) mapped a series of aphidicolin-induced chromosome 3 breakpoints to the same region, and identified two clusters of breaks flanking the region studied by Wilke et al. (1996). By cloning sequences surrounding pSV2neo-plasmid DNA integrated into FRA3B after being transfected into cells treated with aphidicolin, Rassool et al. (1996) identified sequences within the fragile site region ~350 kb distal to the t(3;8) breakpoint. Boldog et al. (1997) cloned a 300 kb region spanning an aphidicolin-induced chromosome 3 translocation breakpoint and have sequenced over 110 kb of this region. This sequence matched the HPV16 integration site, the aphidicolin-induced breakpoints and the pSV2neo integration sites in the FRA3B region. Finally, in an approach aimed at investigating regions of loss of heterozygosity (LOH) in tumors, Ohta et al. (1996) cloned the *FHIT* (for fragile histadine triad) gene from the same region, and it is now known that *FHIT* spans FRA3B.

The results of these studies show that the common fragile sites, and FRA3B in particular, differ from FRAXA and other rare fragile sites in many ways. First, gaps, breaks and instability occur over a very large genomic region relative to FRAXA. FRA3B extends from approximately the t(3;8) breakpoint to roughly 500 kb telomeric. Whether this represents a single unstable region or multiple unstable regions is unknown. Secondly, trinucleotide repeats have not been identified in the region (Wilke et al. 1996; Pardee et al. 1995; Boldog et al. 1997). Thus, while all fragile sites appear similar on the level of the metaphase chromosome, there are significant differences on the molecular level.

Are common fragile sites associated with genes as are at least some rare fragile sites? Given their apparent instability, this might have been considered doubtful not long ago. However, FRA3B, the only common fragile site to so far be characterized at the molecular level, lies within a gene that is highly unstable in tumor cells. The identification of this gene followed from searches for regions that might contain tumor suppressor genes in tumor cell lines.

Based on representational difference analysis (RDA) of genomic DNA, Lisitsyn et al. (1995) identified a region on 3p which showed homozygous deletions in gastrointestinal tumor cell lines. Kastury et al. (1996) defined homozygous deletions encompassing these sequences in a variety of epithelial tumor cell lines. Focusing on this deleted region, Otha et al. (1996) used exon trapping to identify an exon of what is now known as the *FHIT* gene from a cosmid contig spanning this region. The region of homozygous deletion and the *FHIT* gene were subsequently found to map exactly at FRA3B.

The *FHIT* gene spans approximately 1 mb of 3p14.2, and spans both FRA3B and the t(3;8) familial renal cell carcinoma breakpoint. It contains ten exons, five of which are coding. In contrast to its large genomic size, it encodes only a 1.1-kb transcript that is ubiquitously expressed at relatively low levels (Ohta et al. 1996). The product of the *FHIT* gene is a 147 amino acid

(16.8 kDa) protein with identity to diadenosine 5′,5‴-P1,P4-tetraphosphate hydrolase (Ap4A) from *Schizosacchramyces pompe* which functions in the cleavage of diadenosine tetraphosphates (Barnes et al. 1996). Both proteins have sequence homology to the HIT family of proteins. These proteins are characterized by four conserved histidines, three of which comprise a histidine triad (HxHxH), or HIT sequence which is encoded by exon 8 for the human protein. Barnes et al. (1996) have recently demonstrated that the preferred substrate for the *FHIT* protein is a diadenosine triphosphate, rather than tetraphosphate, thus *FHIT* functions as a 5′5‴-P1,P3-diadenosine triphosphate (Ap3A) hydrolase (EC3.6.1.29).

The biological significance of the *FHIT* gene is not clearly understood. Diadenosine tri- and tetra-phosphates are ubiquitous small molecules produced from ATP and consist of two adenosine molecules bridged by two or three phosphate groups. They have been implicated in cell cycle arrest and are synthesized in response to cellular stress such as starvation and heat shock conditions in prokaryotes, leading to their being termed "alarmones" (Segal and Le Pecq 1986; Garrison et al. 1986). This possible role is of particular interest when considering fragile sites given that they are induced under conditions of cellular stress or nucleotide starvation. Besides this, the significance of diadenosine phosphates as modulators of physiological processes such as hemostasis and neurotransmission has been the focus of intensive research interest for many years.

The FHIT/FRA3B Region is Frequently Deleted in Tumor Cells

Because of its location in a region of frequent LOH in many tumors, and the fact that a homozygous deletion in an esophageal tumor provided a foothold into 3p14.2 for the identification of *FHIT*, Ohta et al. (1996) and others from this group studied the *FHIT* gene in a number of tumors and tumor cell lines. Using RT-PCR to study RNA from cell lines as well as primary squamous cell esophageal, stomach, and colon carcinomas, aberrant *FHIT* transcripts, suggesting deletions, were identified in many of the tumors and most of the cell lines. The cell lines were also shown to have homozygous deletions within *FHIT* and the *FHIT* protein was shown to be absent or reduced in some of these cell lines. Based on these findings, Ohta et al. (1996) suggested that *FHIT* is a frequently mutated tumor suppressor gene.

Aberrant transcripts have subsequently been identified by RT-PCR in numerous tumors or tumor cell lines including breast (Negrini et al. 1996), lung (Sozzi et al. 1996), head and neck (Virgilio et al. 1996), cervical (Muller et al. 1948) and Barrett's esophageal tumors (Michael et al. 1997). While the nature of the aberrant transcripts is not completely understood, genomic deletions have been identified in many of the cell lines and some of the primary tumors. In our study of premalignant metaplasia and adenonocarcinomas of Barrett's esophagus (Michael et al. 1997) deletions of exon 5 and within intron 5 of *FHIT*, both within FRA3B by FISH, were observed. The results of genomic deletion analysis coincided with the RT-PCR results in some, but not all, cases, suggesting that other factors such as aberrant splicing in tumor cells may also contribute to the appearance of aberrant transcripts.

In addition to deletions and aberrant transcripts, the FRA3B region and *FHIT* gene have so far been found to be involved in two chromosome translocations associated with cancer. The first is the hereditary t(3;8) translocation breakpoint, mentioned earlier, that was found in a family segregating a genotype conferring high risk for renal cell carcinoma (Cohen et al. 1979). This translocation breaks the chromosome in intron 3 of the *FHIT* gene. The second is a tumor-specific translocation found in a pleomorphic adenoma of the thyroid gland (Geurts et al. 1997). In this latter case, *FHIT* forms a chimeric transcript with the *HMGIC* tumor supressor gene on chromosome 12. Whether these translocations are related to instability of FRA3B is not known, but as mentioned above, translocations in FRA3B can be induced at a high frequency in vitro (Glover and Stein 1988; Wang et al. 1993).

These and other studies (see Huebner et al. this volume) have firmly shown a relationship between deletions and instability at the *FHIT*/FRA3B locus and cancer cells. Questions that remain include whether these deletions are a cause or an effect of cancer, whether *FHIT* is a classic tumor suppressor gene, and whether FRA3B is truly the cause of the instability. Siprashvili et al. (1997) have recently presented functional data in which transfected *FHIT* constructs suppressed tumor growth, supporting the tumor suppressor hypothesis. Arguments against the *FHIT* gene acting as a classical tumor suppressor gene include the fact that the known function of *FHIT* is not obviously related to tumor suppressor activity. In addition, some primary tumors and cancer cell lines were found to harbor allelic and homozygous deletions only in intronic regions (Boldog et al. 1997; Sozzi et al. 1996; Thiagalingam et al. 1996), thus presumably not affecting *FHIT* function. Also, under certain conditions, "aberrant" *FHIT* transcripts have been seen in normal cells (Boldog et al. 1997; Thiagalingam et al. 1996). Therefore, alternative hypotheses for the unusual findings with the *FHIT* gene include aberrant or alternative splicing, selection for another mutated gene tumor suppressor gene in the region, perhaps in the large *FHIT* intron 5, and genomic instability at FRA3B which lies at the center of the frequently deleted regions of *FHIT*.

Genomic instability is a frequent characteristic of tumor cells and common fragile sites may be particularly sensitive to such instability. Thus, as now suggested by many investigators, *FHIT* deletions and aberrant splicing and aberrant transcripts may arise through FRA3B leading to genomic instability and possibly interfering with *FHIT* transcription and/or splicing with or without providing a selective advantage to the affected cell (Boldog et al. 11997; Michael et al. 1997; Thiagalingam et al. 1996). However, the hypothesis that FRA3B is responsible for the high frequency of *FHIT* deletions is not mutually exclusive with the tumor suppressor gene hypothesis. Regardless of the function of the *FHIT* gene, it represents a highly unstable gene in cancer, and it contains a common fragile site that may cause the instability. It is possible that similarly unstable genes could be associated with the 80 or so other common fragile sites, and such associations would lend support to this hypothesis. Huang et al. (1997) have recently identified yeast artificial chromosomes (YACs) spanning the common fragile site at 7q32.1 (FRA7G). This fragile site region also appears large, over 300 kb, and contains markers that are frequently lost in breast, prostate and ovarian cancers. My laboratory has recently identified YAC clones spanning common fragile sites at Xp22.3 (FRAXB) and 16q23.1 (FRA16D) and has begun their analysis. FRAXB lies in a region of frequent deletions at Xp22.3, while the region in which FRA16D maps has been identified as a region of frequent LOH in prostate and breast cancer (Cleton-Jansen et al. 1994). Whether these fragile sites are mechanistically related to the deletions noted in these regions is unknown at present.

Mechanism of Instability: Genetic and Environmental Influences

The mechanism underlying instability at all fragile sites, including the trinucleotide repeats, is not well understood. The mechanism for induction of all fragile sites appears to involve interruptions of normal DNA synthesis. DNA repair mechanisms may also play a role, since caffeine, an inhibitor of G2 repair, increases the number of cells expressing fragile sites (Yunis and Soren 1984; Glover et al. 1986). Based on the fact that fragile sites are induced by agents that retard DNA replication or repair, and the high frequency of sister chromatid exchanges and chromosome rearrangements, it was proposed many years ago that fragile sites were associated with unreplicated DNA or DNA strand breaks (Glover et al. 1984; Glover and Stein 1987, 1988).

For the majority of rare fragile sites, the same events that lead to instability at CCG repeats during meiosis or mitosis in vivo also likely lead to the manifestation of fragile sites on metaphase chromosomes. Richards and Sutherland have suggested that the massive expansion seen at trinucleotide repeats may be due to the occurrence of more than one single-strand DNA break causing slippage of unanchored Okazaki fragments during replication (Richards and Sutherland 1995). Instability in related tandem repeat sequences has been shown by Jeffreys et al. (1994) to involve a complex process involving strand breaks, gene conversion or internal reduplication, and gap repair. Interestingly, mutations in these repeats tend to occur at one end of the repeat, i.e. they are polar, and this has led to the suggestion that sequences adjacent to the repeats may play a role in the instability. In recent years, investigators have demonstrated an association of trinucleotide repeats with exclusion of nucleosomes (Wang and Griffith 1996), DNA hairpin structures (Gracy et al. 1995) and pausing of DNA synthesis (Kang et al. 1995).

Less is known about the mechanism responsible for common fragile sites. No trinucleotide or other simple repeat sequence motif has yet been identified that could be responsible for the instability (Wilke et al. 1996; Boldog et al. 1977). The common fragile site region so far examined in greatest detail,

FRA3B, is very large and a complete sequence is not yet available. Boldog et al. (1997) have sequenced approximately 110 kb of the centromeric portion of FRA3B within intron 5 of the *FHIT* gene and have found the region to be high in AT content and in LINE and MER repeats, with few alu repeats. Interestingly, they identified a small polydispersed circular DNA (spc-DNA) sequence in this region. Such sequences have been shown to be associated with clustered repeats such as *β*-satellites and are elevated in Fanconi's anemia patients. They are also induced by DNA damaging agents, including the fragile site inducer aphidicolin.

If fragile sites are indeed regions of unreplicated DNA, this could arise from a number of reasons in addition to repeats leading to blocks to DNA replication, such as late replication or a paucity of replication origins in the region. Laird et al. (1987) have proposed a model for fragile sites wherein they occur at alleles whose replication is delayed relative to nonfragile alleles. Le Beau et al. (1998) have recently shown that FRA3B is a late replicating region and that replication is further delayed or inhibited by aphidicolin, used to induce expression of FRA3B. While late replication alone does not result in a fragile site, fragile site sequences may not be able to recover from a further delay in DNA synthesis. Such regions of unreplicated DNA persisting in G2 and M could explain why caffeine, an inhibitor of G2 repair, increases fragile site expression. A largely unexplored possibility is that common fragile site expression is related to transcriptional timing of associated late replicating genes, such as *FHIT* or other genes at FRA3B.

In addition to *cis*-acting sequences, there are undoubtedly other genetic and environmental factors that influence fragile site expression and associated genomic instability. Candidates for genes influencing expression are those involved in DNA replication and repair, and those involved in cell cycle checkpoints such as p53. It is clear that one of the defining features of cancer cells is an increase in genome instability. Mutations in the p53 gene are known to result in polyploidy and widespread karyotypic instability, amplifications and deletions (Donehower et al. 1995; Huang et al. 1996). Loss of p53 function by mutation or inactivation of the protein leads to an inability of the cell to interrupt its cell division cycle in response to many types of DNA damage, perhaps including DNA damage at fragile sites. It is very possible that fragile site regions, and any associated genes (such as *FHIT* at FRA3B), may be especially sensitive to the effects of such instability. This could in part explain why the *FHIT* gene is so frequently deleted and rearranged in many tumors. Boldog et al. (1997) have recently found a correlation between tumors with *FHIT* deletions and their p53 mutation status, supporting this suggestion. The recent findings, that fragile sites are associated with intrachromosomal gene amplification in CHO cells, may relate to their deficiency in p53 or related genes.

Environmental factors also may influence fragile site expression or stability. As mentioned above, caffeine treatment of cells in vitro increases fragile site expression. Ban et al. (1995) have provided data indicating that cigarette smokers show increased frequencies of fragile site expression in their cul-

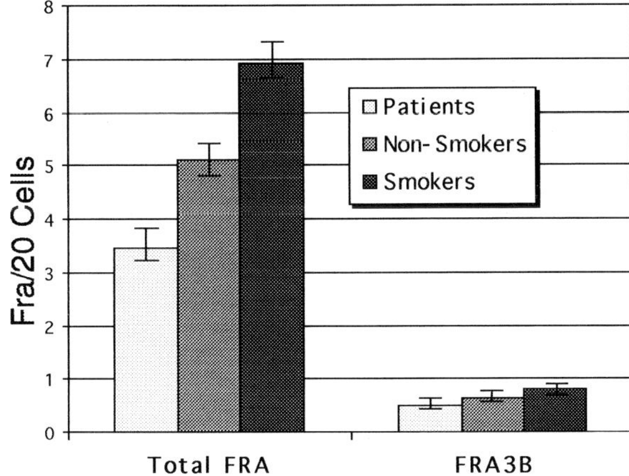

Fig. 2. Summary of fragile site expression in cultured lymphocytes from nonsmoking lung cancer patients, nonsmoking controls and smokers. Values are presented as least squares means ± std. error. Both total fragile site and FRA3B expression are significantly higher in smokers (from Stein et al., submitted)

tured lymphocytes. In our own studies (Stein et al., submitted) of fragile site expression in lung cancer patients vs controls, we also found this to be the case. Current cigarette smokers showed a significantly increased frequency of expression of FRA3B and other fragile sites as compared to nonsmoking cancer patients or controls (Fig. 2). In what could be related to these findings, Sozzi et al. (1997) have recently reported loss of alleles on chromosome 3p, specifically at the *FHIT* locus, occurs in tumors from cigarette smokers at a higher frequency than in tumors from nonsmokers. How cigarette smoking can lead to increased expression of a fragile site, even after lymphocytes are cultured for 3–4 days, is presently unknown, as is the effect on *FHIT* or other genes at the molecular level. However, theses studies point to the possibility that FRA3B and other common fragile sites may be targets for common carcinogens such as those found in cigarette smoke.

Conclusions

The phenomenon of fragile sites has intrigued a handful of investigators for over two decades, but has become increasingly of interest with findings over the past few years. Some, like FRAXA seen in the *FMR1* gene, are caused by expansion of CCG trinucleotide repeats. The majority of fragile sites, however, are the common fragile sites about which much less is known regarding their biological significance or mechanism of instability. Although a number of early reports attempted to link fragile sites with chromosome breakpoints found in cancer cells, until recently there was no direct molecular evidence to support this association. It now appears from studies of FRA3B and the *FHIT* gene that this is a large genomic region that is particularly unstable in cancer cells. A number of interesting questions are now approachable, including the mechanism of this instability, the genetic and environmental influences affecting instability and the functional significance of instability at FRA3B and other fragile sites.

Acknowledgments. I am grateful to the Deutsche Krebshilfe, Dr. Mildred Scheel Foundation. I thank Diane Miller for producing Fig. 1. TWG is supported by grant CA 43222 from the National Cancer Institute (USA).

References

Austin MJF, Collins JM, Corey LA, Nance WE, Neale MC et al (1992) Aphidicolin-inducible common fragile-site expression: results from a population survey of twins. Am J Hum Genet. 50:76–83

Ban S, Cologne JB, Neriishi K (1995) Effect of radiation and cigarette smoking on expression of FUdR-inducible common fragile sites in human peripheral lymphocytes. Mutat Res 334:197–203

Barnes LD, Garrison PN, Siprashvili Z, Guranowski A, Robinson AK, Ingram SW, Croce CM, Ohta M, Huebner K. (1996) *FHIT*, a putative tumor suppressor in humans, is a dinucleoside 5′,5′′′-P1,P3-triphosphate hydrolase. Biochemistry 35:11529–11535

Boldog F, Gemmill R, West J, Robinson M, Li E (1997) Chromosome 3p14 homozygous deletions and sequence analysis of FRA3B. Hum Mol Genet 6:193–203

Cleton-Jansen AM, Moerland EW, Kuipers-Dijkshoorn NJ, Callen DF, Sutherland GR et al (1994) At least two different regions are involved in allelic imbalance on chromosome arm 16q in breast cancer. Genes Chromosomes Cancer 9:101–107

Cohen AJ, Li FP, Berg S, Marchetto DJ, Tsai S et al (1979) Hereditary renal-cell carcinoma associated with a chromosomal translocation. New Engl J Med 301:592–595

Coquelle A, Pipiras E, Toledo F, Buttin G, Debatisse M (1997) Expression of fragile sites triggers intrachromosomal mammalian gene amplification and sets boundaries to early amplications. Cell 89:215–225

De Braekeleer M, Sreekantaiah C, Haas O (1992) Herpes simplex virus and human papillomavirus sites correlate with chromosomal breakpoints in human cervical carcinoma. Cancer Genet Cytogenet 59:135–137

Donehower LA, Godley LA, Aldaz CM, Pyle R, Shi YP, Pinkel D, Gray J, Bradley A, Medina D, Varmus HE (1995) Deficiency of p53 accelerates mammary tumorigenesis in Wnt-1 transgenic mice and promotes chromosomal instability. Genes & Development 9:882–895

Fu YH, Kuhl DPA, Pizzut A, Pierett M, Sutcliffe JS et al (1991) Variation of the CGG repeat at the fragile X site results in genetic instability: resolution of the Sherman paradox. Cell 67:1047–1058

Gacy AM, Goellner G, Juranic N, Macura S, McMurray CT (1995) Trinucleotide repeats that expand in human disease form hairpin structures in vitro. Cell 81:533–540

Garrison PN, Mathis SA, Barnes LD (1986) In vivo levels of diadenosine tetraphosphate and adenosine tetraphospho-guanosine in Physarum polycephalum during the cell cycle and oxidative stress. Mol Cell Biol 6:1179–1186

Geurts JMW, Schoenmakers EFPM, Roijer E, Stenman G, Van de Ven WJM (1997) Expression of reciprocal hybrid transcripts of HMGIC and FHIT in a pleomorphic adenoma of the parotid gland. Cancer Res 57:13–17

Glover TW (1998) Common fragile sites. In: Wells RD, Warren ST (eds) Genetic instabilities and neurological diseases. Academic Press, San Diego, pp 75–83

Glover TW, Stein CK (1987) Induction of sister chromatid exchanges at common fragile sites. Am J Hum Genet 41:882–890

Glover TW, Stein CK (1988) Chromosome breakage and recombination at fragile sites. Am J Hum Genet 43:265–273

Glover TW, Berger C, Coyle J, Echo B (1984) DNA polymerase α inhibition by aphidicolin induces gaps and breaks at common fragile sites in human chromosomes. Hum Genet 67:136–142

Glover TW, Coyle-Morris J, Morgan R (1986) Fragile sites: overview, occurrence in acute nonlymphocytic leukemia-M4 and effects of caffeine on expression. Cancer Genet Cytogenet 19:141–150

Glover TW, Coyle-Morris JF, Li, FP, Brown RS, Berger CS (1988) Translocation t(3;8) (p14.2;q24.1) in renal cell carcinoma affects expression of the common fragile site at 3p14 (FRA3B) in lymphocytes. Cancer Genet Cytogenet 31:69–73

Hecht F, Sutherland GR (1984) Fragile sites and cancer breakpoints. Cancer Genet Cytogenet 12:179–181

Hecht F (1988) Fragile sites, cancer chromosome breakpoints, and oncogenes all cluster in light G-bands. Cancer Genet Cytogenet 31:17–24

Hecht F, Glover TW (1984) Cancer chromosome breakpoints and common fragile sites induced by aphidicolin. Cancer Genet Cytogenet 13:185–188

Hibi K, Takahashi T, Yamakawa K, Ueda R, Sekido Y et al (1992) Three distinct regions involved in 3p deletion in human lung cancer. Oncogene 7:445–449

Huang H, Qian C, Jenkins R, Smith D (1998) FISH mapping of YAC clones at human chromsomal band 7q31.2: Identification of YACs spanning FRA7G within the common region of LOH in breast and prostate cancer. Genes Chromosomes Cancer 21:152–159

Huang LC, Clarkin KC, Wahl GM (1996) Sensitivity and selectivity of the DNA damage sensor responsible for activating p53-dependent G1 arrest. Proc Natl Acad Sci 93:4827–4832

Jalal SM, Lindor NM, Michels VV, Buckley DD, Hoppe DA, Sarkar G, Dewald GW (1993) Absence of chromosome fragility at 19q13.3 in patients with myotonic dystrophy. Am J Med Genet 46:441–439

Jeffreys AJ, Tamaki K, MacLeod A, Monckton DG, Neil DL et al (1994) Complex gene conversion events in germline mutation at human satellites. Nat Genet 6:136–145

Jones C, Penny L, Mattina T, Yu S, Baker E, Voullaire L, Langdon WY, Sutherland GR, Richards RI, Tunnacliffe A (1995) Association of a chromosome deletion syndrome with a fragile site within the proto-oncogene *CBL2*. Nature 376:145–149

Kang S, Ohshima K, Shimizu M et al (1995) Pausing of DNA synthesis in vitro at specific loci in CGT and CGG triplet repeats from human hereditary disease genes. J Biol Chem 270:27014–27021

Kastury K, Baffa R, Druck, T, Ohta M, Cotticelli MG, Inoue H, Negrini M, Rugge M., Huang D, Croce CM, Palazzo J, Huebner K (1996) Potential gastrointestinal tumor suppressor locus at the 3p14.2 FRA3Bsite identified by homozygous deletions in tumor cell lines. Cancer Res 56:978–983

Knight SJL, Flannery AV, Hirst AC, Campbell L, Christodoulou Z et al (1993) Trinucleotide repeat amplification and hypermethylation of a CpG island in FRAXE mental retardation. Cell 74:1–20

Kuo MT, Vyas RC, Jiang LX, Hittelman WN (1994) Chromosome breakage at a major fragile site associated with P-glycoprotein gene amplification in multidrug-resistant CHO cells. Mol Cell Biol 14:5202–5211

Kremer EJ, Pritchard M, Lynch M, Yu S, Holman K et al (1991) Mapping of DNA instability at the fragile X to a trinucleotide repeat sequence p(CCG)n. Science 252:1711–1718

Laird C, Jaffe E, Karpsen G, Lamb M, Nelson R (1987) Fragile sites in human chromosomes as regions of late-replicating DNA. Trends Genet 3:274–281

Le Beau MM, Rowley JD (1984) Heritable fragile sites and cancer. Nature 308:607–608

Le Beau MM, Rassool FV, Neilly ME, Espinosa R, Glover TW, Smith DI, McKeithan TW (1998) Replication of a common fragile site, FRA3B, occurs late in S phase and is delayed further upon induction: implications for the mechanism of fragile site induction. Hum Mol Genet 7:755–761

Lisitsyn NA, Lisitsina NM, Dalbagni G, Barker P, Sanchez CA, Gnarra J, Linehan WM, Reid BJ, Wigler MH (1995) Proc Natl Acad Sci USA 92:151–155

Michael D, Beer DG, Wilke CM, Miller DM, Glover TW (1997) Frequent deletions of *FHIT* and FRA3B in Barrett's metaplasia and esophageal adenocarcinomas. Oncogene 15:1653–1659

Muller CY, O'Boyle JD, Fong KM, Wistuba II, Biesterveld E, Ahmadian M, Miller DS, Gazdar AF, Minna JD (1998) Abnormalities of FHIT genomic and cDNAs in human cervical cancer with HPV subtype correlation. J Natl Cancer Inst (in press)

Nancarrow JK, Kremer E, Holman K, Eyre H, Dogget NA, Le Paslier D, Callen DF, Sutherland GR, Richards RI (1994) Implications of FRA16A structure for the mechanism of chromosomal fragile site genesis. Science 264:1938–1941

Negrini M, Monaco C, Vorechovsky I, Ohta M, Druck T, Baffa R., Huebner K, Croce CM (1996) The *FHIT* gene at 3p14.2 is abnormal in breast carcinomas. Cancer Res 56:3173–3179

Oberle I, Rousseau F, Heitz D, Kretz C, Deveys D et al (1991) Instability of a 550-base pair DNA segment and abnormal methylation in fragile X syndrome. Science 252:1097–1102

Ohta M, Inoue H, Cotticelli MG, Kastury K, Baffa R, Palazzo J, Siprashvili Z, Mori M, McCue P, Druck T, Croce CM, Huebner K (1996) The FHIT gene, spanning the chromosome 3p14.2 fragile site and renal carcinoma-associated t(3;8) breakpoint, is abnormal in digestive tract cancers. Cell 84:587–597

Pardee W, Mullins C, He Z, Glover TW, Wilke C, Opalka B, Schutte J, Smith DI (1995) Precise localization of aphidicolin-induced breakpoints on the short arm of human chromosome 3. Genomics 27:358–361

Pardee W, Wilke CM, Hoge A, Glover TW, Smith DI (1996) A 350 Kb cosmid contig in 3p14.2 that crosses the t(3;8) hereditary renal cell carcinoma translocation breakpoint and 17 aphidicolin-induced FRA3B breakpoints. Genomics 35:87–93

Parrish P, Oostra BA, Verkerk AJMH, Richards, CS et al (1994) Isolation of a GCC repeat showing expansion in FRAXF, a fragile site distal to FRAXA and FRAXE. Nature [Genet] 8:229–235

Popescu NC, DiPaolo JA (1989) Preferential sites for viral integration on mammalian genome. Cancer Genet Cytogenet 42:157–171

Rassool FV, McKeithan TW, Neilly ME, van Melle E, Espinosa R III, Lebeau MM (1991) Preferential integration of marker DNA into the chromosomal fragile site at 3p14: An approach to cloning fragile sites. Proc Natl Acad Sci USA 88:6657–6661

Rassool FV, Le Beau MM, Shen ML, Neilly ME, Espinosa R III, Ong ST, Boldog F, Drabkin H, McCarroll R, McKeithan TW (1996) Direct cloning of DNA sequences from the common fragile site region at chromosome band 3p14.2. Genomics 35:109–117

Richards RI, Sutherland GR (1994) Simple repeat DNA is not replicated simply. Nat Genet 6:114–116

Segal E, Le Pecq JB (1986) Relationship between cellular diadenosine 5', 5'''-P1, P4-tetraphosphate level, cell density, cell growth stimulation and toxic stresses. Exp Cell Res 167:119–126

Siprashvili Z, Sozzi G, Barnes LD, McCue P, Robinson AK Eryomin V, Sard L, Tagliabue E, Greco A, Fusetti L, Schwartz G, Pierotti MC, Croce CM, Huebner K (1997) Replacement of Fhit in cancer cells supresses tumorigenicity. Proc Natl Acad Sci USA 94:13771–13776

Smith PP, Friedman C, Bryant EM, McDougall JK (1992) Viral integration and fragile sites in human papillomavirus-immortalized human keratinocyte cell lines. Genes Chromosomes Cancer 5:150–157

Sozzi G, Veronese ML, Negrini M, Baffa R, Cotticelli MG, Inoue H, Tornielli S, Pilotti S, De Gregorio L, Pastorino U, Pierotti MA, Ohta M, Huebner K, Croce CM (1996) The *FHIT* gene 3p14.2 is abnormal in lung cancer. Cell 85:7–26

Sozzi G, Sard L, De Gregorio L, Marchetti A, Musso K et al (1997) Association between cigarette smoking and FHIT gene alterations in lung cancer. Cancer Res. 57:2121–2123

Sutherland GR, Hecht F (1985) Fragile sites on human chromosomes Oxford University Press, Oxford (Oxford Monographs on Medical Genetics)

Tedeschi B, Vernole P, Sanna ML, Nicoletti B (1992) Population cytogenetics of aphidicolin-induced fragile sites. Hum Genet 89:543–547

Thiagalingam S, Lisitsyn, NA, Hamaguchi M, Wigler MH, Willson JK, Markowitz SD, Leach FS, Kinzler KW, Vogelstein B (1996) Evaluation of the FHIT gene in colorectal cancers. Cancer Res 56:2936–2939

Verkerk AJM, Pieretti M, Sutcliffe JS, Fu YH, Kuhl DP et al (1991) Identification of a gene (FMR-1) containing a CGG repeat coincident with a breakpoint cluster region exhibiting length variation in fragile X syndrome. Cell 65:905–914

Virgilio L, Shuster M, Gollin SM, Veronese ML, Ohta M, Huebner K, Croce CM (1996) *FHIT* gene alterations in head and neck squamous cell carcinomas. Proc Natl Acad Sci USA 93:9770–9775

Wang ND, Testa JR, Smith DI (1993) Determination of the specificity of aphidicolin-induced breakage of the human 3p14.2 fragile site. Genomics 17:341–347

Wang YH, Griffith J (1996) Methylation of expanded CCG triplet repeat DNA from fragile X syndrome patients enhances nucleosome exclusion. J Biol Chem 271:22937–22940

Warren ST (1996) The expanding world of trinucleotide repeats. Science 271:1374–1375

Wilke CM, Hall BK, Buldog F, Gemmill RM, Chandrasekharappa C, Drabkin H, Glover TW (1994) Multicolor FISH mapping of YAC clonec in 3p14 and isolation of a YAC spanning both FRA3B and the t(3;8) translocation associated with heritable renal cell Carcinoma. Genomics 22:319–326

Wilke CM, Hall BK, Hoge A, Pardee W, Smith DI, Glover TW (1996) FRA3B extends over a broad region and contains a spontaneous HPV integration site: Direct evidence for the coincidence of viral integration sites and fragiles sites. Hum Mol Genet 5:187–195

Wistuba II, Montellano FD, Milchgrub S, Virmani AK, Behrens C, Chen H, Ahmadian M, Nowak JA, Muller C, Minna JD, Gazdar AF (1997) Deletions of chromosome 3p are frequent and early events in the pathogenesis of uterine cervical carcinoma. Cancer Res 57:3154–3158

Yunis JJ, Soreng AL (1984) Constitutive fragile sites and cancer. Science 226:1199–1204

Yu S, Mangelsforf M, Hewett D, Hobsen L et al (1997) Human chromosomal fragile site FRA16B is an amplified AT-rich minisatellitte repeat. Cell 88:367–374

Yamakawa K, Morita R, Takahashi E, Hori T, Ishikawa J et al (1991) A detailed deletion mapping of the short arm of chromosome 3 in sporadic renal cell carcinoma. Cancer Res 51:4707–4711

The Role of Deletions at the *FRA3B/FHIT* Locus in Carcinogenesis

K. Huebner[1], T. Druck[1], Z. Siprashvili[1], C. M. Croce[1], A. Kovatich[2], and P. A. McCue[2]

[1] Department of Microbiology and Immunology, Kimmel Cancer Center,
Thomas Jefferson University, 233 South 10th Street,
Bluemle Life Sciences Building, Room 1008, Philadelphia, PA 19107, USA
[2] Department of Pathology, Anatomy and Cell Biology,
Division of Surgical Pathology, Thomas Jefferson University,
132 South 10th Street, Main Building, Room 28SD, Philadelphia, PA 19107, USA

Abstract

The *FHIT* gene, which encodes a 1-kb message and a 16.8-kDa protein that hydrolyses diadenosine triphosphate (ApppA) to ADP and AMP in vitro, covers a megabase genomic region at chromosome band 3p14.2. The gene encompasses the most active of the common human chromosomal fragile regions, *FRA3B*. Over the years, it has been suggested that fragile sites might be especially susceptible to carcinogen damage and that chromosomal regions of nonrandom alterations in cancer cells may coincide with defined fragile sites. Within the *FRA3B* region, the characteristic induced chromosome gaps can occur across the entire region, but 60% of the gaps are centered on a 300-kb region flanking *FHIT* exon 5, the first protein-coding exon. Numerous hemizygous and homozygous deletions, translocations and DNA insertions occur within *FHIT* in cancer cell lines, uncultured tumors, and even in preneoplastic lesions, especially in tissues such as lung that are targets of carcinogens. This supports the proposed cancer–fragile site connection and suggests that the *FHIT* gene, expression of which is frequently altered in cells showing *FHIT* locus damage, is a tumor suppressor gene whose inactivation may drive clonal expansion of preneoplastic and neoplastic cells. Replacement of Fhit expression in Fhit-negative cancer cells abrogates their tumorigenicity in nude mice.

Analysis of the approximately 300-kb DNA sequence encompassing *FHIT* exon 5 in the *FRA3B* epicenter has provided clues to the mechanism of repair of the fragile site double strand breaks. The mechanism involves recombination between LINE 1 elements with deletion of the intervening sequence, often including *FHIT* exons. These studies have also shown that *FHIT* alterations generally entail independent deletion of both *FHIT* alleles.

Future studies will focus on two objectives: study of (1) the in vivo function of the Fhit protein and (2) mechanisms of break and repair in the *FRA3B* fragile region.

Recent Results in Cancer Research, Vol. 154
© Springer-Verlag Berlin · Heidelberg 1998

Background

With the mapping of the *PTPRG* (receptor protein tyrosine phosphatase gamma or PTPγ gene) locus to 3p14–21 centromeric to a chromosome translocation break (LaForgia et al. 1991) associated with familial clear cell renal carcinoma in a family carrying a t(3;8)(p14.2; q24), translocation (Li et al. 1993), we began a search for the gene at 3p14.2 which was disrupted or dysregulated by the translocation and thus might be a tumor suppressor gene important for kidney cancer. It was already known that alterations on the short arm of chromosome 3 (3p), usually involving loss of portions of 3p, were extensive in a number of important types of human cancers, notably lung and kidney cancer; it has subsequently been shown that 3p rearrangements resulting in loss of 3p alleles are among the most frequent alterations in human cancer. There are at least four target regions for loss of alleles on 3p – at 3p12, 3p14, 3p21, and 3p25 – and tumor suppressor genes were being sought for each of these loci. A number of laboratories had been interested in the 3p14.2 region because of the familial kidney cancer translocation and because the most active of human chromosome fragile sites was also in 3p14.2, perhaps coincident with the t(3,8) chromosome translocation (Glover et al. 1988). We studied the relationship of the PTPγ gene and the t(3;8) flanking region to loss of heterozygosity (LOH) in sporadic human cancers, with the ultimate goal of isolation and characterization of the tumor suppressor gene at the translocation break. We have shown that the PTPγ gene maps closely centromeric to the 3p14.2 breakpoint and that the breakpoint region is involved in LOH in more than 80% of clear cell renal carcinomas (Druck et al. 1995) and a substantial fraction of stomach, colon, lung (Kastury et al. 1996; Ohta et al. 1996; Sozzi et al. 1996) and other tumors. We have also shown that the remaining PTPγ allele in kidney tumors is not altered (Druck et al. 1995). We thus moved to the telomeric side of the translocation break, showed that numerous homozygous deletions in cancer cell lines mapped closely telomeric to the translocation break, and isolated a gene which encompassed the translocation break, the common fragile site, and the homozygous deletions. The gene, designated the fragile histidine triad or *FHIT* gene, has now been further characterized to strengthen its credentials as a multiple tumor suppressor gene that, by virtue of its inclusion of the common fragile site, is especially sensitive to disruption by environmental carcinogens, such as those found in cigarette smoke (Mao et al. 1997; Wistuba et al. 1997b). Additionally, expression of Fhit protein has been assessed by immunohistochemistry in small cell lung cancers (SCLC) and the related lung carcinoids.

Materials and Methods

Tissue Specimens and DNA Isolation

Tumor specimens and matched normal controls were obtained from the archival files or frozen tissue bank of Thomas Jefferson University Hospital. Slides and tissue sections were reviewed to confirm the diagnosis and check conformity with standard histologic criteria. Carcinoid tumors were microdissected prior to DNA preparation. SCLC samples were taken from biopsies of less than 3 mm and were not microdissected. Slides used for immunohistochemistry were coated with neoprene. Dissected tissues were placed in sterile microcentrifuge tubes, deparaffinized with xylene, and incubated overnight at 37 °C in Tris-ethylenediaminetetraacetate (EDTA), pH 7.8, and proteinase K (50 µg). DNA from sections, biopsies, and frozen or fresh tissue was isolated by standard phenol-chloroform extraction and ethanol precipitation.

Loss of Heterozygosity Analysis

LOH at microsatellite loci was detected using a polymerase chain reaction (PCR)-based approach. Primers which amplify polymorphic microsatellite-containing alleles from numerous 3p loci were prepared in the Kimmel Cancer Institute core sequencing and synthesis facility or were purchased from Research Genetics. Map order and position were established on the basis of data from the Genome Data Base (GDB) and the Human Cooperative Linkage Center Database and were confirmed, where possible, by analysis of a panel of rodent–human hybrids containing portions of 3p. Band positions were estimated from a combination of genetic and physical positions. For informative cases, allelic loss was scored visually if the radiographic signal of one allele was reduced by at least 50% in the tumor DNA when compared to its corresponding normal allele. Altered alleles observed in tumors displaying apparent microsatellite instability were not scored for allelic loss.

Microsatellite loci from tumor and normal DNA templates were amplified by PCR with the appropriate oligonucleotides. PCR amplification reactions were carried out in 12.5-µl final volume with 100 ng template DNA, 20 ng primers, 10 mM Tris-HCl pH 8.3, 50 mM KCl, 0.1 mg/ml gelatin, 1.5 mM $MgCl_2$, 0.1 mM each deoxynucleoside triphosphate (dNTP), 0.5 units Taq polymerase (ABI), and 1 µCi [a^{32}P]-deoxycytidine triphosphate (dCTP). The amplification reactions were performed in a Perkin-Elmer Cetus thermal cycler for 30 cycles at 94 °C for 30 s, at 57 °C (varied for specific primer pairs) for 30 s, and at 72 °C for 30 s. PCR product (1 µl) was mixed with 9 µl sequencing stop buffer (95% formamide, 10 mM NaOH, 0.05% bromphenol blue, 0.05% xylene cyanol FF) and denatured at 94 °C for 5 min. For LOH, analysis 5 µl of this mixture was loaded onto a 6% acrylamide:bis (19:1), 8 M urea gel for electrophoresis at 80 W for 2–3 h. Gels were dried and exposed to X-ray film for 1–14 h.

Immunohistochemical Methods

Routine deparaffinization from xylene to 95% alcohol and rehydration prior to microwave antigen recovery were carried out on a Leica Autostainer (Leica Inc., Deerfield, IL). The deparaffinization process included a 30-min methanolic peroxide block for endogenous peroxidase activity. The antigen recovery step was carried out in an 800-W microwave oven in 200 ml heat-induced epitope retrieval ChemMate (HIER) Buffer, pH 5.5–5.7 (Ventana Medical Systems, Tucson, AZ). The holder and slides were then removed from the oven and cooled for 20 min prior to continuing the immunostaining procedure.

Slides were washed in dH_2O and placed in ChemMate Buffer 1 (phosphate-buffered solution containing carrier protein and sodium azide). Immunostaining was performed on a Techmate 1000 (Ventana Medical Systems, Tucson, AZ) using capillary gap technology. Tissue sections were exposed for 10 min to normal horse serum (1:50) followed by overnight primary antibody incubation (1:2000), as described by Kovatich et al. (1998). The primary antibody was a polyclonal rabbit immunoglobulin raised against GSTFhit protein (Barnes et al. 1996; Druck et al. 1997). The next day, slides were washed, incubated for 30 min with a biotinylated goat anti-rabbit IgG secondary antibody (1:200), and exposed to avidin biotinylated complex (ABC) for 45 min. After washing, slides were subjected to three consecutive 8-min applications of diaminobenzidine (DAB)/peroxide solution. Treated slides were counterstained with hematoxylin and coverslipped prior to evaluation.

Tumorigenicity Studies

Preparation of mammalian expression vectors, transfection of Fhit-negative cancer cell lines, and evaluation of tumorigenicity of Fhit-expressing transfected clones have been described (Siprashvili et al. 1997).

Sequencing and Sequence Analysis

Preparation of plasmid templates from the cosmid contig, sequencing, assembly, and analysis of the 210-kb region flanking *FHIT* exon 5 has been described (Inoue et al. 1997). Sequencing and analysis of the overlapping 110-kb region in *FHIT* intron 4 has been described by Boldog et al. (1997).

Results

Isolation of the *FHIT* Gene

To begin the search for a tumor suppressor gene encompassing the t(3;8) break, we had several valuable reagents. First, we had somatic cell hybrids carrying the derivative 8 chromosome, der 8 (8qter → 8q24::3p14.2 → 3pter), without chromosome 3 or the der 3; we also had the entire PTPγ gene cloned in yeast artificial chromosomes (YACs) and phages and had markers derived from within PTPγ. Figure 1 shows a karyotype of lymphoblasts from a member of the t(3;8) family. The derivative 3 (der 3 (3qter → 3p14.2::8q24 → 8qter) is duplicated as indicated by the arrows, while the der 8 is present in one copy. Available 3p markers were used to evaluate up to 50 renal cell carcinomas for LOH within the PTPγ locus and flanking markers and it was found that approximately 85% of these sporadic tumors showed LOH using markers flanking the t(3;8) break (Druck et al. 1995); thus we could be sure that the locus was important both in sporadic kidney tumors and in familial tumors. Since the remaining PTPγ allele in tumors was intact and apparently normal (Druck et al. 1995) and we knew the PTPγ 5′ end was within a few hundred kilobases of the t(3;8) break, we assumed that the suppressor gene might be telomeric to the t(3;8) and began assembling a map of this region.

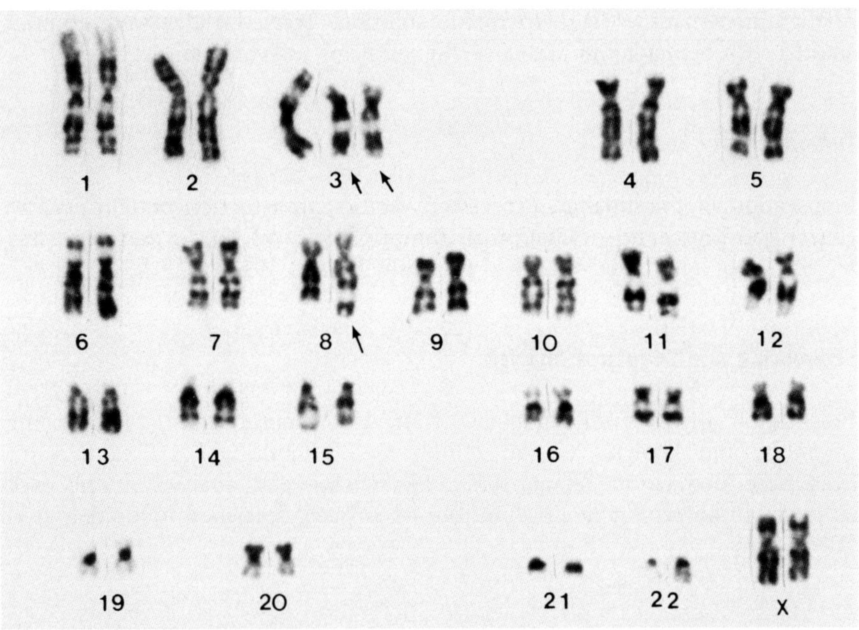

Fig. 1. The t(3;8)(p14.2;q24) reciprocal chromosome translocation associated with familial clear cell renal carcinoma. G-banded karyotype of an Epstein-Barr virus (EBV)-transformed lymphoblast from a member of the family carrying the t(3;8) constitutional reciprocal translocation. *Arrows* mark the derivative chromosomes, der 3 (two copies) and der 8

About this time, in early 1995, Lisitsyn et al. reported that a novel 3p marker isolated by representational difference analysis from a Barret's esophagus metaplasia was homozygously deleted in a number of cancer cell lines. We mapped this marker, BE758-6, into our region telomeric to the t(3;8), defined the size of the common homozygous deletion, and were able to isolate the cDNA for a gene which encompassed the homozygous deletions, the translocation break, a region of hemizygous loss and the common fragile site that flanked exon 5 of the gene, the first protein-coding exon (Ohta et al. 1996). The cDNA encoded the *FHIT* gene, a fragile histidine triad gene which is translated into a 17-kDa protein, with Ap_3A hydrolase activity (Barnes et al. 1996; Fig. 2).

Delineation and Sequencing of the Fragile Region

A number of laboratories, notably that of Thomas Glover (see chapter by Glover, this volume), had defined the position of the *FRA3B* fragile region. Thus we knew that the chromosome gaps in this fragile region were telomeric to the t(3;8) and were within YAC 850A6, which extended from $PTP\gamma$ to within the large *FHIT* intron 5 (see Fig. 3). Using cosmid probes from within the large contiguous cloned region surrounding *FHIT* exon 5, we were thus able to determine that the gaps induced in *FRA3B* by aphidicolin treatment were distributed over a broad region of at least 1 Mb with about 60% of the gaps occurring within a 300-kb region surrounding exon 5 (Zimonjic et al. 1997). Using cosmid templates (cosmids c63, cP4, cS8, c76, and cB4; Fig. 3), we sequenced 210 kb of this fragile region (Inoue et al. 1997); our sequenced region overlapped the 110 kb intron 4 sequence of Boldog et al (1997), resulting in a total sequenced region of 276 kb. This sequence was analyzed for repeated sequences (alu, LINE, MIR), for positions of cancer cell deletion breakpoints, and for the position of an HPV16 integration site, pSV2 integration sites, and somatic cell hybrid breakpoints. Significant features of the sequence were a GC content of approximately 38% with minimal deviation from this mean over the region; no apparent CpG islands; no confirmed exons other than *FHIT* exon 5; and the presence of 43 LINE elements, mostly of the L1 subtype, that were clustered in two subregions. Sequence analysis of 22 cancer cell deletion breakpoints showed that the sequenced region was a frequent target of homologous recombination between LINE sequences, resulting in *FHIT* gene internal deletions, probably as a result of carcinogen-induced damage at *FRA3B* fragile sites. Individual cancer cell lines exhibited overlapping-independent deletions of the two *FHIT* alleles, with clustering of end points in subregions of high LINE content (Inoue et al. 1997). This clustering of breakpoints may allow the design of primers and probes which will detect *FHIT* alterations in primary tumors.

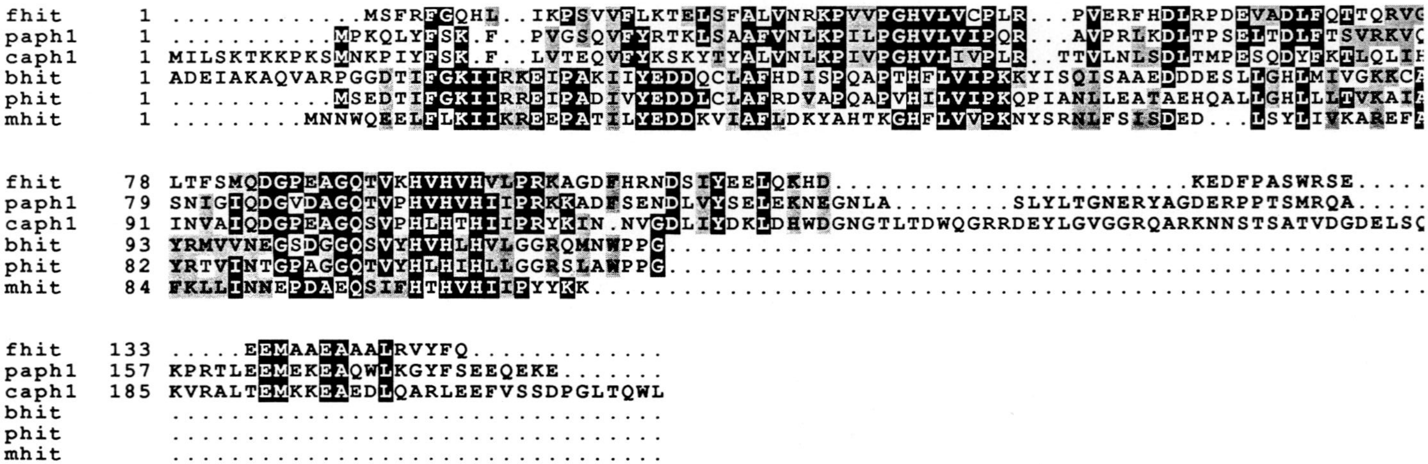

```
fhit      1  ...........MSFRFGQHL..IKPSVVFLKTELSFALVNRKPVVPGHVLVCPLR...PVERFHDLRPDEVADLFQTTQRVC
paph1     1  ..........MPKQLYFSK.F..PVGSQVFYRTKLSAAFVNLKPILPGHVLVIPQR...AVPRLKDLTPSELTDLFTSVRKVC
caph1     1  MILSKTKKPKSMNKPIYFSK.F..LVTEQVFYKSKYTYALVNLKPIVPGHVLIVPLR..TTVLNLSDLTMPESQDYFKTLQLIF
bhit      1  ADEIAKAQVARPGGDTIFGKIIRKEIPAKIIYEDDQCLAFHDISPQAPTHFLVIPKKYISQISAAEDDDESLLGHLMIVGKKCA
phit      1  ..........MSEDTIFGKIIRREIPADIVYEDDLCLAFRDVAPQAPVHILVIPKQPIANLLEATAEHQALLGHLLLTVKAIA
mhit      1  .........MNNWQEELFLKIIKREEPATILYEDDKVIAFLDKYAHTKGHFLVVPKNYSRNLFSISDED...LSYLIVKAREFA

fhit     78  LTFSMQDGPEAGQTVKHVHVHVLPRKAGDFHRNDSIYEELQKHD..................KEDFPASWRSE.....
paph1    79  SNIGIQDGVDAGQTVPHVHVHIIPRKKADFSENDLVYSELEKNEGNLA........SLYLTGNERYAGDERPPTSMRQA.....
caph1    91  INVAIQDGPEAGQSVPHLHTHIIPRYKIN.NVGDLIYDKLDHWDGNGTLTDWQGRRDEYLGVGGRQARKNNSTSATVDGDELSC
bhit     93  YRMVVNEGSDGGQSVYHVHLHVLGGRQMNWPPG...................................
phit     82  YRTVINTGPAGGQTVYHLHIHLLGGRSLAWPPG...................................
mhit     84  FKLLINNEPDAEQSIFHTHVHIIPYYKK...................................

fhit    133  .....EEMAAEAAALRVYFQ.............
paph1   157  KPRTLEEMEKEAQWLKGYFSEEQEKE.......
caph1   185  KVRALTEMKKEAEDLQARLEEFVSSDPGLTQWL
bhit         ................................
phit         ................................
mhit         ................................
```

Fig. 2. The Fhit protein. The 1.1-kb *FHIT* cDNA encodes a 16.8-kDa protein with an amino acid sequence very similar to the amino acid sequence of *Schizosaccharomyces pombe* diadenosine tetraphosphate hydrolase ($A_{p4}A$, paph1, accession number U32615) and the *Saccharomyces cerevisiae* $A_{p3}A$ hydrolase (caph1, U28374). bhit, phit, and mhit are histidine triad (HIT) gene family members from bovine (Acc. No. P16436), cyanobacterium (P30284), and mycoplasma hyorhinis (M37339), as described previously (Ohta et al. 1996). Note the overall conservation (*filled squares*, identical amino acids; *gray squares*, similar), especially at the histidine triad (fhit amino acids 94–98)

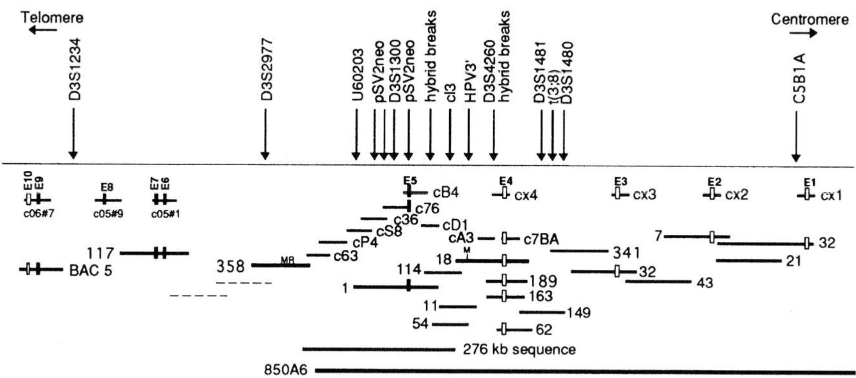

Fig. 3. The *FHIT* locus. The *FHIT* gene at chromosome region 3p14.2 is represented by the *top line* with associated markers. *FHIT* exons are shown below the line within individual cosmids as *filled bars* for protein coding exons and *open bars* for noncoding exons. Other *thick lines* represent cosmids and bacterial artificial chromosome (BAC) clones covering most of the 1-Mb megabase *FHIT* locus. Cosmids B4, 76, 36, S8, P4, and 63 covering mid intron 4 through mid-intron 5 have been fully sequenced. This sequence combined with the overlapping 110-kb partial intron 4 sequence (Boldog et al. 1997) gives a fully sequenced 276-kb region, encompassing *FHIT* exon 5 and most of the fragile gaps which can be induced in lymphocytes

Replacement of Fhit Expression Suppresses Tumorigenicity

The structure and expression of the *FHIT* gene at chromosome region 3p14.2, encompassing the *FRA3B* common fragile site, are frequently altered in primary or cultured esophageal, head and neck, lung, gastric, breast and cervical carcinomas (Ohta et al. 1996; Virgilio et al. 1996; Sozzi et al. 1996; Fong et al. 1997; Negrini et al. 1996; Druck et al. 1997; Boldog et al. 1997; Hendricks et al. 1997; Greenspan et al. 1997). Structural alterations tend to be due to deletion within both *FHIT* alleles, resulting in loss of exons and concomitant absence of full-length *FHIT* transcript and protein (Druck et al. 1997; for review, Huebner et al. 1997). Because loss of Fhit activity involves mechanisms unlike the classical mechanisms for loss of tumor suppressor activity, it has been argued that the *FHIT* gene may be altered in cancer cells simply because it encompasses the fragile region that flanks the first *FHIT* protein-coding exon and is likely to be very susceptible to breakage (Boldog et al. 1997). The locus is highly susceptible to carcinogen damage, explaining why deletion is much more frequent than point mutation in the gene, but we argue that loss of Fhit function provides a selective advantage for the tumor cell; otherwise, such frequent expansion of the deleted *FHIT* clones in tumors and tumor-derived cell lines would be difficult to explain.

Although the gene is a member of a well conserved gene family, the sequence of the *FHIT* gene and protein do not give obvious clues to the biological function of the protein or to its possible role in tumor suppression. In vitro the wild-type Fhit protein, like its yeast homologue, hydrolyzes dinucleoside $5'5'''$-P^1,P^3-triphosphate (Ap$_3$A) to yield ADP and AMP; mutation of the central histidine of the histidine triad (HxHxH or HIT) domain reduces the hydrolase activity by six orders of magnitude, while reducing substrate binding minimally (L. Barnes, personal communication).

To study the biological functions of the Fhit protein, epitope-tagged wild-type and mutant *FHIT* open reading frames were inserted into a mammalian expression vector and transfected into gastric, kidney, and lung cancer cell lines which lacked endogenous Fhit due to genomic deletions within the *FHIT* gene. For each of the cancer cell lines, numerous neomycin-resistant colonies were obtained, and about one in 30 colonies expressed detectable Fhit. Fhit-expressing cancer cell clones hydrolyzed Ap_3A in vitro, while clones expressing mutant Fhit did not. Cancer cell clones expressing exogenous wild-type and mutant Fhit were tested for growth in liquid and semi-solid media and for tumorigenicity in nude mice (Siprashvili et al. 1997). A consistent effect of exogenous Fhit on growth in liquid medium and soft agar was not observed. The Fhit-expressing gastric and kidney cancer cell clones grew as well as the control Fhit-negative parental cancer cells, while Fhit expressing H460 lung cancer clones showed reduced growth in soft agar. However, each transfected Fhit-expressing clone showed reduced tumorigenicity in nude mice. In addition, gastric cancer cell clones expressing mutant Fhit which lacks Ap_3A hydrolase activity also showed reduced tumorigenicity, indicating that the Ap_3A hydrolytic activity is not involved in Fhit tumor suppressor activity.

A possible conclusion to be drawn from these studies is that the tumor suppressive signal is transmitted by the enzyme–substrate complex. We are pursuing this hypothesis by studying suppressor function of Fhit mutant proteins that cannot bind substrate.

Fhit Expression in Human Tumors

We have shown that Fhit protein is expressed in normal lung epithelium but is undetectable in most SCLCs and is reduced or absent in dysplastic lesions (Sozzi et al. 1997 b), suggesting that the *FHIT* gene undergoes inactivation in parallel with genomic alterations at the *FHIT* locus detected by studies of allele loss. Point mutations in the *FHIT* gene are rare in sporadic cancers of various types (Gemma et al. 1997) and we have shown that *FHIT* inactivation occurs through independent deletions within both *FHIT* alleles (Druck et al. 1997; Inoue et al. 1997), triggered by misrepair of sequential double strand breaks within the carcinogen-sensitive common fragile site *FRA3B* (Inoue et al. 1997). Sometimes, the independent allelic deletions partially overlap, allowing detection of homozygously deleted markers within the 1-MB *FHIT* gene. Since nonoverlapping regions of allelic deletions would be detected as LOH, loss of portions of both *FHIT* alleles could be assessed as hemizygous loss at the DNA level, but could be distinguished at the protein level, since deletion within both *FHIT* alleles should result in loss of Fhit expression.

In a study of Fhit expression in cervical carcinomas by immunohisto-chemistry, Greenspan et al. (1997) scored the tumors for both intensity and extent of Fhit staining from a score of 1–3. A composite score was obtained by multiplying the scores for intensity and extent. They observed marked reduction or loss of Fhit protein in 76% of cervical tumors. More than 50% of the lesions had fewer than 10% positive cells, and 36% showed absent to weak intensity of staining. Thus it was not a question of "all or none" Fhit expression for cervical tumors, perhaps because of intratumoral heterogene-ity with respect to alteration of one or both *FHIT* alleles, as previously ob-served for head and neck tumor cell lines (Virgilio et al. 1996). We have found similar patterns of Fhit expression in the atypical lung carcinoids and suggest that the extent of Fhit expression is secondary to heterogeneity of molecular alterations of the *FHIT* locus in individual cells within these neuroendocrine tumors. We demonstrated strong Fhit protein expression in typical lung carcinoids, tumors which rarely progress (Kovatich et al. 1998).

The features that distinguish typical carcinoids, atypical carcinoids, and SCLCs place atypical carcinoids intermediate to typical carcinoids and SCLCs. The results of the Fhit expression study confirm the proposed clinical continuum, suggesting that when they progress and metastasize, atypical car-cinoids, may show alteration of both *FHIT* alleles and complete loss of Fhit expression.

An interesting finding was that a few typical carcinoids showed LOH with-in the *FHIT* gene. All the atypical carcinoids also showed loss of a *FHIT* al-lele, suggesting that *FHIT* alteration is an early event. Typical carcinoids, on the basis of loss of *FHIT* locus markers and lack of reduction in Fhit expres-sion, exhibited minimal damage to the *FHIT* gene, while atypical carcinoids may have sustained loss of one *FHIT* allele and SCLCs loss of both, based on the reduction in extent and intensity of Fhit staining in all atypical tumors compared with the uniform absence of Fhit staining in SCLCs.

Ongoing studies of both clear cell renal carcinoma and colon carcinoma show complete absence of Fhit expression in a significant fraction of these cancers as well; examples are shown in Fig. 4).

Discussion

In setting out to clone and characterize a gene that was important in familial and sporadic renal cancer, we have described a locus and gene, the *FRA3B/ FHIT* locus, which is involved in allele loss in a large fraction of the most important human cancers (Huebner et al. 1997; Shridhar et al. 1996; Michael et al. 1997) and in many preoplastic tissues (Sozzi et al. 1997b; Wistuba et al. 1997a; Larson et al. 1997). We have suggested that the frequent alterations to this locus result from carcinogen damage, possibly in the form of double strand breaks. Repair may occur through homologous recombination with concomitant deletion, in the most inducible common fragile site, *FRA3B*, which is within the 1-Mb *FHIT* gene. Corroboration of this hypothesis has

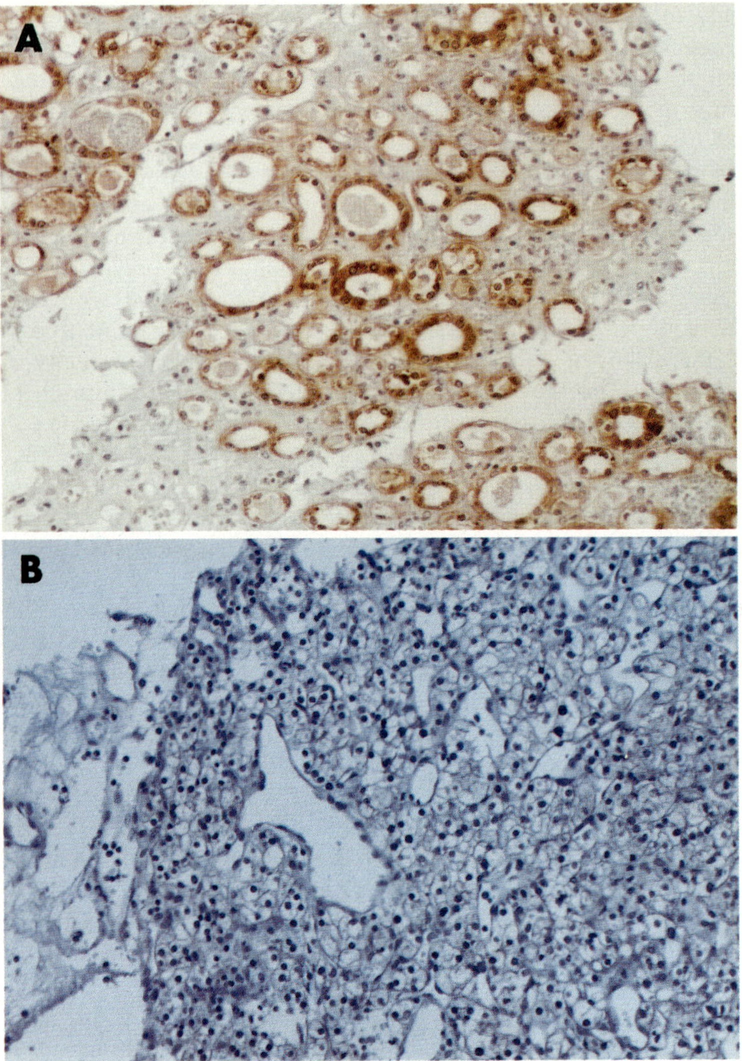

Fig. 4A–D. Immunohistochemical evaluation of Fhit expression in tumor tissues. **A** Normal renal medulla. **B** Clear cell renal carcinoma. **C** Well-differentiated colon carcinoma. **D** High-grade colon carcinoma. Tissue sections were deparaffinized and Fhit expression (*brown stain*) detected using rabbit anti-gstFhit antiserum (1:2000). Sections were counterstained with hematoxylin and eosin (H & E)

come from studies of allele loss at various tumor suppressor or putative tumor suppressor loci in bronchial biopsies of smokers and former smokers compared to nonsmokers (Mao et al. 1997; Wistuba et al. 1997b). Genetic changes at 3p, including markers within the *FHIT* gene, were detected in the nonmalignant bronchial epithelia of current and former smokers and can persist for years after smoking cessation (Wistuba et al. 1997b; Mao et al.

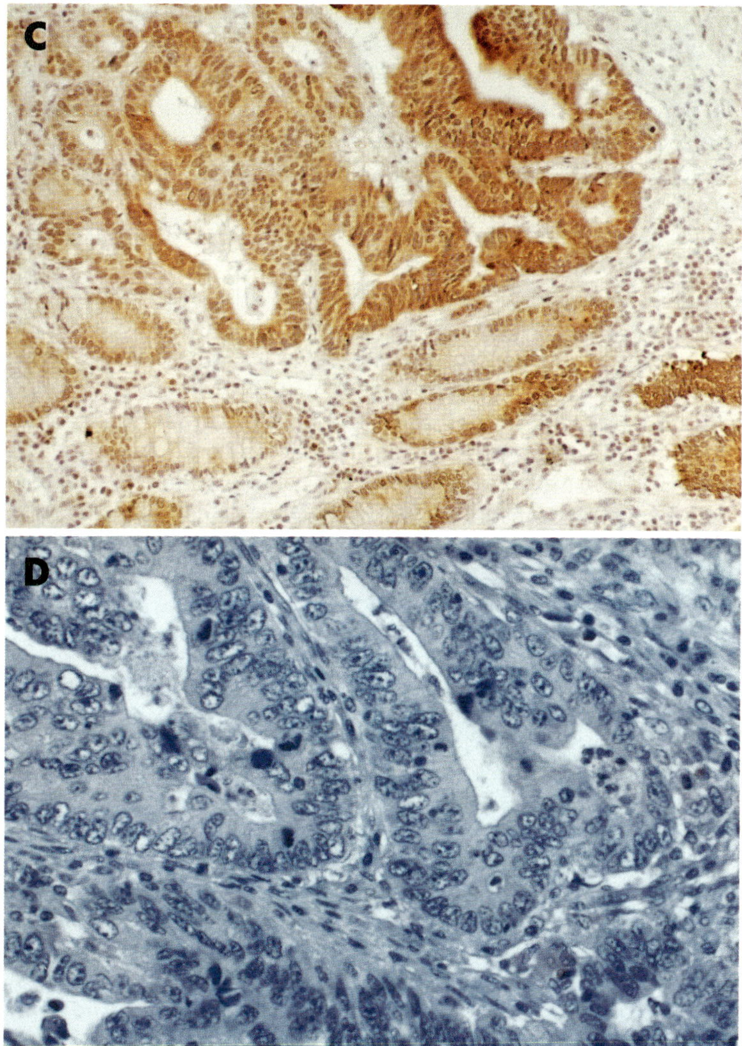

Fig. 4 C, D

1997). Additionally, although human papillomavirus (HPV) infection is the earliest molecular event in cervical carcinogenesis, deletions at 3p14.2 are also frequent and occur early in this process (Wistuba et al. 1997b; Larson et al. 1997), possibly following HPV DNA integration at the *FRA3B*.

Since point mutations in the small Fhit open reading frame (147 amino acids) are rare (Gemma et al. 1997) and rearrangements and deletions are difficult to detect in primary tumor DNA, we have used a reverse-transcriptase (RT)-PCR strategy to look for alterations in the *FHIT* gene in cancers. Using this method, we noted that RNA from a large fraction of many tumor types yielded aberrant, usually shorter RT-PCR amplification products, often but not always accompanied by the expected size product. The normal-sized product may derive from normal contaminating cells, cancerous cells within the population that have not sustained a *FHIT* deletion, cancer cells in which one allele has been deleted and one allele is intact, or a combination of these. If loss of only one *FHIT* allele within a cell does indeed impart a growth advantage due to a reduction in expression of Fhit protein, as suggested by the immunohistochemical studies of cervical carcinoma and atypical lung carcinoids, then it is not surprising that many tumors and cancer cell lines express some normal *FHIT* transcript and protein.

In our initial report, we proposed that the aberrant RT-PCR products might encode shorter proteins lacking for example, exon 8. Because we have been unable to detect expression of such proteins, even after in vitro transcription–translation of cloned short RT-PCR products or after transfection into Cos cells, we now believe that the aberrant RT-PCR products which lack coding exons are meaningless in the cellular context. In other words, they are infrequently transcribed from partially deleted *FHIT* alleles, are not translated, and only serve as markers for a deleted allele. Some investigators have observed aberrant RT-PCR products in normal cells (van den Berg et al. 1997; Panagopoulos et al. 1997). However, most investigators have reported consistently normal RT-PCR products from normal control cells compared to frequent aberrant products in paired tumor RNAs.

With the availability of anti-Fhit polyclonal antisera which detect Fhit protein by western blot or by immunohistochemistry on frozen and paraffin sections, it will be possible to determine the frequency of Fhit-negative cancers for many organs which have been reported to exhibit *FHIT* gene abnormalities. Already, lung (Sozzi et al. 1997b), cervical (Greenspan et al. 1997) and stomach cancers (R. Baffa, personal communication) have been studied by immunohistochemical methods. All show a high frequency of Fhit-negative tumors.

The *FHIT* gene has been expressed by transfection in four cancer cell lines, derived from two gastric carcinomas, a clear cell kidney carcinoma and a lung carcinoma. Subsequent growth of tumors in nude mice was suppressed by expression of exogenous wild-type Fhit. The tumorigenicity assay is now being used to analyze mutant Fhit genes which may be defective in tumor suppression.

Nearly 300 kb of the *FHIT/FRA3B* locus surrounding *FHIT* exon 5 have been fully sequenced and searched for characteristics which may explain the regional fragility (Inoue et al. 1997; Boldog et al. 1997). This 300-kb segment of the *FRA3B* region exhibits a high AT content, a low Alu sequence content, and several clusters of L1 LINE elements which are involved in recombination in cancer cell lines exhibiting deletions in both *FHIT* alleles. Although a number of fragile region landmarks, such as plasmid integration sites, an HPV integration site, and rodent–human hybrid cell breakpoints, have been precisely positioned within the sequence, comparison of these sequences does not suggest mechanisms for generation of gaps or breaks at these

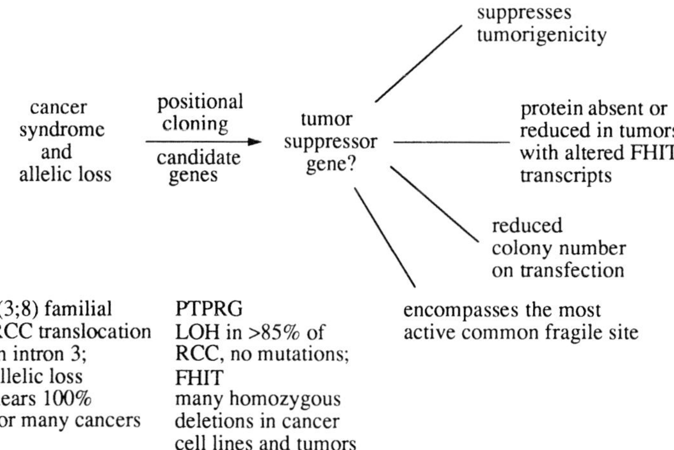

Fig. 5. *FHIT* tumor suppressor credentials. One *FHIT* allele is interrupted between exons 3 and 4 by a constitutional chromosome translocation in a familial kidney cancer syndrome; allelic loss of one *FHIT* gene nears 100% in sporadic lung, kidney, and cervical cancers; numerous cancer-derived cell lines exhibit homozygous deletions within the *FHIT* gene, usually due to independent overlapping deletions of the two *FHIT* alleles; very rare point mutations have been found in sporadic tumors, reexpression of Fhit protein in tumorigenic cancer cell lines suppresses tumorigenicity; and Fhit protein is reduced or absent in a large fraction of lung, stomach, kidney and cervical cancers. *RCC*, renal cell carcinoma; *LOH*, loss of heterozygosity

"fragile sites" (Inoue et al. 1997). Completion of the remaining several hundred kilobases of intron 4 and intron 5 regions may yet provide insight into mechanisms of carcinogen damage to this chromosome region.

Conclusion

Figure 5 illustrates in summary form the status of the investigation of the *FRA3B* locus and the *FHIT* gene which encompasses it. The *FHIT* gene is interrupted by translocation in a family with hereditary multifocal renal cell carcinoma; at least one *FHIT* allele and frequently both are partially or completely deleted in a large fraction of cancers of many types, including esophageal, lung, gastric, breast, cervix, and kidney. Other cancers will no doubt join this list. Replacement of Fhit expression in tumorigenic cancer cell lines results in suppression of tumor growth in nude mice and reduction in the number of selectable transfected colonies. Immunohistochemical studies of lung and cervical tumors have demonstrated reduction or absence of Fhit expression relative to strong expression in the appropriate normal controls. Continued examination of the relationship between carcinogen-induced alteration of the *FRA3B* region and *FHIT* inactivation should provide important insights into the role of this fragile region in cancer. In parallel, the study of the in vivo function of Fhit protein will provide the basis to understand the role of this protein in normal cells and in tumor progression.

Acknowledgment. This work was supported by USPHS grants CA21124 and CA56336 from the National Cancer Institute and by a gift from R. R. M. Carpenter III and M. K. Carpenter.

References

Barnes LD, Garrison PN et al (1996) Fhit, a putative tumor suppressor in humans, is a dinucleoside 5,5′′′P^1,P^3-triphosphate hydrolase. Biochemistry 35:11529–11535

Boldog F, Gemmill RM, West J et al (1997) Chromosome 3p14 homozygous deletions and sequence analysis of FRA3B. Hum Mol Genet 6:193–205

Druck T, Kastury K et al (1995) Loss of heterozygosity at the familial RCC t(3;8) locus in most clear cell renal carcinomas. Cancer Res 55:5348–5353

Druck T, Hadaczek P et al (1997) Structure and expression of the human *FHIT* gene in normal and tumor cells. Cancer Res 57:504–512

Fong KM, Biesterveld EJ et al (1997) *FHIT* and *FRA3B* 3p14.2 allele loss are common in lung cancer and preneoplastic bronchial lesions and are associated with cancer-related *FHIT* cDNA splicing aberrations. Cancer Res 57:2256–2267

Gemma A, Hagiware K et al (1997) *FHIT* mutations in human primary gastric cancer. Cancer Res 57:1435–1437

Glover TW, Coyle-Morris JF et al (1988) Translocation t(3;8)(p14.2;q24) in renal cell carcinoma affects expression of the common fragile site at 3p14 (*FRA3B*) in lymphocytes. Cancer Genet Cytogenet 31:69–73

Greenspan DL, Connolly DC et al (1997) Loss of *FHIT* expression in cervical carcinoma cell lines and primary tumors. Cancer Res 57:4692–4698

Hendricks DT, Taylor R et al (1997) *FHIT* gene expression in human ovarian, endometrial, and cervical cancer cell lines. Cancer Res 57:2112–2115

Huebner K, Hadaczek P et al (1997) The *FHIT* gene, a multiple tumor suppressor gene encompassing the carcinogen sensitive chromosome fragile site, *FRA3B*. Biochim Biophys Acta 1332:M65–M70

Inoue H, Ishii H et al (1997) Sequence of the *FRA3B* common fragile region: Implications for the mechanism of *FHIT* deletion. Proc Natl Acad Sci USA 94:14584–14589

Kastury K, Baffa R et al (1996) Potential gastrointestinal tumor suppressor locus at the 3p14.2 FRA3B site identified by homozygous deletions in tumor cell lines. Cancer Res 56:978–983

Kovatich A, Friedland DM et al (1998) Molecular alterations to human chromosom 3p loci in neuroendocrine lung tumors. Cancer (in press)

LaForgia SK, Morse B et al (1991) Receptor protein-tyrosine phosphatase gamma is a candidate tumor suppressor gene at human chromosome region 3p21. Proc Natl Acad Sci USA 81:5036–5040

Larson AA, Liao S-Y et al (1997) Genetic alterations accumulate during cervical tumorigenesis and indicate a common origin for multifocal lesions. Cancer Res 57:4174–4176

Li FP, Decker H-JH et al (1993) Clinical and genetic studies of renal cell carcinomas in a family with a constitutional chromosome 3;8 translocation. Ann Intern Med 118:106–111

Lisitsyn NA, Lisitsina NM et al (1995) Comparative genomic analysis of tumors: detection of DNA losses and amplification. Proc Natl Acad Sci USA 92:151–155

Mao L, Lee JS et al (1997) Clonal genetic alterations in the lungs of current and former smokers. J Natl Cancer Inst 89:857–862

Michael D, Beer DG et al (1997) Frequent deletions of *FHIT* and *FRA3B* in Barrett's metaplasia and esophageal adenocarcinomas. Oncogene 15:1553–1559

Negrini M, Monaco C et al (1996) The *FHIT* gene at 3p14.2 is abnormal in breast carcinomas. Cancer Res 56:3173–3179

Ohta M, Inoue H et al (1996) The *FHIT* gene, spanning the chromosome 3p14.2 fragile site and renal carcinoma-associated t(3;8) breakpoint, is abnormal in digestive tract cancers. Cell 84:587–597

Panagopoulos I, Thelin S, Mertens F e al (1997) Variable FHIT transcripts in non-neoplastic tissues. Genes Chromosome Cancer 19:215–219

Paradee W, Wilke CM et al (1996) A 350-kb cosmid contig in 3p14.2 that crosses the t(3;8) hereditary renal cell carcinoma translocation breakpoint and 17 aphidicolin-induced *FRA3B* breakpoints. Genomics 35:87–93

Shridhar R, Shridhar V et al (1996) Frequent breakpoints in the 3p14.2 fragile site, *FRA3B*, in pancreatic tumors. Cancer Res 56:4347–4350

Siprashvili Z, Sozzi G et al (1997) Replacement of Fhit in cancer cells suppresses tumorigenicity. Proc Natl Acad Sci USA 94:13771–13776

Sozzi G, Veronese ML et al (1996) The *FHIT* gene at 3p14.2 is abnormal in lung cancer. Cell 85:17–26

Sozzi G, Sard L et al (1997a) Association between cigarette smoking and *FHIT* gene alterations in lung cancer. Cancer Res57:2121–2123

Sozzi G, Tornielli S et al (1997b) Absence of Fhit protein in primary lung tumors and cell lines with *FHIT* gene abnormalities. Cancer Res. 57:5207–5212

van den Berg A, Draaijers TG, Kok K et al (1997) Normal FHIT transcripts in renal cell cancer- and lung cancer-derived cel llines, including as cell line with a homozygous deletion in the FRA3B Region. Genes Chromosome Cancer 19:220–227

Virgilio L, Schuster M et al (1996) *FHIT* gene alterations in head and neck squamous cell carcinomas. Proc Natl Acad Sci USA 93:9770–9775

Wilke MC, Hall BK et al (1996) *FRA3B* extends over a broad region and contains a spontaneous HPV integration site: direct evidence for the coincidence of viral integration sites and fragile sites. Hum Mol Genet 5:187–195

Wistuba II, Montellano FD et al (1997a) Deletions of chromosome 3p are frequent and early events in the pathogenesis of uterine cervical carcinoma. Cancer Res 57:3154–3158

Wistuba II, Lam S et al (1997b) Molecular damage in the bronchial epithelium of current and former smokers. J Natl Cancer Inst 89:1366–1373

Zimonjic DB, Druck T et al (1997) Positions of chromosome 3p14.2 fragile sites (*FRA3B*) within the *FHIT* gene. Cancer Res 57:1166–1170

Gene Amplification Mechanisms:
The Role of Fragile Sites

M. Debatisse, A. Coquelle, F. Toledo, and G. Buttin

Unité de Génétique Somatique (URA CNRS 1960), Institut Pasteur,
25 rue du Dr. Roux, 75724 Paris Cédex 15, France

Abstract

We studied the early stages of gene amplification in a Chinese hamster cell line and identified two distinct amplification mechanisms, both relying on an unequal segregation of gene copies at mitosis. In some cases, a sequence containing the selected gene is looped out, generating an acentric circular molecule, and amplification proceeds through unequal segregation of such extrachromosomal elements in successive cell cycles. In other cases, the accumulation of intrachromosomally amplified copies is driven by cycles of chromatid breakage, followed by fusion of sister chromatids devoid of a telomere, which leads to bridge formation and further break in mitosis (BFB cycles). We showed that some clastogenic drugs specifically trigger the intrachromosomal amplification pathway and strictly correlated this induction of BFB cycles to the ability of these drugs to activate fragile sites. In three model systems, we also established, that the location of centromeric and telomeric fragile sites relative to the selected genes determines the size and sequence content of the early amplicons.

Background

Gene amplification is a genetic alteration through which a cell gains additional copies of a small part of its genome. In mammalian cells, such mutations make an important contribution to tumor progression, and possibly to tumorigenesis, through overexpression of many different cellular oncogenes (Brison 1993; Schwab and Amler 1990). Gene amplification and translocations, inversions or deletions are genetic abnormalities commonly found in tumor but not in normal cells. It has been demonstrated that the permissivity of tumor cells for chromosomal aberrations and genome remodeling depends on the loss of cell cycle check points (Hartwell 1992; Livingstone et al. 1992; Yin et al. 1992).

Because of this high level of genome instability, the reconstitution of the mechanisms responsible for amplification in cells recovered from advanced

Recent Results in Cancer Research, Vol. 154
© Springer-Verlag Berlin · Heidelberg 1998

tumors is often obscured by a variety of secondary rearrangements. To overcome this difficulty, model systems of in vitro cultured cells were used to design experimental protocols allowing mutant cells to be recovered and analyzed as early as 10 to 20 generations after the initial event triggering the amplification process (Smith et al. 1990). Such studies were made possible by the development of the fluorescence in situ hybridization technique (FISH) (Pinkel et al. 1988), which permits cell-by-cell analysis of very small cell populations.

Results

Our goal was to understand the mechanisms and the initiating events leading to gene amplification in mammalian cells. Working with Chinese hamster cells, we focused our study on two genes located on chromosome 1q: the adenylate deaminase 2 gene (AMPD2) and the multidrug resistance 1 gene (MDR1). In both cases, it is possible to select mutants that overcome the toxic action of specific drugs through amplification of one or the other gene. Moreover, several cytogenetic markers are available that permit a precise analysis of the rearrangements taking place on this chromosome (Toledo et al. 1993). When early amplified mutants were analyzed by FISH, the extra copies were found on acentric extrachromosomal elements (double-minute chromosomes, DMs) or within expanded chromosomal regions (ECRs) also referred to as homogeneously staining regions (HSRs) as previously described for established mutant lines (Cowell 1982).

Gene Amplification Driven by Two Different Mechanisms

In all the clones with extrachromosomally amplified copies of the AMPD2 or the MDR1 genes, the telomeric parts of both chromosomes 1q are normal (Coquelle et al. 1997; Toledo et al. 1993; Fig. 1A, B). These clones can be classified into two categories depending on the characteristics of their chromosome 1. In some of them, cells have one normal chromosome 1, while the homologue is deleted for the selected gene; in other clones, cells have two completely normal chromosome 1 homologues (Fig. 1B). To explain these

---

Fig. 1 A–F (see page 218). Amplified structures **A, B**. DMs containing cell. **A** Diamidino-phenylindol (DAPI) staining, the *arrows* point to double-minute chromosomes (DMs). **B** The same metaphase plate hybridized with a MDR1 probe (*green*) and a probe identifying the telomeric part of chromosome 1q (*red*). The *arrowheads* point to the normal chromosomal copies of the MDR1 gene. **C–F** Intermediates of the chromatid type of Breakage – fusion – bridge (BFB) cycles. **C, D** Fused sister chromatids. **C** Phase contrast picture before fluorescence *in situ* hybridization (FISH) treatment. **D** Same metaphase plate after hybridization with an AMPD2 probe (*red*) and a probe for a coamplifiable marker (*green*). The *long arrows* point to the fusion and the *short arrows* to the normal chromosome 1. **E** Bridge between two son nuclei. **F** FISH with an AMPD2 probe (*red*) and a probe for a coamplifiable marker as in **D** (*white*) showing symmetrically organized inverted repeats along an amplified chromosome 1q

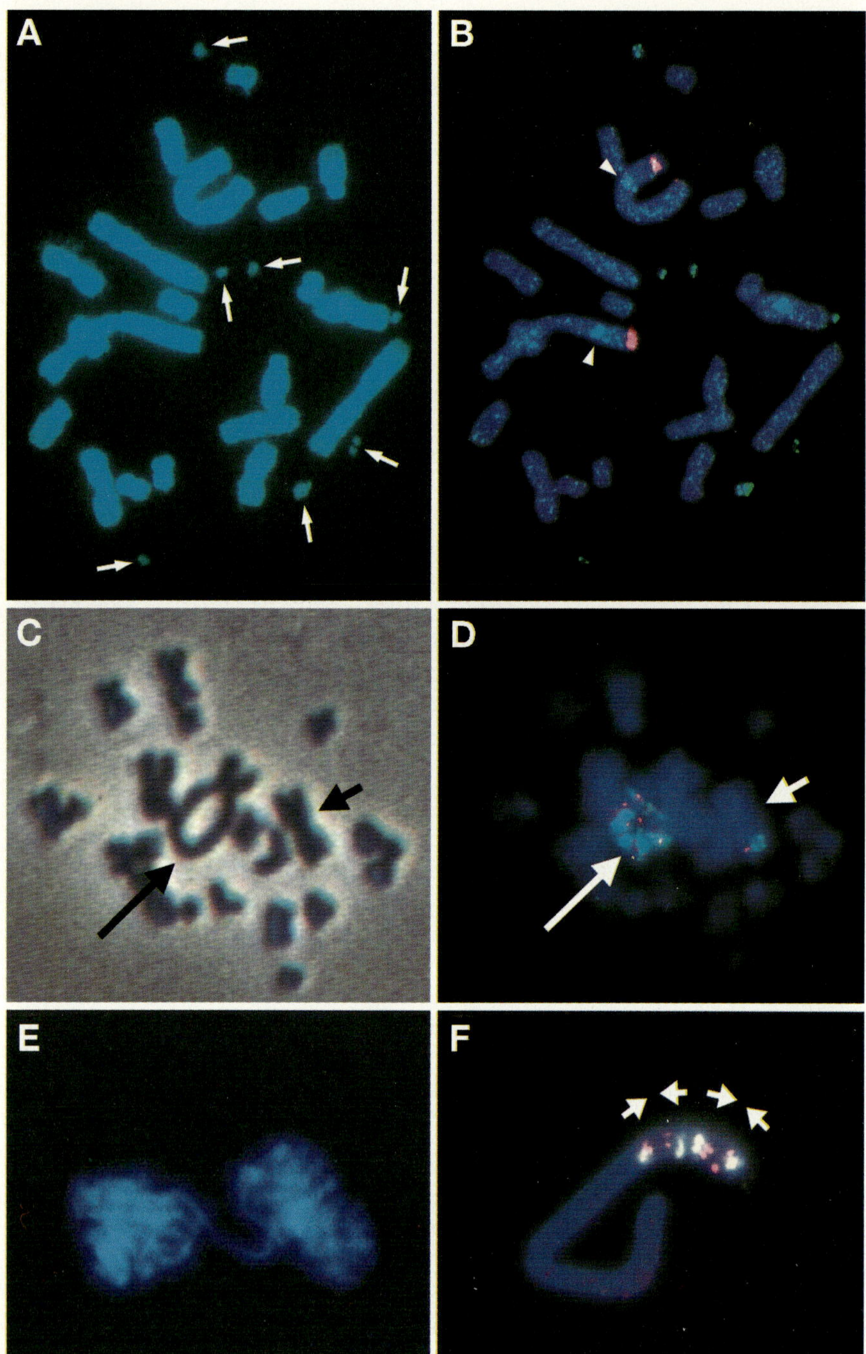

Fig. 1 A–F.

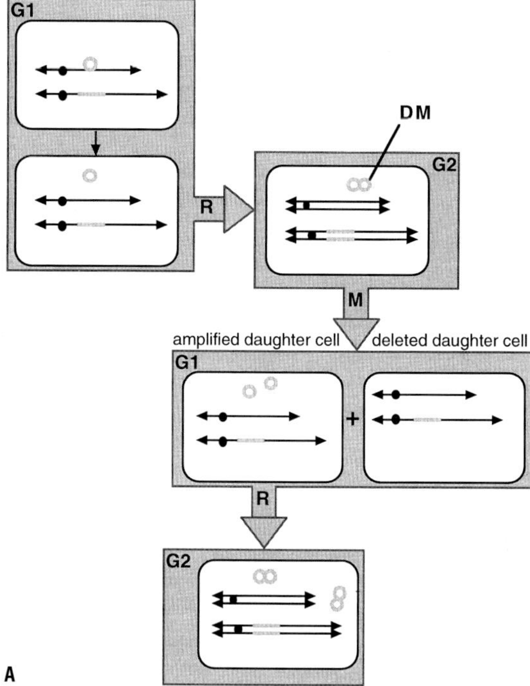

Fig. 2 A, B (B see page 220). Looping out mechanism of extrachromosomal amplification. **A** Looping out in a cell in phase G₁. At the following G₁ phase, after one step of replication (*R*) and mitosis (*M*), one daughter cell (*right*) receives a single copy of the *gray sequence* (sequence to be amplified) which is lethal in selective medium, while three copies are present in the other daughter cell (*left*). The uneven segregation of the extrachromosomal acentric molecules during subsequent cell cycles might lead to higher levels of amplification. The cells of the resulting amplified clone are characterized by an interstitial deletion corresponding to the excised sequence. **B** Looping out in a cell in phase G₂. Among the four chromatids of the cell, only one is deleted. At mitosis, in half the cases, the acentric molecule segregates within a cell with two normal chromosomes (*left*). Such a cell can later give rise to an amplified clone devoid of chromosomal abnomalies. In the other cases, the acentric molecule segregates within a cell with one normal and one deleted chromosome (*right*), a situation indistinguishable from the one depicted in **A**. *Arrowheads*, telomeres; *black circles*, centromeres

features, we proposed that DMs are formed without chromosome breakage but rather by looping out of a sequence a few megabases long (Toledo et al. 1993; Fig. 2). If such an event occurs in a cell in phase G₁ (Fig. 2A), a chromosome 1 deleted for this sequence on both sister chromatids is generated after replication. The second chromosome 1 remains completely normal. At mitosis, each daughter cell receives a normal and a deleted chromosome. If looping out of the same sequence occurs in a cell in phase G₂ (Fig. 2B), a single chromatid of one homologue is deleted. After mitosis, one daughter cell has two normal copies of chromosome 1, and the other, as above, contains one normal and one deleted homologue. The acentric circle has a 50% chance of segregating in the daughter cell that received two normal chromosome 1 homologues. Because DMs are acentric, their unequal segregation at

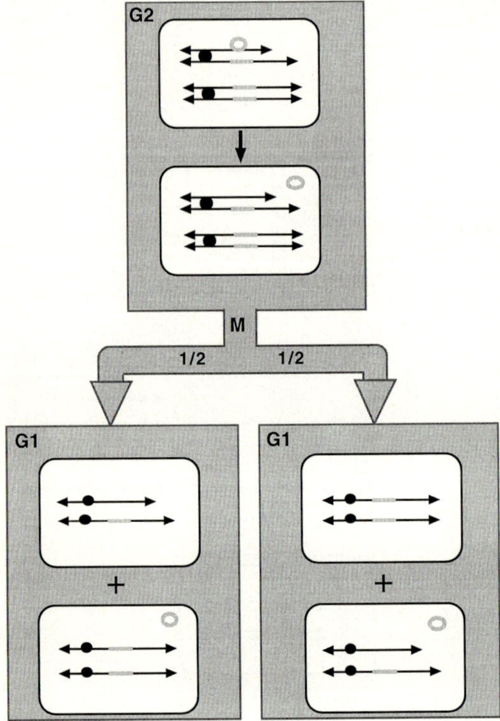

Fig. 2 B

mitosis is expected to allow one daughter cell to gain more copies of the gene, while the other one loses copies and dies in selective medium. This model accounts for both categories of DM-containing clones and for the absence of rearrangement of the telomeric part of the chromosomes. Stahl et al. (1992) also obtained results supporting this model by comparing the map of the MDR1 chromosomal locus and of the DMs present in a mutant line amplified for this gene. They showed that both maps are similar, with the exception of a novel junction present on the DMs, which probably reflects the recombination event responsible for excision.

At early steps of the process, in clones with an intrachromosomal amplification of the dihydrofolate reductase (DHFR), carbamyl-P-synthetase, aspartate transcarbamylase, dihydro-orotase (CAD), AMPD2, or MDR1 genes, the amplified copies were found on one of the chromosome arms that bear a normal copy of the gene in unamplified cells (Coquelle et al. 1997; Smith et al. 1990; Toledo et al. 1992b; Trask and Hamlin 1989). In striking contrast to DM-containing cells, the telomeric part of the amplified chromosome is deleted in cells of these clones (Coquelle et al. 1997; Ma et al. 1993; Toledo et al. 1992a; 1993) (see Fig. 4, *left*). This feature constitutes the landmark of intrachromosomal amplification. In the case of early mutants amplified for the AMPD2 gene, we showed for the first time that the selected gene and a passively coamplified marker alternate in symmetrically arranged inverted repeats a few megabases- long (Fig. 1F; Toledo et al. 1992 a). Characteristic structures bearing amplified copies of the selected gene, such as fusion between two 1q sister chromatids (Fig. 1C, D) or bridges between late anaphase and telophase nuclei were also frequently observed (Fig. 1E; Toledo et al. 1993). All these features are perfectly explained by the chromatid type of BFB cycles (Fig. 3). According to this model, the whole process can be triggered by a double strand break. After replication, the two broken sister chromatids fuse. At anaphase, the centromeres of the dicentric chromatid move to opposite poles of the mitotic spindle, creating a bridge which is later broken. Each daughter cell receives a normal and a broken chromosome which forms another bridge after replication, perpetuating the cycles until the broken end is healed. This model accounts for the main features observed in cell populations undergoing the intrachromosomal mechanism. The same mechanism was later shown to operate in at least three other model systems (Bertoni et al. 1994; Coquelle et al. 1997; Kuo et al. 1994; Ma et al. 1993; Smith et al. 1992).

Initiation of BFB Cycles

To test the hypothesis that a double strand break is able to trigger the whole process of intrachromosomal amplification, we tried to identify agents able to induce gene amplification. For this purpose, we concentrated on the MDR1 gene, because several drugs can be used to select for its amplification (Biedler and Meyers 1989). Some of these drugs are well-known inducers of DNA breaks (adriamycin and actinomycin D), while others are spindle poisons (vinblastine). Table 1 shows the results obtained in parallel experiments differing only in the drug utilized to select the mutants (Coquelle et al. 1997). We recovered independent clones resistant to each of these three drugs; because it is well known that resistance can be achieved through mechanisms other than MDR1 gene amplification, we first determined the MDR1 copy number in each of them. Surprisingly, the percentages of amplified clones recovered in adriamycin or vinblastine are low and relatively similar. The products of the intrachromosomal and extrachromosomal mechanisms of amplification are equally frequent in these cases. In contrast, amplified clones represent the large majority of the clones recovered in actinomycin D, and the products of the breakage – fusion – bridge (BFB) cycle mechanism were observed in all the clones. We concluded that only actinomycin D induces gene amplification and that only the BFB cycle mechanism is triggered by the drug. Such a result confirms that different mechanisms, initiated by different types of primary events, drive the early steps of extra- or intrachromosomal amplification.

However, the differential effect of the two clastogenic drugs was unexpected. In order to clarify this point, we undertook a cytogenetic analysis of the chromosome damage resulting from treatment of the cells by each drug

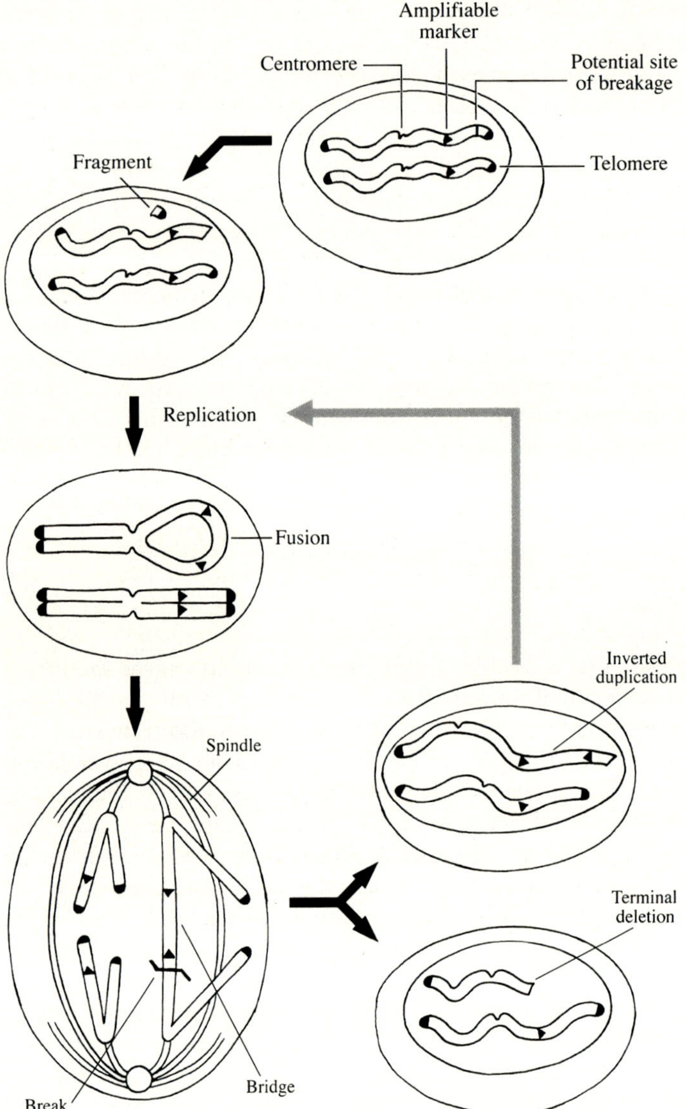

Fig. 3. The chromatid type of breakage – fusion – bridge (BFB) cycles. The phenomenon is postulated to result from a chromosome break: the fragment corresponding to the part of the chromosome telomeric to the break is lost and, after replication, the two broken chromatids fuse. At mitosis, the fused chromatids form a bridge. If this structure is asymmetrically broken, one daughter cell receives an additional copy of the corresponding sequence, while the other one has a terminal deletion and is expected to die in selective medium. In the amplified daughter cell, the third copy of the considered sequence lies in an inverted orientation relative to the normal one on the broken chromosome arm. After replication, the broken chromatids can fuse again, perpetuating the amplification cycles

Table 1. Mechanism of resistance in independent mutant clones

Selective agent	Analyzed clones (n)	Clones not amplified for MRD1		Clones amplified for MDR1			
				Total		DMs	BFBs
		(n)	%				
				(n)	(%)	(n)	(n)
Vinblastine	37	35	95	2	5	1	1
Adriamycin	28	25	89	3	11	1	2
Actinomycin D	16	6	37	10	63	0	10

DM, double-minute chromosome; BFB, breakage – fusion – bridge.

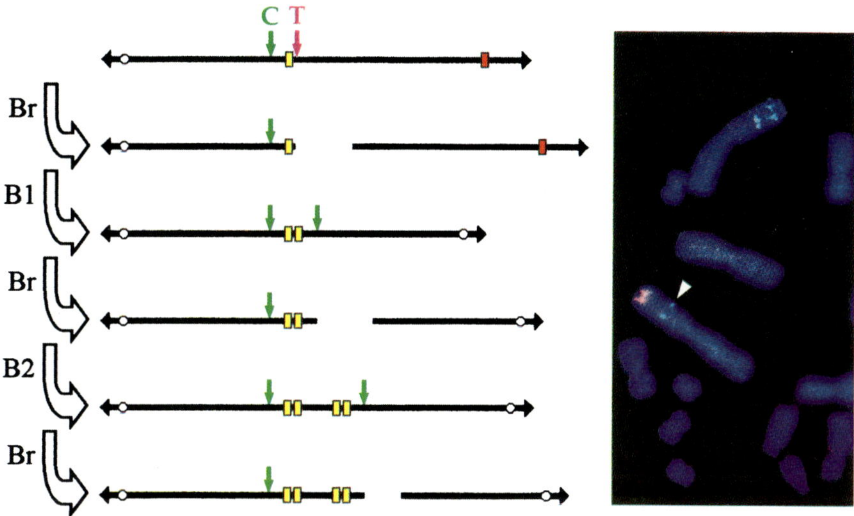

Fig. 4. Role of fragile sites in the early stages of intrachromosomal amplification. *Left.* model involving a centromeric (*C*) and a telomeric (*T*) fragile site in MDR1 amplification. *Black triangles*, telomeres; *white circles*, centromeres, *yellow squares*, MDR1 genes; *red squares*, telomeric marker; *Br*, breakage; *B1, B2*, bridges of the first and the second cycles, respectively. *Right*, fluorescence in situ hybridization (FISH) with a probe for the MDR1 gene (*green*) and a telomeric marker (*red*). The *arrowhead* points to the normal copy of the MDR1 gene on the unamplified chromosome 1q. The homologue is deleted for the telomeric marker and bears two doublets of the MDR1 gene

at the concentration used to select mutants. We found that adriamycin induces chromosome breaks very efficiently at random locations. In contrast, actinomycin D induces breaks targeted to specific loci. With the help of the cytogenetic markers available on chromosome 1, we identified and localized at least six hotspots of breakage along this chromosome. One of them lies close to and telomeric to the MDR1 gene, a convenient location to trigger MDR1 amplification. A break at this site has been observed in as many as 14% of the metaphase plates. Experiments were also undertaken with coformycin, and the very same hotspots of breakage were observed. Remarkably, breaks at a site just telomeric to the AMPD2 gene are also efficiently induced by the drug. The same pattern of breakage was also revealed following treatment of the cells with methotrexate, a well-known activator of a particular type of fragile sites. Thus the ability of a drug to induce amplification of a given gene relies directly on its ability to activate adequately located fragile sites. The location of these sites along chromosome 1q suggests that not only is the intrachromosomal amplification process induced by activation of fragile sites telomeric to the selected genes, but that in each case, a centromeric one contributes to determine the sequence content of the early amplified units (Coquelle et al. 1997; Fig. 4). In this work, we were unable to determine clearly whether the breaks per se or some particular sequences or structural features of the fragile sites contribute to initiate the process. More recently, we used a model system allowing a single double strand break to be targeted in a mammalian chromosome to demonstrate that such a break can trigger the intrachromosomal amplification process (Pipiras et al. 1998).

Conclusions

Because of the clinical importance of gene amplification, the initiating events and the nature of the mechanisms responsible for these mutations in mammalian cells have been intensively studied for over 20 years. Recently, development of the FISH technique has provided a powerful tool to study the early stages of the amplification process. The results described here indicate that two independent pathways, both relying on unequal segregation of gene copies at mitosis, drive the initial steps of gene amplification. First, the analysis of DM-containing cells indicated that extrachromosomal amplification results from the looping out of a few megabases-long molecule, generating an initial circular acentric extrachromosomal element (Coquelle et al. 1997; Toledo et al. 1993). We have also shown that a second pathway accumulates copies organized as giant inverted repeats on a chromosome arm where one normal gene copy maps in unamplified cells (Toledo et al. 1992a). These features and the fact that the telomeric part of the amplified chromosome is deleted in such mutant cells correspond to the expected products of the BFB cycles mechanism, first described by McClintock (1942). Moreover, the frequent observation of both the fusion and bridge intermediates of this mechanism in cell populations undergoing intrachromosomal amplification definitely established the involvement of the BFB cycles in intrachromosomal mammalian gene amplification (Coquelle et al. 1997; Toledo et al. 1993).

Until recently, the initial events triggering either of the pathways remained uncertain. Some clue as to the nature of these events can be expected from the identification and properties of agents that can induce the amplification processes. We showed that the drugs behaving as potent activators of fragile sites specifically induce the BFB cycles. Moreover, evidence was obtained at three different loci that breaks at fragile sites telomeric to and centromeric to the selected genes frame the initial intrachromosomal amplicons (Coquelle et al. 1997). Because most drugs used to select mutants in vitro are also used in cancer therapy, our results suggest that knowledge of the ability of chemotherapeutic agents to induce fragile sites in human cells, coupled to precise mapping of these sites relative to oncogenes frequently amplified in tumors, may help to choose among drugs of comparable antiproliferative efficiency those which are not prone to inducing marked genomic instability.

References

Bertoni L, Attolini C, Tessera L, Mucciolo E, Giulotto E (1994) Role of telomeric and non-telomeric (TTAGGG)n sequences in gene amplification and chromosome stability. Genomics 24:53–62

Biedler JL, Meyers MB (1989) Multidrug resistance (vinca alkaloids, actinomycin D, and anthracycline antibiotics). In: Gupta RS (ed) Drug resistance in mammalian cells. CRC, Boca Raton, 2:57–88

Brison O (1993) Gene amplification and tumor progression. Biochim Biophys Acta 1155:25–41

Coquelle A, Pipiras E, Toledo F, Buttin G, Debatisse M (1997) Expression of fragile sites triggers intrachromosomal mammalian gene amplification and sets boundaries to early amplicons. Cell 89:215–225

Cowell J (1982) Double minutes and homogeneously staining regions: gene amplification in mammalian cells. Annu Rev Genet 16:21–59

Hartwell L (1992) Defects in a cell cycle checkpoint may be responsible for the genomic instability of cancer cells. Cell 71:543–546

Kuo MT, Vyas RC, Jiang LX, Hittelman WN (1994) Chromosome breakage at a major fragile site associated with P-glycoprotein gene amplification in multidrug-resistant CHO cells. Mol Cell Biol 14:5202–5211

Livingstone LR, White A, Sprouse J, Livanos E, Jacks T, Tlsty TD (1992) Cell cycle arrest and gene amplification potential accompany loss of wild-type p53. Cell 70:923–935

Ma C, Martin S, Trask B, Hamlin JL (1993) Sister chromatid fusion initiates amplification of the dihydrofolate reductase gene in chinese hamster cells. Genes Dev. 7:605–620

McClintock B (1942) The fusion of broken ends of chromosomes following nuclear fusion. Proc Natl Acad Sci USA 28:458–463

Pinkel D, Landegent J, Collins C, Fuscoe J, Segraves R, Lucas J, Gray J (1988) Fluorescence in situ hybridization with human chromosome-specific libraries: detection of trisomy 21 and translocations of chromosome 4. Proc Natl Acad Sci USA 85:9138–9142

Pipiras E, Coquelle A, Bieth A, Debatisse M (1998) Interstitial deletions and intrachromosomal amplification initiated from a double-strand break targeted to a mammalian chromosome. EMBO J 17:325–333

Schwab M, Amler LC (1990) Amplification of cellular oncogenes: a predictor of clinical outcome in human cancer. Genes Chromosomes Cancer 1:181–193

Smith KA, Gorman PA, Stark MB, Groves RP, Stark GR (1990) Distinctive chromosomal structures are formed very early in the amplification of CAD genes in Syrian hamster cells. Cell 63:1219–1227

Smith KA, Stark MB, Gorman PA, Stark GR (1992) Fusion near telomeres occur very early in the amplification of CAD genes in Syrian hamster cells. Proc Natl Acad Sci USA 89:5427–5431

Stahl F, Wettergren Y, Levan G (1992) Amplicon structure in multi-drug-resistant murine cells: a non-rearranged region of genomic DNA corresponding to large circular DNA. Mol Cell Biol 12:1179–1187

Toledo F, LeRoscouet D, Buttin G, Debatisse M (1992a) Co-amplified markers alternate in megabase long chromosomal inverted repeats and cluster independently in interphase nuclei at early steps of mammalian gene amplification. EMBO J 11:2665–2673

Toledo F, Smith KA, Buttin G, Debatisse M (1992b) The evolution of the amplified adenylate deaminase 2 domains in Chinese hamster cells suggests the sequential operation of different mechanisms of DNA amplification. Mutat Res 276:261–273

Toledo F, Buttin G, Debatisse M (1993) The origin of chromosome rearrangements at early stages of *AMPD2* gene amplification in Chinese hamster cells. Curr Biol 3:255–264

Trask B, Hamlin J (1989) Early dihydrofolate reductase gene amplification events in CHO cells usually occur on the same chromosome arm as the original locus. Genes Dev 3:1913–1925

Yin Y, Tainsky MA, Bischoff FZ, Strong LC, Wahl GM (1992) Wild-type p53 restores cell cycle control and inhibits gene amplification in cells with mutant p53 alleles. Cell 70:937–948

V. Genetic Susceptibility and Environmental Exposure: "The RET Paradigm"

Mechanisms of Development of Multiple Endocrine Neoplasia Type 2 and Hirschsprung's Disease by *ret* Mutations

M. Takahashi, N. Asai, T. Iwashita, H. Murakami, and S. Ito

Department of Pathology, Nagoya University School of Medicine,
65 Tsurumai-cho, Showa-ku, Nagoya 466, Japan

Abstract

The *ret* proto-oncogene encodes a receptor tyrosine kinase whose ligands belong to the glial cell line-derived neurotrophic factor (GDNF) protein family. Its germline mutations are responsible for the development of multiple endocrine neoplasia (MEN) types 2A and 2B and Hirschsprung's disease (HSCR). MEN2A and MEN2B mutations result in the constitutive activation of Ret by different molecular mechanisms. MEN2A mutations involve cysteine residues present in the Ret extracellular domain and induce disulfide-linked Ret dimerization on the cell surface. MEN2B mutations were identified in methionine 918 in the tyrosine kinase domain and activate Ret without dimerization, probably due to a conformational change of its catalytic core region. In contrast to MEN2 mutations, HSCR mutations represent loss of function mutations. We found that most of HSCR mutations detected in the extracellular domain impair the Ret cell surface expression. More interestingly, *ret* mutations in cysteines 618 and 620 were reported in several families who developed both MEN2A and HSCR. It was suggested that these mutations might have two biological effects on Ret function, leading to the development of different clinical phenotypes in the same patients.

Introduction

The *ret* proto-oncogene encodes a receptor tyrosine kinase that contains a cadherin-related sequence in the extracellular domain (Takahashi 1995). It was recently demonstrated that glial cell line-derived neurotrophic factor (GDNF) and neurturin, which define a new protein family, can induce Ret tyrosine phosphorylation, indicating that these two neurotrophic factors represent Ret ligands. It is interesting to note that these factors mediate their actions through a multicomponent receptor system composed of ligand-binding glycosyl-phosphatidylinositol (GPI)-linked proteins and Ret (Buj-Bello et al. 1997; Jing et al. 1996; Klein et al. 1997; Treanor et al. 1996). This unique

Recent Results in Cancer Research, Vol. 154
© Springer-Verlag Berlin · Heidelberg 1998

multicomponent receptor system plays an important role in the survival and/ or differentiation of a variety of central and peripheral neurons.

Germline mutations of the *ret* proto-oncogene are associated with the development of three hereditary neoplastic disorders: multiple endocrine neoplasia (MEN)2A, MEN2B, and familial medullary thyroid carcinoma (FMTC) (Carlson et al. 1994; Donis-Keller et al. 1993; Hofstra et al. 1994; Mulligan et al. 1993). MEN2A and MEN2B share the clinical features of medullary thyroid carcinoma and pheochromocytoma, and FMTC is characterized by the development of medullary thyroid carcinoma alone. MEN2B is distinguished from MEN2A and FMTC by a more complex phenotype including mucosal neuroma, hyperganglionosis of the gastrointestinal tract, and marfanoid habitus. The MEN2A and FMTC mutations resulted mainly in nonconservative substitutions for six cysteines (cysteines 609, 611, 618, 620, 630, and 634) in the Ret extracellular domain, whereas the MEN2B mutation was detected in methionine 918 in the tyrosine kinase domain.

Germline mutations of *ret* are also responsible for Hirschsprung's disease (HSCR), which is characterized by the absence of intrinsic ganglion cells in the distal gastrointestinal tract (Pasini et al. 1996). HSCR mutations, including missense, nonsense, and frameshift mutations, are scattered along the whole coding sequence of *ret* and account for 50% of familial and 10%–20% of sporadic cases of HSCR. Based on the length of the aganglionic segment, HSCR is classified into two subtypes, short-segment HSCR and long-segment HSCR; *ret* mutations appear to be associated with long segment HSCR. In addition, three mutations in cysteine 618 or 620 were reported in several families who developed both MEN2A and HSCR.

To assess the correlation between genotype and phenotype, we introduced most mutations reported in these diseases into *ret* cDNA which was transfected into NIH 3T3 cells. Characterization of the nature of the mutant Ret proteins provided interesting insights into the mechanisms of development of MEN2A, MEN2B, FMTC, and HSCR.

Mechanism of Ret Activation by MEN2A and FMTC Mutations

We investigated the transforming activity of Ret with a MEN2A or FMTC mutation found in cysteine 609, 611, 618, 620, 630, or 634. Of these cysteine mutations, cysteine 634 mutations are known to be strongly associated with the MEN2A phenotype, whereas cysteine 609, 618, and 620 mutations were found in about 70% cases of FMTC (Pander and Smith 1996). We introduced a total of 18 mutations into six cysteine residues (Fig. 1) and found that all mutant *ret* cDNAs had the ability to transform NIH 3T3 cells at variable levels (Ito et al. 1997). The transforming activity of cysteine 634 mutant proteins was approximately three- to five-fold higher than that of cysteine 609, 611, 618, or 620 mutant proteins. The activity of cysteine 630 mutant proteins was slightly lower than that of cysteine 634 mutant proteins. In addition, different amino acid substitution for the same cysteine displayed com-

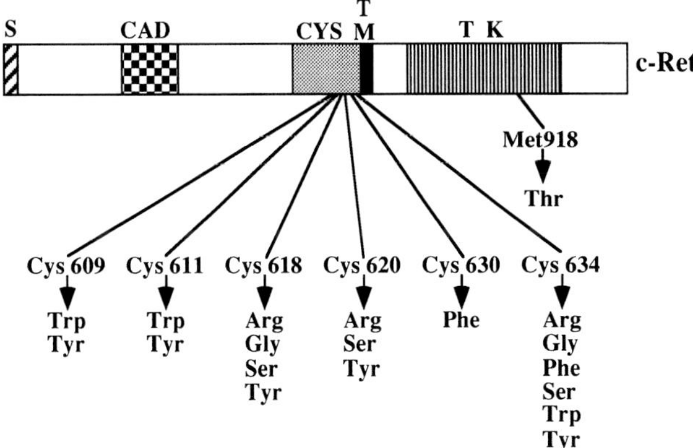

Fig. 1. Ret protein. *S*, signal sequence; *CAD*, cadherin-like domain; *CYS*, cysteine-rich region; *TM*, transmembrane domain; *TK*, tyrosine kinase domain. Eighteen cysteine mutations and a MEN-2B mutation (Met918→Thr) are shown

parable transforming activity, suggesting that the degree of activity depends on the position of cysteine rather than the substituted amino acids. Our results showing that cysteine 634 mutant proteins had the highest transforming activity are consistent with the observation that there is a strong association between cysteine 634 mutations and the development of pheochromocytoma in MEN2A. On the other hand, the low transforming activity of cysteine 609, 618, and 620 mutant proteins appears to correlate with the FMTC phenotype.

Western blot analysis of the mutant Ret proteins revealed that the level of expression of the 175-kDa Ret form present on the cell surface was directly proportional to the transforming activity of each mutant protein [Ito et al. 1997]. The level of expression the 175-kDa Ret form with a cysteine 609, 611, 618, or 620 mutation was approximately five- to ten-fold lower than that of the 175-kDa form with a cysteine 634 mutation. Since the expression of the 155-kDa Ret form present in the cytoplasmic membrane fraction was not affected by each cysteine mutation, this result suggests that cysteine 609, 611, 618, or 620 mutations severely impair the transport of Ret to the plasma membrane or its correct maturation. As we and others have already reported (Asai et al. 1995; Borrello et al. 1995; Iwashita et al. 1996a; Santoro et al. 1995), cysteine 634 mutations are able to activate Ret by inducing homodimers of the 175-kDa Ret form on the cell surface (Fig. 2). Although cysteine 609, 611, 618, and 620 mutations were also able to form homodimers of the 175-kDa form, the amount of homodimers with these mutations was very low. Thus the levels of expression of the 175-kDa Ret form with each cysteine mutation and of its homodimers appear to correlate with both the transforming activity and the clinical phenotype.

Difference in Activation Mechanisms by the MEN2A Versus MEN2B Mutation

Unlike the MEN2A and FMTC mutations, the MEN2B mutation does not induce Ret dimerization. Since the MEN2B mutation is present in the catalytic core region of the Ret kinase domain, it could induce a conformational change of its region, resulting in Ret activation (Fig. 2; Iwashita et al. 1996a). Ret is translated as two isoforms of 1114 amino acids (long isoform) and 1072 amino acids (short isoform). The 51 carboxy-terminal amino acids of the long isoform are replaced by the nine unrelated amino acids of the short isoform by alternative splicing in the 3' region. Interestingly, the transforming activity of the long isoform with the MEN2B mutation was approximately ten fold higher than that of the short isoform, although the transforming activity of both isoforms with the MEN2A mutation showed similar transforming activity (Asai et al. 1996). Thus the carboxy-terminal tail may regulate the transforming activity of Ret with the MEN2B mutation.

To investigate further the different activation mechanisms by MEN2A versus MEN2B mutations, we mutated tyrosine residues present in the tyrosine

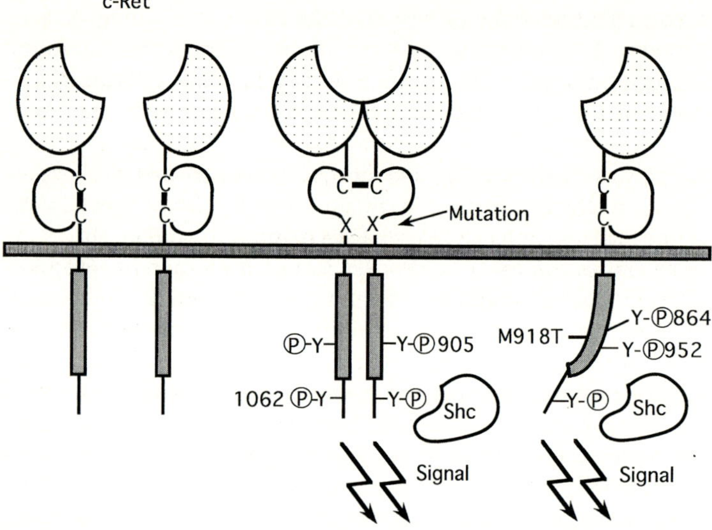

Fig. 2. Mechanisms of Ret activation by the MEN2A (*center*) or MEN2B mutation (*right*). When one cysteine residue (*C*) in the extracellular domain is replaced by other amino acids (*X*) due to a MEN2A mutation, it is anticipated that another cysteine which should form an intramolecular disulfide bond with the mutated cysteine becomes free and forms an aberrant intermolecular disulfide bond, leading to ligand-independent Ret dimerization. However, since the MEN2B mutation (Met918 → Thr) is present in the catalytic core region in the kinase domain, it could induce a conformational change of its region, resulting in Ret activation without dimerization. In addition, tyrosine 905 and tyrosines 864 and 952 are required for the transforming activity of MEN2A-Ret and MEN2B-Ret, respectively. Tyrosine 1062 represents a binding site of Shc adaptor proteins that are crucial for the transforming activity of both MEN2A-Ret and MEN2B-Ret

kinase domain. When tyrosine 905 that is conserved at the same position in all tyrosine kinases was changed to phenylalanine, the transforming activity of Ret with a MEN2A mutation (Cys634 → Arg; designated MEN2A-Ret) was completely abolished, suggesting that phosphorylation of this tyrosine is essential for its activity (Iwashita et al. 1996a). On the other hand, this tyrosine mutation did not affect the transforming activity of Ret with the MEN2B mutation (MEN2B-Ret) at all.

To look for tyrosine residues required for the activity of MEN2B-Ret, we further changed several tyrosines in the kinase domain to phenylalanine. When tyrosine 864 or 952 was replaced with phenylalanine, the transforming activity of MEN2B-Ret significantly decreased. In addition, the double mutation of these two tyrosines completely abolished the activity of MEN2B-Ret, but not of MEN2A-Ret, indicating that tyrosine residues essential for the transforming activity differ between MEN2A-Ret and MEN2B-Ret (Iwashita et al. 1996a). In addition to these tyrosine residues, we identified tyrosine 1062 as a binding site of Shc adaptor proteins that could play an important role in the activity of both MEN2A-Ret and MEN2B-Ret proteins. Possible activation mechanisms of Ret by the MEN2A or MEN2B mutation are summarized in Fig. 2.

Mechanism of Ret Dysfunction by HSCR Mutations

It is known that *ret* is an important gene for the development of enteric neurons because *ret* knockout mice completely lack ganglion cells in the intestine (Schuchardt et al. 1997). To date, a variety of mutations, including missense, nonsense, and frameshift mutations, have been identified in both the extracellular and intracellular domains of Ret in HSCR (Chakravarti 1996). Pasini et al. (1995) reported that some mutations detected in the kinase domain impair the Ret kinase activity as expected. We and others investigated the biological effects of several HSCR mutations reported in the Ret extracellular domain and found that these mutations severely impair Ret cell surface expression (Carlomagno et al. 1996; Iwashita et al. 1996b). Based on its length, the aganglionic segment is classified into two groups: short-segment HSCR and long-segment HSCR. Our results also showed that long-segment HSCR mutations more severely impair transport of Ret to the plasma membrane than a short-segment HSCR mutation, suggesting that the level of its cell surface expression may correlate with the HSCR phenotype (Iwashita et al. 1996b). In addition, the fact that *ret* heterozygous deletions were detected in both familial and sporadic HSCR patients suggests that haploinsufficiency for *ret* is crucial for development of HSCR. Since the cell surface expression of Ret with long-segment HSCR mutations was very low, a haploinsufficiency effect might be also postulated in the cases of missense mutations found in the Ret extracellular domain. Thus it seems likely that sufficient GDNF binding to Ret on the cell surface of enteric neuroblasts is required for their full differentiation during embryogenesis.

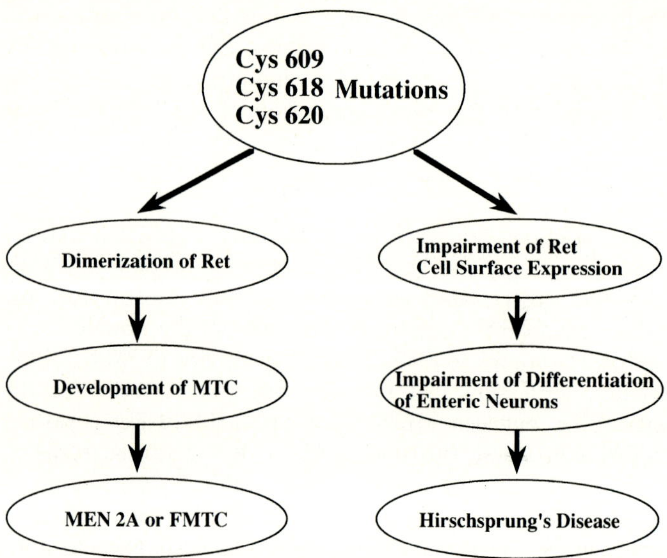

Fig. 3. Biological effects of cysteine 609, 618, and 620 mutations on Ret function. These mutations might have different biological effects on Ret function, depending on the cell type expressing Ret. *MTC*, medullary thyroid carcinoma

Another interesting finding is that there are several families who develop both MEN2A and FMTC (Ponder and Smith 1996). In these families, substitution of arginine or serine for cysteine 618 and of arginine for cysteine 620 in *ret* was identified. In addition, mutations of cysteine 609 reported in MEN2A were found in sporadic cases of HSCR. These findings suggest that the same cysteine mutations are able to induce both MEN2A and HSCR. As mentioned already, the transforming activity of Ret with cysteine 609, 618, or 620 mutations was very low compared with the activity of Ret with cysteine 634 mutations (Ito et al. 1997). The low activity of Ret with cysteine 609, 618 or 620 mutations correlated with the low expression of the 175-kDa Ret form present on the cell surface, indicating that these mutations impair the Ret cell surface expression in the same way as HSCR mutations affecting the Ret extracellular domain. These results thus suggest that cysteine 609, 618, and 620 mutations have two biological effects on Ret function (Fig. 3; Ito et al. 1997). First, these mutations induce ligand-independent Ret homodimers at low levels that are sufficient for tumorigenesis of thyroid C cells, leading to the development of MEN2A or FMTC. Second, they also severely impair Ret cell surface expression in enteric neurons. This could result in the premature arrest of differentiation of enteric neuroblasts during embryogenesis, leading to the development of HSCR.

Conclusion

We have studied and elucidated molecular mechanisms of development of MEN2A, MEN2B, FMTC, HSCR, and papillary thyroid carcinoma by *ret* mutations. However, further studies of the intracellular signaling pathway via the mutant Ret proteins could be essential to better understand the correlation between genotype and phenotype correlation observed in these diseases. In addition, *ret* is known to play a crucial role in the development of the enteric nervous system and kidney and in survival of various neurons. In this regard, the recent identification of GDNF and neurturin as Ret ligands may be an important step in promoting the study of Ret signaling in neuronal cells and embryonic kidney.

References

Asai N, Iwashita T, Matsuyama M, Takahashi M (1995) Mechanism of activation of the ret proto-oncogene by multiple endocrine neoplasia 2A mutations. Mol Cell Biol 15:1613–1619

Asai N, Murakami H, Iwashita T, Takahashi M (1996) A mutation at tyrosine 1062 in MEN2A-Ret and MEN2B-Ret impairs their transforming activity and association with Shc adaptor proteins. J Biol Chem 271:17644–17649

Borrello MG, Smith DP, Pasini B, Bongarzone I, Greco A, Lorenzo MJ, Arighi E, Miranda C, Eng C, Alberti L, Bocciardi R, Mondellini P, Scopsi L, Romeo G, Ponder BAJ, Pierotti MA (1995) RET activation by germline MEN 2A and MEN 2B mutations. Oncogene 11:2419–2427

Buj-Bello A, Adu J, Pinon LGP, Horton A, Thompson J, Rosenthal A, Chinchetru M, Buchman VL, Davies AM (1997) Neurturin responsiveness requires a GPI-linked receptor and the Ret receptor tyrosine kinase. Nature 387:721–724

Carlomagno F, De Vita G, Berlingieri MT, de Franciscis V, Melillo RM, Colantuoni V, Kraus MH, Di Fiore PP, Fusco A, Santoro M (1996) Molecular heterogeneity of RET loss of function in Hirschsprung's disease. EMBO J 15: 2717–2725

Carlson KM, Dou S, Chi D, Scavarda N, Toshima K, Jackson CE, Wells SA, Goodfellow PJ, Donis-Keller H (1994) Single missense mutation in the tyrosine-kinase catalytic domain of the RET proto-oncogene is associated with multiple endocrine neoplasia type 2B. Proc Natl Acad Sci USA 91:1579–1583

Chakravarti A (1996) Endothelin receptor-mediated signaling in Hirschsprung's disease. Hum Mol Genet 5:303–307

Donis-Keller H, Dou S, Chi D, Carlson KM, Toshima T, Lairmore TC, Howe JR, Moley JF, Goodfellow P, Wells SA (1993) Mutations in the RET proto-oncogene are associated with MEN 2A and FMTC. Hum Mol Genet 2:851–856

Hofstra RMW, Landsvater RM, Ceccherini I, Stulp RP, Stelwagen T, Luo Y, Pasini B, Hoppener JWM, van Amstel HKP, Romeo G, Lips CJM, Buys CHCM (1994) A mutation in the RET proto-oncogene associated with multiple endocrine neoplasia type 2B and sporadic medullary thyroid carcinoma. Nature 367:375–376

Ito S, Iwashita T, Asai N, Murakami H, Iwata Y, Sobue G, Takahashi M (1997) Biological properties of Ret with cysteine mutations correlate with multiple endocrine neoplasia type 2A, familial medullary thyroid carcinoma and Hirschsprung's disease phenotype. Cancer Res 57:2870–2872

Iwashita T, Asai N, Murakami H, Matsuyama M, Takahashi M (1996a) Identification of tyrosine residues that are essential for transforming activity of the ret proto-oncogene with MEN2A or MEN2B mutation. Oncogene 12:481–487

Iwashita T, Murakami H, Asai N, Takahashi M (1996b) Mechanism of Ret dysfunction by Hirschsprung mutations affecting its extracellular domain. Hum Mol Genet 5:1577–1580

Jing S, Wen D, Yu Y, Holst PL, Luo Y, Fang M, Tamir R, Antonio L, Hu Z, Cupples R, Louis JC, Hu S, Altrock BW, Fox GM (1996) GDNF-induced activation of the Ret protein tyrosine kinase is mediated by GDNFR-α, a novel receptor for GDNF. Cell 85:1113–1124

Klein RD, Sherman D, Ho W-H, Stone D, Bennett GL, Moffat B, Vandlen R, Simmons L, Gu Q, Hongo J-A, Devaux B, Poulsen K, Armanini M, Nozaki C, Asai N, Goddard A, Phillips H, Henderson CE, Takahashi M, Rosenthal A (1997) A GPI-linked protein that interacts with Ret to form a candidate neurturin receptor. Nature 387:717–721

Mulligan LM, Kwok JBJ, Healey CS, Elsdon MJ, Eng C, Gardner E, Love DR, Mole SE, Moore JK, Papi L, Ponder MA, Telenius H, Tunnacliffe A, Ponder BAJ (1993) Germ-line mutations of the RET proto-oncogene in multiple endocrine neoplasia type 2A. Nature 363:458–460

Pasini B, Borrello MG, Greco A, Bongarzone I, Luo Y, Mondellini P, Alberti L, Miranda C, Arighi E, Bocciardi R, Seri M, Barone V, Radice MT, Romeo G, Pierotti MA (1995) Loss of function effect of RET mutations causing Hirschsprung disease. Nature [Genet] 10:35–40

Pasini B, Ceccherini I, Romeo G (1996) RET mutations in human disease. Trends Genet 12:138–144

Ponder BAJ, Smith D (1996) The MEN II syndromes and the role of the ret proto-oncogene. Adv Cancer Res 70:179–222

Santoro M, Carlomagno F, Romano A, Bottaro DP, Dathan NA, Grieco M, Fusco A, Vecchio G, Matoskova B, Kraus MH, Di Fiore PP (1995) Activation of RET as a dominant transforming gene by germline mutations of MEN2A and MEN2B. Science 267:381–383

Schuchardt A, D'Agati V, Larsson-Blomberg L, Costantini F, Pachnis V (1997) Defects in the kidney and enteric nervous system of mice lacking the tyrosine kinase receptor Ret. Nature 367:380–383

Takahashi M (1995) Oncogenic activation of the ret protooncogene in thyroid cancer. Crit Rev Oncog 6:35–46

Treanor JJS, Goodman L, de Sauvage F, Stone DM, Poulsen KT, Beck CD, Gray C, Armanini MP, Pollock RA, Hefti F, Phillips HS, Goddard A, Moore MW, Buj-Bello A, Davies AM, Asai N, Takahashi M, Vandlen R, Henderson CE, Rosenthal A (1996) Characterization of a multicomponent receptor for GDNF. Nature 382:80–83

Rearrangements of RET and NTRK1 Tyrosine Kinase Receptors in Papillary Thyroid Carcinomas

M. A. Pierotti, P. Vigneri, and I. Bongarzone

Division of Experimental Oncology A, Istituto Nazionale per lo Studio e la Cura del Tumori, 1 Via Venezian, 20133 Milan, Italy

Abstract

A combined cytogenetic and molecular analysis of thyroid tumours has indicated that these neoplasms might represent a significant model for analysing human epithelial cell multi-step cancerogenesis. Thyroid tumours comprise a broad spectrum of lesions with different phenotypes and variable biological and clinical behaviour. Molecular analysis has detected specific genetic alterations in these different tumour types. In particular, the well-differentiated carcinomas of the papillary type are characterised by the activation of the tyrosine kinase receptors (TKRs) RET and NTRK1 proto-oncogenes. Cytogenetic analysis of these tumours has contributed to defining the chromosomal mechanisms leading to the TKRs' oncogenic activation. The results have shown that, in the majority of the cases, intra-chromosomal inversions of chromosome 10 and of chromosome 1 lead to the formation of RET-derived and NTRK1-derived oncogenes, respectively. Exposure to ionizing radiation is associated with papillary carcinomas, and RET activation has been suggested to be related to this event. All these findings are contributing to the definition of genetic and environmental factors relevant to the pathogenesis of thyroid tumours. Moreover, the molecular characterisation of specific genetic lesions could provide significant information about the association between ionising radiation and RET oncogene activation.

Introduction

Thyroid tumours comprise medullary thyroid carcinoma (MTC) developing from neural crest-derived C cells and tumours originating from epithelial follicular cells. The latter include several tumour types with different phenotypic characteristics and variable biological and clinical behaviours. Thyroid adenomas are benign neoplasms, although some are capable of malignant growth and progression. Papillary and follicular carcinomas are the most common forms of thyroid cancer. Although originating from the same follicular cell, papillary and follicular carcinomas are regarded as different bio-

Recent Results in Cancer Research, Vol. 154
© Springer-Verlag Berlin · Heidelberg 1998

logical entities. Follicular carcinoma, which is solitary and encapsulated, is associated with endemic goitre, and low iodine intake and metastatises almost exclusively via the blood stream, often to bones. In contrast, papillary carcinoma is multifocal, is associated with previous radiation exposure and high iodine intake and metastatises by lymphatic spread to regional lymphnodes. Anaplastic or undifferentiated thyroid carcinomas are almost invariably fatal, representing the most aggressive form of thyroid tumours.

In particular, papillary thyroid carcinomas (PTCs) account for about 80% of tumours originating from the epithelium of the thyroid gland, and their prognosis correlates with the initial extent of the primary tumour (occult, intrathyroid or extrathyroid). Furthermore, this parameter is closely related to the histological pattern of the various papillary carcinoma subtypes, which are graded according to their level of differentiation. These tumours provided the first evidence for an activated oncogene in thyroid tumours; a review of their molecular characterisation will follow.

RET/NTRK1 Rearrangements

Over the last 10 years, several reports have demonstrated the alternative involvement of the *RET* and *NTRK1* tyrosine kinase (TK) receptors (TKRs) in the development of a consistent fraction of PTCs. Somatic rearrangements of both *RET* and *NTRK1* produce several forms of oncogenes (Pierotti et al. 1996). In all cases, *RET* or *NTRK1* TK domains are fused to the amino terminus of different gene products (Table 1).

In particular, the *RET* proto-oncogene encodes for the TKR of glial cell-derived neurotrophic factor (GDNF) and neurturin (NTN) (Baloh et al. 1997; Creedon et al. 1997; Durbec et al. 1996; Jing et al. 1996; Sanicola et al. 1997; Suvanto et al. 1997, Treanor et al. 1996; Trupp et al. 1996). Activation of *RET* by GDNF or NTN has been shown to require one of two accessory proteins, *GDNFR-α* and *GDNFR-β* (Buj-Bello et al. 1997, Jing et al. 1996; Klein et al. 1997; Sanicola et al. 1997; Treanor et al. 1996). In humans, *RET* is expressed in the thyroid by normal C cells and their pathologic counterpart, MTC. Moreover, *RET* expression can be detected in normal adrenal medulla and pheochromocytomas (Santoro et al. 1990). Germline mutations of proto-*RET* result in human diseases, including familial MTC, multiple endocrine neo-

Table 1. Oncogenic version of RET and NTRK1 tyrosine kinases

Tyrosine kinase	Activating gene	Oncogene
RET	H4(D10 5170)	RET/PTC1
	RIα	RET/PTC2
	ELE1	RET/PTC3
NTRK1	Tropomyosin	TRK
	TPR	TRK/T1 (T2; T4)
	TFG	TRK/T3

plasia types 2A and 2B (MEN2A and MEN2B) and Hirschprung's disease (Donis-Keller at al. 1993; Hofstra et al. 1994; Mulligan et al. 1994; Pasini et al. 1996; Romeo et al. 1994). The human *RET* locus maps to 10q11.2.

The RET/PTC1 oncogene represents the first report of oncogene activation in solid tumours due to an acquired chromosomal abnormality. RET/PTC1 is a chimeric transforming sequence generated by the fusion of the TK domain of RET to the 5'-terminal sequence of the gene *H4/D10S170* (Griew et al. 1990). The latter has been shown to display a coiled-coil sequence which confers to the oncoprotein the ability to form dimers, resulting in a constitutive activation of the TK function. Both partners in the fusion have been localised to chromosome 10q.

We subsequently found a second example of *RET* activation: the RET/PTC2 oncogene. In this case, the rearrangement involved the gene of the regulatory subunit *RI-a* of protein kinase A, which maps to chromosome 17q23 (Bongarzone et al. 1993; Sozzi et al. 1994). Interestingly, like the *H4* gene, *RI-a* also contains a dimerisation domain, and the construction of RET/PTC2 mutants with deletions in *RI-a* has demonstrated that the formation of dimers is necessary to express the activity of the oncogene. Cytogenetic analysis of one case of RET/PTC2-positive carcinoma revealed that this oncogene arises from a t(10;17)(q11.2;q23) reciprocal translocation (Minoletti et al. 1994). Finally, a third example of *RET* activation in PTCs has been reported: RET/PTC3. In this oncogene, the TK domain of *RET* is fused to sequences derived from a previously unknown gene named *ELE1* (also known as RFG; Bongarzone et al. 1994; Santoro et al. 1994). Interestingly, we have localised *ELE1* to the same chromosomal region of RET, 10q11.2. In this case, too, a paracentric inversion of the long arm of chromosome 10 was identified.

The *NTRK1* proto-oncogene is a component of the high-affinity receptor for nerve growth factor (NGF) (Kaplan et al. 1993). *NTRK1* is primarily expressed in the nervous system, and mice carrying a germline mutation that eliminates *NTRK1* show severe sensory and sympathetic neuropathies and most die within 1 month of birth (Smeyne et al. 1994). Thus NGF signalling via *NTRK1* appears essential for the development of both the peripheral and central nervous systems. *NTRK1* is expressed in neuroblastoma, and its expression correlates with a good prognosis (Borrello et al. 1993; Nagakawara et al. 1992). The human *NTRK1* locus has been mapped to 1q22 (Weier et al. 1995).

In our analysis of PTCs, several cases showed an activation of the *NTRK1* proto-oncogene. In three specimens, we identified a chimeric sequence generated by the rearrangement of an isoform of non-muscle tropomyosin *(TPM3)* and *NTRK1* (Martin-Zanca et al. 1986). We mapped the former to chromosome 1q31. Therefore, *NTRK1* localisation to 1q22 suggested that a 1q intrachromosomal rearrangement could have generated the TRK oncogene. Molecular analysis of TRK-positive PTCs revealed the presence not only of the product of the oncogenic rearrangement (5'TPM3-3'NTRK1), but also of that related to the reciprocal event (5'NTRK1-3'TPM3). This finding indicates that an intrachromosomal inversion, inv(1q), provided the mechanism of the *NTRK1* oncogenic activation in these tumours (Pierotti et al. 1996).

In the remaining cases, different genes provided the 5′terminus of the on-cogene; we therefore designated the latter as TRK-T (Greco et al. 1992, 1995).

Three cases showed the fusion of the NTRK1 TK domain to sequences of the *TPR* (*T*ranslocated *P*romoter *R*egion) gene, originally identified as part of the MET oncogene. The first of these cases, TRK-T1, is encoded by a hybrid mRNA containing 598 nucleotides of TPR and 1148 nucleotides of NTRK1. We have localised the TPR locus on chromosome 1q25 (Miranda et al. 1994). Therefore, as for TRK, an intrachromosomal rearrangement, molecularly de-fined as an inversion of 1q, is responsible for its formation. A rearrangement involving the same two genes, *TPR* and *NTRK1,* has been found in two other papillary thyroid tumours, and the relative oncogenes have been designated TRK-T2 and TRK-T4 (Grew et al. 1993). Although the two rearrangements involve different genomic regions of the partner genes, they occur in the same intron of both *TPR* and *NTRK1.* As a consequence, the same mRNA and 1323 amino acid oncoprotein are produced in both cases. Similarly to TRK-T1, the molecular characterisation of these rearrangements indicated the chromosomal mechanism leading to the oncogenic activation as an inv(1q) (Grew et al. 1993). As for the last two oncogenes derived from NTRK1 activation, one is still uncharacterised, whereas the other, designated TRK-T3, has recently been analysed (Grew et al. 1995). Sequence analysis re-vealed that TRK-T3 contains 1412 nucleotides of NTRK1 preceded by 598 nu-cleotides belonging to a novel gene named *TFG* (*TRK Fused Gene*) encoding a 68-kDa cytoplasmic protein. The latter displays a coiled-coil region in the TFG part, that could endow the oncoprotein with the capability to form com-plexes as shown by sedimentation gradient experiments. The *TFG* gene is ubiquitously expressed and is located on chromosome 3, thus suggesting that a still undetected t(1q;3) occurred in this tumour. Molecular analysis of the rearranged fragments supported this conclusion by indicating that the chromosomal rearrangement is reciprocal and balanced, involving the loss of only a few nucleotides of germline sequences.

The relative frequency of *RET* and *NTRK1* activation has been found to be different in PTCs collected from various geographical areas. We have demon-strated the formation of oncogene sequences from *RET* and *NTRK1* in about 50% of PTCs collected at the National Cancer Institute in Milan (Italy). In a total of 76 PTCs, there were 26 (34%) oncogenic versions of RET (13 RET/PTC1, two RET/PTC2 and 11 RET/PTC3) and nine (12%) oncogenic versions of NTRK1 (three TRK, one TRK-T1, two TRK-T2, one TRK-T3 and two as yet uncharacterised. However, lower percentages have been described, rang-ing from 2.5% in Saudi Arabia to 8% in Japan (Table 2). In order to deter-mine whether their diversity is due to different methodologies or to the in-volvement of different genetic and/environmental factors, we tested the pres-ence of *RET/NTRK1* oncogenes in other cases from different Italian regions. The presence of oncogenic versions of *RET* and *NTRK1* was assessed in 14 samples of PTC from Pisa and in 39 samples from Catania using different ex-

Table 2. RET activation

References	Country	Positive		Total (n)
		(n)	(%)	
Sporadic tumors:				
Bongarzone[a]	Italy	27	21	129
Santoro et al. (1992)	USA	15	15	101
Jhiang et al. (1992)				
Santoro et al. (1992)	France	8	11	70
Ishizaka et al. (1991)	Japan	2	4	49
Wajjwalku et al. (1992)				
Zou et al. (1994)	Saudi Arabia	1	2.5	40
Radiation-related tumours:				
Fugazzola et al. (1995)	Belarus	12	66	18
Klugbauer et al. (1995)				
Bounacer et al. (1997)	France	16	84	19

[a] see Table 3.

Table 3. RET activation in different Italian locactions

Source	Cases (n)	RET/PTC and NTRK1 positivity	
		(n)	(%)
Istituo Nazionale Tumori (Milan)	76	35	46
Pisa University	14	1	7[a]
Catania University	39	1	2.6[b]

[a] NTRK1 activation.
[b] RET activation.

perimental procedures, including transfection, Southern blotting, extra-long polymerase chain reaction (PCR) (XL-PCR) and reverse transcriptase (RT)-PCR (Table 3). In these samples, we observed a very low frequency of *RET/NRTK1* activation, corresponding to 7% in the Pisa cases and 2.5% in those from Catania. Considering the fact that, in Italy, ethnical differences are unlikely to significantly influence these events, a possible explanation for these results might lie in exposure to diverse environmental factors. The primary role of environmental factors has already been shown in tumours in children exposed to high levels of radiation following the Chernobyl disaster (Shore et al. 1985) and in thyroid lesions associated with radiation therapy of the head and neck (Kazakov et al. 1992). Although uncertainties remain about the dose – response relationship, a history of radiation exposure, particularly in childhood, is probably the best characterised risk factor for thyroid cancer and for *RET* oncogenic rearrangements. In fact, molecular studies both from our laboratory and by Klugbauer's group have found *RET* rearrangements in 67% of post-Chernobyl PTCs. Interestingly, in these cases, RET/PTC3 was the most frequently observed rearrangement. Little is known about the mechanism of *RET* damage by ionising radiation. Random breaks due to incomplete replication or exogenously introduced mutagens may cause a large number of broken ends that can represent potential recombination substrata (Nelson and Kastan 1997). As a consequence, illegitimate recombination can occur and produce genetic rearrangements. In keeping with this concept, RET/PTC1 oncogenic activation has been induced by high-doses of X-irradiation in cell lines in thyroid tissues transplanted into severe combined immunodeficient (SCID) mice following X-ray radiations (Ho et al. 1993; Mizuno et al. 1997). In addition, most importantly, about 80% of PTCs from patients who received external radiation for benign or malignant conditions showed *RET* oncogenic rearrangements (Bounacer et al. 1997). In contrast with the results obtained with Chernobyl tumours, the most frequently observed chimaeric gene was not RET/PTC3, but RET/PTC1. It has been suggested that the predominance of RET/PTC1 or RET/PTC3 rearrangements may be due to a different preferential target of the damage produced by external therapeutical ionising radiation or by accidental exposure to radioisotopes which could also act via an intra-body irradiation mechanism.

Role of Age

Age appears to be the main factor related to an excess risk of thyroid cancer associated with radiation exposure. In fact, risk is greatest if irradiation occurs in the first two decades of life, when thyroid cells display a significant mitotic rate. In view of the fact that *RET* activation is frequently involved in PTCs related to radiation exposure, we examined a possible relationship between *RET/NTRK1* oncogenic activation and age in a sample of 92 consecutive patients (Bongarzone et al. 1996). The results showed that the frequency of *RET* and *NTRK1* activation was significantly higher in the group of PTC patients aged 4–30 years ($p=0.02$), thus supporting the concept that age might contribute to this specific carcinogenic process.

Correlation Between *RET/NTRK1* Rearrangements and Clinico-Pathological Features

Having obtained the above-mentioned results, we investigated the age-independent correlations between *RET* and *NTRK1* activation and the clinico-pathologic features of 76 sporadic (i.e. non-radiation-associated) PTCs. Among the 76 tumours analysed, 35 (46%) were positive for RET/PTC or NTRK1 oncogenic rearrangements. Specifically, RET/PTC oncogenes were detected in 34.2% (26 of 76) and NTRK1 oncogenes in 11.8% (nine of 76) of the evaluated patients. The presence or absence of *RET/NTRK1* oncogenic activation was then correlated to gender, age and the clinico-pathologic fea-

Table 4. RET/NTRK1 oncogenic activation accorting to pT stage

Stage	Negative cases (n)	Positive cases (n)	Cramer's V	p
pT1–pT3	33	18	–	–
pT4	9	17	0.280	0.015

tures (in terms of pTNM) of the patients. Statistical testing yielded a significant p-value for age (Bongarzone et al. 1996) and pT stage (Table 4). Results from a multivariate analysis showed that unfavourable disease characteristics, such as pT4 stage, presence of nodal (pN1) or distant metastases (pM1) or poorly differentiated and undifferentiated histologies, were placed close to *RET/NTRK1* oncogenic expression, thus suggesting the existence of an association between the latter feature and the presence of unfavourable disease characteristics. Due to the modest number of RET/PTC2- and NTRK1-positive cases, it was not possible to distinguish any biological feature specifically conferred by these two rearrangements on the basis of their statistical analysis. Conversely, both RET/PTC1 and RET/PTC3 rearrangements occurred with higher frequencies (13 and 11 of 26 positive cases, respectively). Interestingly, in this case, RET/PTC3 oncogenes seemed to be associated with a more aggressive tumour. Taken as two homogeneous groups, RET/PTC and NTRK1 oncogenic rearrangements were topologically strictly related and therefore did not imply a different pattern of association with pTNM or histological characteristics. Finally, young age (≤ 20 years) and male sex also tend to imply less favourable disease characteristics. In our analysis, RET/PTC and NTRK1 rearrangements were not associated with the degree of tumour differentiation. In fact, all the histological variants (with the exception of tall cell carcinomas) had similar frequencies of RET/PTC and NTRK1 activation with no particular imbalance in the frequencies of the oncogene subtypes. Unfortunately, due to the lack of follow-up in our patients, we cannot interpret these results in a prognostic context.

Conclusions

A comparative analysis of the oncogenes originating from the rearrangement of the two RTK proto-oncogenes *RET* and *NTRK1* allowed us to identify a common cytogenetic and molecular mechanism for their activation.

In all cases, chromosomal rearrangements fuse the TK portion of the TKRs to the 5′end of different genes, which we have designated as "activating" genes. Furthermore, although functionally different, the various activating genes share three properties:

1. They are ubiquitously expressed.
2. They have demonstrated or predicted domains able to form dimers or multimers.

3. They translocate the TKR-associated enzymatic activity from the membrane to the cytoplasm.

These characteristics are in agreement with the following scenario. After the fusion of their TK domain to the activating gene, *RET* and *NTRK1*, whose tissue-specific expression is restricted to subsets of neural cells, become expressed in the epithelial thyroid cells. Their dimerisation triggers a constitutive, ligand-independent *trans*-autophosphorylation of the TK domains. In this condition, the latter can recruit SH2- and SH3-containing cytoplasmic effector proteins. The relocalisation in the cytoplasm of *RET* and *NTRK1* enzymatic activity could allow their interaction with unusual substrates, perhaps modifying their functional properties. Therefore, following chromosomal rearrangements in PTCs, the oncogenic activation of *RET* and *NTRK1* proto-oncogenes can be defined as an ectopic, constitutive and topologically abnormal expression of their enzymatic (TK) activity. Moreover, the possibility that other carcinogenic factors may produce the same genetic changes remains to be determined. It seems likely that specific, as yet undetermined environmental factors are important in the aetiology of *RET/NTRK1*-positive PTCs. Direct evidence for this concept stems from the observation that PTCs from different geographical areas within the same country (Italy) or among different countries show a significantly different frequency of *RET/NTRK1* oncogenic expression. In addition, we must consider the possibility of a strong association between ionising radiation exposure and *RET* oncogenic activation.

References

Baloh RH, Tansey MG, Golden JP, Creedon DJ, Heuckeroth RO, Keck CL, Zimonjic DB, Popescu NC, Johnson EMJ, Milbrandt J (1997) TrnR2, a novel receptor that mediates neurtrin and GDNF signaling through Ret. Neuron 18:793–802

Bongarzone I, Monzini N, Borrello MG, Carcano C, Ferraresi G, Arighi E, Mondellini P, Della Porta G, Pierotti MA (1993) Molecular characterization of a thyroid tumor-specific transforming sequence formed by the fusion of ret tyrosine kinase and the regulatory subunit RIa of cyclic AMP-dependent protein kinase A. Mol Cell Biol 13:358–366

Bongarzone I, Butti MG, Coronelli S, Borrello MG, Santoro M, Mondellini P, Pilotti S, Fusco A, Della Porta G, Pierotti MA (1994) Frequent activation of *ret* protooncogene by fusion with a new activating gene in papillary thyroid carcinomas. Cancer Res 54:2979–2985

Bongarzone I, Fugazzola L, Vigneri P, Mariani L, Mondellini P, Pacini F, Basolo F, Pinchera A, Pilotti S, Pierotti MA (1996) Age-related activation of the tyrosine kinase receptor protooncogenes RET and NTRK1 in papillary thyroid carcinoma. J Clin Endocrinol Metab 81:2006–2009

Borrello MG, Bongarzone I, Pierotti MA, Luksch R, Gasparini M, Collini P, Pilotti S, Rizzetti MG, Mondellini P, De Bernardi B, Di Martino D, Garaventa A, Brisigotti M, Tonini GP (1993) trk and ret proto-oncogene expression in human neuroblastoma specimens: high frequency of trk expression in non-advanced stages. Int J Cancer 54:540–545

Bounacer A, Wicker R, Caillou B, Cailleux AF, Sarasin A, Schlumberger M, Suarez HG (1997) High prevalence of activating *ret* proto-oncogene rearrangements in thyroid tumors from patients who had received external radiation. Oncogene 5:1263–1273

Buj-Bello A, Adu J, Pinon LG, Horton A, Thompson J, Rosenthal A, Chinchetru M, Buchman VL, Davies AM (1997) Neurturin responsiveness requires a GPI-linked receptor and the Ret receptor tyrosine kinase. Nature 387:721–724

Creedon DJ, Tansey MG, Baloh RH, Osborne PA, Lampe PA, Fahrner TJ, Heuckeroth RO, Milbrandt J, Johnson EMJ (1997) Neurturin shares receptor and signal transduction pathways with glial cell line-derived neurotrophic factor in sympathetic neurons. Proc Natl Acad Sci USA 94:7018–7023

Donis-Keller H, Dou S, Chi D, Carlson KM, Toshima K, Lairmore TC, Howe JR, Moley JF, Goodfellow P, Wells SAJ (1993) Mutations in the RET proto-oncogene are associated with MEN2A and FMTC. Hum Mol Genet 2:851–856

Durbec P, Marcos-Gutierrez CV, KilKenny C, Grigoriou M, Wartiowaara K, Suvanto P, Smith D, Ponder B, Costantini F, Saarma M, Sariola H, Pachnis V (1996) *GDNF* signalling through the Ret receptor tyrosine kinase. Nature 381:789–793

Fugazzola L, Pilotti S, Pinchera A, Vorontsova TV, Mondellini P, Bongarzone I, Greco A, Astakhova L, Butti MG, Demidchik EP, Pacini F, Pierotti MA (1995) Oncogenic rearrangements of the RET proto-oncogene in papillary thyroid carcinomas from children exposed to Chernobyl nuclear accident. Cancer Res 55:5617–5620

Greco A, Pierotti MA, Bongarzone I, Pagliardini S, Lanzi C, Della Porta G (1992) TRK-T1 is a novel oncogene formed by the fusion of TPR and TRK genes in human papillary thyroid carcinomas. Oncogene 7:237–242

Greco A, Mariani C, Miranda C, Pagliardini S, Pierotti MA (1993) Characterization of the NTRK1 genomic region involved in chromosomal rearrangements generating TRK oncogenes. Genomics 18:397–400

Greco A, Mariani C, Miranda C, Lupas A, Pagliardini S, Pomati M, Pierotti MA (1995) The DNA rearrangement that generates the TRK-T3 oncogene involves a novel gene on chromosome 3 whose product has a potential coiled-coil domain. Mol Cell Biol 15:6118–6127

Grieco M, Santoro M, Berlingieri MT, Melillo RM, Donghi R, Bongarzone I, Pierotti MA, Della Porta G, Fusco A, Vecchio G (1990) PTC is a novel rearranged form of the ret proto-oncogene and is frequently detected in vivo in human thyroid papillary carcinomas. Cell 60:557–563

Hofstra RM, Landsvater RM, Ceccherini I, Stulp RP, Stelwagen T, Luo Y, Pasini B, Hoppener JWM, Ploos van Hamstel HK, Romeo G, Lips CJM, Buys CHCM (1994) A mutation in the *RET* proto-oncogene associated with multiple endocrine neoplasia type 2B and sporadic medullary thyroid carcinoma. Nature 367:375–376

Ishizaka Y, Kobayashi S, Ushijima T, Hirohashi S, Sugimura T, Nagao M (1991) Detection of retTPC/PTC transcripts in thyroid adenomas and adenomatous goiter by an RT-PCR method. Oncogene 6:1667–1672

Ito T, Seyama T, Iwamoto KS, Hayashi T, Mizuno, T, Tsuyama N, Dohi K, Nakamura N, Akiyama M (1993) In vitro irradiation is able to cause RET oncogene rearrangement. Cancer Res 53:2940–2943

Jhiang SM, Caruso DR, Gilmore E, Ishizaka Y, Tahira T, Nagao M, Chiu IM, Mazzaferri EL (1992) Detection of the PTC/retTPC oncogene in human thyroid cancers. Oncogene 7:1331–1337

Jing S, Wen D, Yu Y, Holst PL, Luo Y, Fang M, Tamir R, Anatonio L, Hu Z, Cupples R, Louis J-C, Hu S, Altrock BW, Fox GM (1996) GDNF-induced activation of the Ret protein tyrosine kinase is mediated by GDNFR-alpha, a novel receptor for GDNF. Cell 85:1113–1124

Kaplan DR, Hempstead BL, Martin-Zanca D, Chao MV, Parada LF (1991) The trk proto-oncogene product: a signal transducing receptor for nerve growth factor. Science 252:554–558

Kazakov VS, Demidchik EP, Astakhova LN (1992) Thyroid cancer after Chernobyl. Nature 359:21

Klein RD, Sherman D, Ho WH, Stone D, Bennett GL, Moffat B, Vandlen R, Simmons L, Gu Q, Hongo JA, Devaux B, Poulsen K, Armanini M, Nozaki C, Asai N, Goddard A, Phillips H, Henderson CE, Takahashi M, Rosenthal A (1997) A GPI-linked protein that interacts with Ret to form a candidate neurturin receptor. Nature 387:717–721

Klugbauer S, Lengfelder E, Demidchik EP, Rabe HM (1995) High prevalence of *RET* rearrangement in thyroid tumors of children from Belarus after the Chernobyl reactor accident. Oncogene 11:2459–2467

Martin-Zanca D, Hughes SH, Barbacid M (1986) A human oncogene formed by the fusion of truncated tropomyosin and protein tyrosine kinase sequences. Nature 319:743–748

Minoletti F, Butti MG, Coronelli S, Miozzo M, Sozzi G, Pilotti S, Tunnacliffe A, Pierotti MA, Bongarzone I (1994) The two genes generating RET/PTC3 are localized in chromosomal band 10q11.2. Genes Chromosomes Cancer 11:51–57

Miranda C, Minoletti F, Greco A, Sozzi G, Pierotti MA (1994) Refined localization of the human TPR gene to chromosome 1q25 by in situ hybridization. Genomics 23:714–715

Mizuno T, Kyoizumi S, Suzuki T, Iwamoto KS, Seyama T (1997) Continued expression of a tissue specific activated oncogene in the early steps of radiation-induced human thyroid carcinogenesis. Oncogene 15:1455–1460

Mulligan LM, Eng C, Healey CS, Clayton L, Kwok JBJ, Gardner E, Ponder MA, Frilling A, Jackson CE, Lehnert H, Neumann HPH, Thibodeau SN, Ponder BAJ (1994) Specific mutations of the *RET* proto-oncogene are related to disease phenotype in MEN 2A and FMTC. Nature [Genet] 6:70–74

Nagakawara A, Arima M, Azar CG, Scavarda NJ, Brodeur GM (1992) Inverse relationship between *trk* expression and N-*myc* amplification in human neuroblastomas. Cancer Res 52 :1364–1368

Nelson WG, Kastan MB (1997) DNA strand breaks: the DNA template alterations that trigger p53-dependent DNA damage response pathways. Mol Cell Biol 14:1815–1823

Pasini B, Ceccherini I, Romeo G (1996) RET mutations in human disease. Trends Genet 12(4):138–144

Pierotti MA, Bongarzone I, Borrello MG, Greco A, Pilotti S, Sozzi G (1996) Cytogenetics and molecular genetics of the carcinomas arising from the thyroid epithelial follicular cells. Genes Chromosomes Cancer 16:1–14

Romeo G, Ronchetto P, Luo Y, Barone V, Seri M, Ceccherini I, Pasini B, Bocciardi R, Lerone M, Kaariainen H, Martucciello G (1994) Point mutations affecting the tyrosine kinase domain of the RET proto-oncogene in Hirschsprung's disease. Nature 367:377–378

Sanicola M, Hession C, Worley D, Carmillo P, Ehrenfels C, Walus L, Robinson R, Jaworski G, Wei H, Tizard R, Whitty A, Pepinski RB, Cate RL (1997) Glial cell line-derived neurotrophic factor-dependent RET activation can be mediated by two different cell-surface accessory proteins. Proc Natl Acad Sci USA 94:6238–6243

Santoro M, Rosati R, Grieco M, Berlingieri MT, Colucci-D'Amato GL, de Franciscis V, Fusco A (1990) The ret proto-oncogene is consistently expressed in human pheochromocytomas and thyroid medullary carcinomas. Oncogene 5:1595–1598

Santoro M, Carlomagno F, Hay ID, Herrmann MA, Grieco M, Melillo R, Pierotti MA, Bongarzone I, Della Porta G, Berger N, Peix JL, Paulin C, Fabien N, Vecchio G, Jenkins RB, Fusco A (1992) Ret oncogene activation in human thyroid neoplasms is restricted to the papillary cancer subtype. J Clin Invest 89:1517–1522

Santoro M, Dathan NA, Berlingieri MT, Bongarzone I, Paulin C, Grieco M, Pierotti MA, Vecchio G, Fusco A (1994) Molecular characterization of *RET*/PTC3; a novel rearranged version of the *RET* proto-oncogene in a human thyroid papillary carcinoma. Oncogene 9(2):509–516

Shore RE, Woodard E, Hildreth N, Dvoretsky P, Hempelmann L, Pasternack B (1985) Thyroid tumors following thymus irradiation. J Natl Cancer Inst 74:1177–1184

Smeyne RJ, Klein R, Schnapp A, Long LK, Bryant S, Lewin A, Lira SA, Barbacid M (1994) Severe sensory and sympathetic neuropathies in mice carrying a disrupted Trk/NGF receptor gene. Nature 368:246–249

Sozzi G, Bongarzone I, Miozzo M, Borrello MG, Butti MG, Pilotti S, Della Porta G, Pierotti MA (1994) A t(10;17) translocation creates the RET/ptc2 chimeric transforming sequence in papillary thyroid carcinoma. Genes Chromosomes Cancer 9:244–250

Suvanto P, Wartiovaara K, Lindhal M, Arumae U, Moshnyakov M, Horelli-Kuitunen N, Airaksinen MS, Palotie A, Sariola H, Saarma M (1997) Cloning, mRNA distribution and chromosomal localisation of the gene for glial cell line-derived neurotrophic factor receptor beta, a homologue to GDNFR-alfa. Hum Mol Genet 6:1267–1273

Treanor JJS, Goodman L, de Sauvage F, Stone DM, Poulsen KT, Beck CD, Gray C, Armanini MP, Pollock RA, Hefti F, Phillips HS, Goddard A, Moore MW, Buj-Bello A, Davies AM, Asai N, Takahashi M, Vandlen R, Henderson CE, Rosenthal A (1996) Characterization of a multicomponent receptor for GDNF. Nature 382:80–83

Trupp E, Arenas E, Fainzilber M, Nilsson AS, Sieber BA, Grigoriou M, KilKenny C, Salazar-Grueso F, Pachnis V, Arumae U, Sariola H, Saarma M, Ibanez CF (1996) Functional receptor for *GDNF* encoded by the c-ret proto-oncogene. Nature 381:785–789

Wajjwalku W, Nakamura S, Hasegawa Y, Miyazaki K, Satoh Y, Funahashi H, Matsuyama M, Takahashi M (1992) Low frequency of rearrangements of the *ret* and *trk* proto-oncogenes in Japanese thyroid papillary carcinomas. Jpn J Cancer Res 83:671–675

Weier H-UG, Rhein AP, Shadravan F, Collins C, Polikoff D (1995) Rapid physical mapping of the human *trk* protooncogene (NTRK1) to human chromosome 1q21-q22 by P1 cldone selection, fluorescence *in situ* hybridization (FISH), and computer-assisted microscopy. Genomics 26:390–393

Zou M, Shi Y, Farid NR (1994) Low rate of *ret* proto-oncogene activation (PTC/ret TPC) in papillary thyroid carcinomas from Saudi Arabia. Cancer 73:176–180

Molecular Genetics of Childhood Papillary Thyroid Carcinomas After Irradiation: High Prevalence of RET Rearrangement

H. M. Rabes and S. Klugbauer

Institute of Pathology, Ludwig Maximilians University, Thalkirchner Strasse 36, 80337 Munich, Germany

Abstract

Epidemiological studies have revealed a connection between thyroid carcinogenesis and a history of radiation. The molecular mechanisms involed are not well understood. It has been claimed that RAS, p53 or GSP mutations and RET or TRK rearrangements might play a role in adult thyroid tumors. In childhood, the thyroid gland is particularly sensitive to ionizing radiation. The reactor accident in Chernobyl provided a unique chance to study molecular genetic aberrations in a cohort of children who developed papillary thyroid carcinomas after a short latency time after exposure to high doses of radioactive iodine isotopes. According to the concepts of molecular genetic epidemiology, exposure to a specific type of irradiation might result in a typical molecular lesion. Childhood papillary thyroid tumors after Chernobyl exhibit a high prevalence of RET rearrangement as almost the only molecular alteration. The majority showed RET/PTC3 (i.e., ELE/RET rearrangements), including several subtypes. Less frequently, RET/PTC1 (i.e., H4/ RET rearrangements), and a novel type (RET/PTC5, i.e., RFG5/RET) were observed. Proof of reciprocal transcripts suggests that a balanced intrachromosomal inversion leads to this rearrangement. Breakpoint analyses revealed short homologous nucleotide stretches at the fusion points. In all types of rearrangement, the RET tyrosine kinase domain becomes controlled by 5′ fused regulatory sequences of ubiquitously expressed genes that display coiled-coil regions with dimerization potential. Oncogenic activation of RET is apparently due to ligand-independent constitutive ectopic RET tyrosine kinase activity. The analysis of this cohort of children with radiation-induced thyroid tumors after Chernobyl provides insights into typical molecular aberrations in relation to a specific mode of environmental exposure and may serve as a paradigm for molecular genetic epidemiology.

Recent Results in Cancer Research, Vol. 154
© Springer-Verlag Berlin · Heidelberg 1998

Background

The identification of genomic fingerprints that reflect a specific interaction of target cells with a defined class of carcinogens in human tumors is an important new tool available to molecular epidemiology. Recent work on types and patterns of p53 mutations in various human tumors revealed the feasibility of this concept (Harris 1993). Examples are G-T transversion mutations at codon 249 of p53 in hepatocellular carcinomas developing in aflatoxin B_1-contaminated areas (Bressac et al. 1991; Hsu et al. 1991). In many other groups of tumors, a specific molecular lesion that might be related to a certain class of carcinogens is missing, probably due to the multiplicity of factors acting in concert in tumor induction and progression. In radiation-induced human tumors, a typical molecular genetic aberration has not yet been found. Reports on a p53 mutation hotspot (G-T transversion mutation at codon 249) in radon-associated lung cancer (Taylor et al. 1994) have not been confirmed by others (Bartsch et al. 1995). Because of the wealth of epidemiological data on the association between radiation exposure and thyroid cancer, this tumor is a most interesting type of cancer for such an approach. Ionizing radiation, particularly during childhood, increases the risk of thyroid cancer. Head, neck, or thorax irradiation administered in childhood to treat tinea capitis (Ron et al. 1989), lymphoid hyperplasia of the tonsils (Favus et al. 1976; Schneider et al. 1993), enlarged thymus gland (Shore et al. 1985, 1993) and Hodgkin's disease (Hancock et al. 1991) and exposure during the atomic bomb explosions in Japan (Prentice et al. 1982; Thompson et al. 1994) increased the risk of thyroid carcinogenesis. In a comprehensive evaluation, an average excess relative risk of 7.7 per Gy was reported. It was concluded that, in children, the thyroid gland has one of the highest risk coefficients observed in any organ, with convincing evidence for an increased risk even at a level of approximately 0.10 Gy (Ron et al. 1995).

When searching for typical molecular genetic alterations, thyroid carcinomas occurring after the atomic bomb explosions or nuclear tests are, in principle, a valuable source of information, as large populations have been exposed for a known period of time at a defined dose range. However, not much is yet known about critical genetic changes which would provide a clue to characterizing a typical radiation-related molecular lesion in such cohorts of radiation-exposed individuals.

The Chernobyl Reactor Accident and Thyroid Cancer

A similar case of radiation exposure as that caused by atomic bombs, but on a much larger scale, was the explosion of the nuclear reactor in Chernobyl on April 26, 1986. The released radioactivity led to a very high population exposure (Balonov et al. 1996). Certain areas in Belarus, the oblast Gomel in particular, were most severely contaminated by radioactive fallout. Immediately after the reactor accident, various short-lived iodine radioisotopes, especially ^{131}I, accounted for the largest fraction of contamination (Balonov et al. 1996). As the southern part of Belarus is an iodine-deficient area and iodine supplementation was incomplete, large doses of radioactive iodine were incorporated by inhalation or in food and led to high thyroid doses. Children were most affected. As early as 1990, an increased incidence of thyroid carcinomas was observed in children from the most severely contaminated regions (Baverstock et al. 1992; Kazakov and Demidchick 1992). The annual incidence of thyroid cancer rose steeply to more than 20 per 100 000 children in the oblast Gomel. The morbidity rates increased in Belarus by a factor of 55.7 as compared with the 10-year pre-accident period (Demidchik et al. 1996). Almost exclusively papillary thyroid carcinomas were detected, including solid and follicular variants of papillary carcinomas (Furmanchuk et al. 1992; Nikiforov and Gnepp 1994). The majority of these early-developing carcinomas revealed lymphatic spread and lymph node mestastasis at the time of thyroidectomy suggesting aggressive growth behavior (Demidchik et al. 1996). In a comparison of a large series of thyroid cancers from Belarus with naturally occurring thyroid carcinomas from Italy and France, a lower female to male ratio, a higher proportion of papillary tumors, a more frequent extrathyroidal extension, and lymph node metastasis were observed in the tumors from Belarus (Pacini et al. 1997). A similar histology and cytology has been reported in childhood thyroid cancers in England and Wales (Harach and Williams 1995).

Inadvertent simultaneous irradiation exposure of a large population to specific carcinogenic factors provides a unique possibility for molecular studies. A large number of children were exposed to a high dose of internal ionizing radiation, particularly radioactive iodine, during a short period of time, as determined by the limited period of radioactive release from the reactor and by the short half-life of [131]I. Papillary thyroid carcinomas developed as a typical tumor after a very short latency period. The majority of tumors revealed the same biological behavior with aggressive growth and early metastatic spread. In this model-like system, molecular studies can be performed in order to reveal critical genomic aberrations that might be typical for radiation-induced thyroid carcinomas in childhood.

Molecular Genetics: RAS, p53, GSP

Molecular genetic studies of sporadic thyroid carcinomas in adults with unknown carcinogen exposure revealed point mutations in genes of the RAS family, mostly in follicular carcinomas; p53 mutations, preferentially in anaplastic types of thyroid carcinomas; mutations at the GTP-binding α-subunit of the adenylate cyclase stimulatory protein $G_s\alpha$; mutations at the TSH receptor; overexpression of c-met; and rearrangements of genes coding for the receptor tyrosine kinases RET and TRK (for reviews, see Said et al. 1994; Santoro et al. 1995; Wynford-Thomas 1997).

Table 1. H-, K-, and N-RAS mutations (codons 12, 13, and 61) in adult papillary thyroid carcinomas

Total investigated PTC (*n*)	Tumors with mutant RAS	
	(*n*)	(%)
173	29	16.8

Data from Lemoine and Mayall 1988; Wright et al. 1989; Suarez et al. 1990; Namba et al. 1990; Karga et al. 1991; Shi et al. 1991; Hara et al. 1994

Table 2. Results of studies on p53, RAS, and GSP mutations in childhood thyroid carcinomas after the reactor accident in Chernobyl

p53 mutations (exons 5–8)	RAS mutations (H-, K-, and N-RAS, codons 12, 13, and 61	GSP mutations (exons 8, 9, codons 201, 227)	Reference
6/26[a]	–	–	Hillebrandt et al. (1996)
2/33[b]	0/33	–	Nikiforov et al. (1996)
5/24[c]	–	–	Smida et al. (1997)
–	–	0/20	Waldmann and Rabes (1997)
0/22[d]	0/34[e]	–	Suchy et al. (1998)

The numbers after the slashes give the total number of investigated tumors in each group.
[a] TGGE pattern, no sequencing.
[b] One missense mutation (ATGmet-GTGval, codon 160); one silent mutation (TGCcys-TGTcys, codon 182).
[c] Five silent mutations: neutral CGA/CGG dimorphism in exon 6, codon 213 (Bhatia et al. 1992).
[d] Exons 5, 7, and 8.
[e] One missense mutation in codon 15 (GGCgly-AGCser); one silent mutation in codon 14 (GTGval-GTAval).

Table 3. p53 mutations in adult thyroid carcinomas

	With mutation		Total (*n*)
	(*n*)	(%)	
Well differentiated	11	11.1	99
Poorly or not differentiated	21	52.5	40

Data from Ito et al. 1992, 1993a; Nakamura et al. 1992; Fagin et al. 1993; Zou et al. 1993; Dobashi et al. 1994.

While RAS mutations have been described in about 17% of thyroid carcinomas in adults (Table 1), similar mutations at the critical codons 12, 13, or 61 of H-, K-, or N-RAS were not observed in a large series of childhood carcinomas after Chernobyl in two independent studies (Nikoforov et al. 1996; Suchy et al. 1998; Table 2).

p53 mutations have been observed in undifferentiated thyroid carcinomas in adults (Table 3). As no tumors of this type have yet occurred in children, it is not surprising that p53 missense mutations have rarely been found in post-Chernobyl tumors (Table 2). A recent report on a cluster of silent muta-

Table 4. GSP mutations in adult thyroid tumors

Total tumors (*n*)	Tumors with wild-type GSP (*n*)	Tumors with mutant GSP	
		(*n*)	(%)
257	215	42	16.3

Data from Lyons et al. 1990; O'Sullivan et al. 1991; Suarez et al. 1991; Goretzki et al. 1992; Matsuo et al. 1993; Yoshimoto et al. 1993; Russo et al. 1995.

tions in codon 213 (Smida et al. 1997) might reflect clonality or polymorphism rather than a carcinogenic effect.

In about 16% of thyroid tumors, preferentially hyperfunctioning adenomas in adults, the $G_s\alpha$ gene shows missense mutations at codon 201 or 227 (Table 4). In contrast, in a series of 20 childhood papillary thyroid carcinomas after Chernobyl, mutations at these critical sites have never been found (Waldmann and Rabes 1997; Table 2).

It is evident that these molecular changes which prevail in thyroid tumors in adults do not play a significant role in thyroid carcinogenesis in children exposed to irradiation.

Molecular Genetics: RET

Studies on papillary thyroid carcinomas in adults revealed that, in a minority of cases (about 16%), an oncogenic rearrangement of the proto-oncogene c-RET occurs, with striking geographical variations (Ishizaka et al. 1991; Jhiang et al. 1992; Santoro et al. 1992, 1994, 1995; Wajjwalku et al. 1992; Wynford-Thomas 1993; Bongarzone et al. 1994; Said et al. 1994; Zou et al. 1994; Sugg et al. 1996; Bounacer et al. 1997).

c-RET (Takahashi et al. 1988) codes for a receptor tyrosine kinase. It is expressed in a developmental stage-specific pattern (Avantaggio et al. 1994; Tsuzuki et al. 1995). Recently, glial cell line-derived neurotrophic factor (GDNF) was found as its ligand. The RET receptor acts in a multicomponent complex with GDNFR-α (Durbec et al. 1996; Jing et al. 1996; Treanor et al. 1996; Trupp et al. 1996). RET tyrosine kinase activity is essential for the development of the kidney and the cells of the enteric nervous system and the neural crest. In the normal thyroid, a strong expression is found in parafollicular C cells. c-RET mutations have been detected in medullary thyroid carcinomas (see Marsh et al. 1997), but in papillary thyroid carcinomas the oncogenic activation involves chromosomal rearrangements. The chromosomal location of the c-RET proto-oncogene is 10q11.2 (Minoletti et al. 1994).

Three different forms of rearrangements have been found: RET/PTC1, RET/PTC2, and RET/PTC3 (Grieco et al. 1990; Ishizaka et al. 1991; Bongarzone et al. 1993, 1994; Jhiang et al. 1994). In all three, the tyrosine kinase domain is fused at its 5′ end to another gene, thereby losing the ligand binding

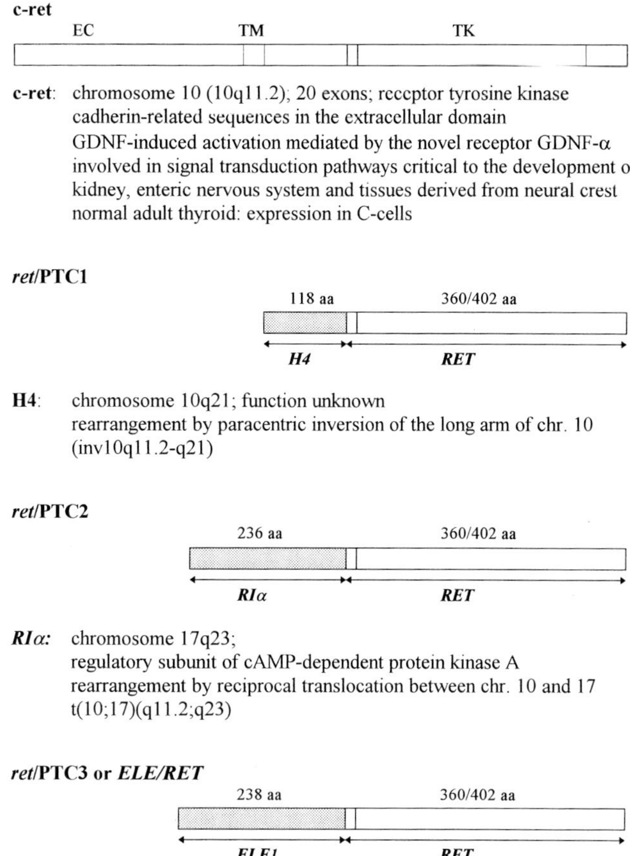

c-ret: chromosome 10 (10q11.2); 20 exons; receptor tyrosine kinase
cadherin-related sequences in the extracellular domain
GDNF-induced activation mediated by the novel receptor GDNF-α
involved in signal transduction pathways critical to the development of the
kidney, enteric nervous system and tissues derived from neural crest
normal adult thyroid: expression in C-cells

H4: chromosome 10q21; function unknown
rearrangement by paracentric inversion of the long arm of chr. 10
(inv10q11.2-q21)

RIα: chromosome 17q23;
regulatory subunit of cAMP-dependent protein kinase A
rearrangement by reciprocal translocation between chr. 10 and 17
t(10;17)(q11.2;q23)

ELE1 chromosome 10q11.2; function unknown
rearrangement by paracentric inversion in locus 10q11.2

Fig. 1. Different forms of oncogenic activation of RET; ret proto-oncogence and rearranged forms. *GDNF,* glial cell line-derived neurotrophic factor; *EC* extracellular domain; *TM,* transmembrane domain; *TK,* tyrosine kinase domain

and transmembrane domain. Instead, the tyrosine kinase domain becomes
dependent on the regulation by the 5′ fused genes. In RET/PTC1, a fusion to
the H4 gene is found (Grieco et al. 1990). H4 is located at 10q21. Rearrangement involves paracentric chromosomal inversion. RET/PTC1 represents the
prevailing type of rearrangement in adult papillary thyroid carcinomas, but
occurs in only about 16% of patients (see Table 6). RET/PTC2 involves fusion
by interchromosomal translocation t (10;17) (Sozzi et al. 1994) to the regulatory subunit RIα of cyclic adenosine monophosphate (cAMP)-dependent protein kinase A and occurs in very rare cases of adult tumors (Bongarzone et
al. 1993; Pierotti et al. 1996). In RET/PTC3, the RET carboxy terminus is
fused to the amino terminus of the ELE1 gene (Bongarzone et al. 1994;

Jhiang et al. 1994; Santoro et al. 1994). As with RET/PTC1, an intrachromosomal paracentric inversion is observed in RET/PTC3. A schematic summary of the different forms of oncogenic activation of RET is given in Fig. 1.

RET Rearrangement in Childhood Thyroid Carcinomas

Small frozen tissue samples of 59 papillary thyroid carcinomas from children (21 males and 38 females) living in Belarus at the time of the Chernobyl reactor accident were made available to us for a molecular genetic study on the prevalence of RET rearrangement. Their age varied between 7 months and 18 years at the time of the reactor accident. The latency period before thyroidectomy was between 7 and 10 years. Surgery was performed between May 1993 and April 1996. Various TNM stages were included.

Using an approach combining multiplex reverse-transcriptase polymerase chain reaction (RT-PCR), identification PCR with rearrangement-specific PCR primers, direct sequencing, and rapid amplification of 5′-cDNA ends (5′ RACE) in those samples that did not reveal a known type of RET rearrangement (for the description of methods, see Klugbauer et al. 1995, 1996, 1998 a, b), a very high prevalence of RET rearrangements was detected. Among the 59 investigated tumors, 36 showed a RET rearrangement. RET/PTC3 was the most prominent type and almost 64% of all RET rearrangement-positive tumors revealed this form of rearrangement. RET/PTC2 was not found at all. RET/PTC1, the prevailing type in adult papillary thyroid carcinomas, was observed in only eight tumors, i.e., in 22% of all RET rearrangement-positive carcinomas (Table 5). An obvious dependence on age at exposure, gender or TNM stage has not been detected for the different types of RET rearrangement (to be published in detail).

Table 5. *RET* rearrangements in papillary thyroid carcinomas in children from Belarus thyroidectomized in Minsk during the first decade after the Chernobyl rector accident ($n = 59$)

Type of rearrangement	Patients (*n*)	Proportion of total (%)	Proportion of *RET* rearrangement-positive cases (%)
No *RET* rearrangement	23	39.0	–
RET rearrangement (all types)	36	61.0	100
RET/PTC1 (H4/RET)	8	13.6	22.2
RET/PTC2 (RIα/RET)	0	0	0
RET/PTC3 (ELE/RET)	23	39.0	63.9
PTC3 r1	19	32.2	52.8
PTC3 r2	3	5.1	8.3
PTC3 r3	1	1.7	2.8
RET/PTC5 (RFG5/RET)	1	1.7	2.7
RET/PTCx /unidentified)	4	6.8	11.1

Data from Klugbauer et al. 1995, 1996, 1998a,b; Rabes and Klugbauer 1997.

ELE/RET or H4/RET rearrangements are most likely due to radiation-induced double strand breaks with subsequent illegitimate recombination. If this recombination proceeds via reciprocal chromosomal inversion (at 10q11.2), reciprocal chromosomal transcripts might be expected. Using appropriate PCR primer combinations when amplifying cDNA from these tumors, fragments were obtained that represented the reciprocal transcripts (Klugbauer et al. 1996, 1998a). In the majority of RET/PTC3 tumors, both ELE/RET and RET/ELE transcripts were expressed. It has to be concluded that not only does the RET tyrosine kinase domain become irregularly dependent on regulation by the ELE gene, but, conversely, the carboxy terminus of the ELE gene is also regulated by the 5′ RET fusion partner. This implies that, in these cases, the RET promoter, not known to be active in normal thyrocytes, becomes activated in thyroid carcinomas, leading to expression of the reciprocal fusion transcript. It is not known whether the simultaneous expression of both fusion transcripts has an impact on the biology of transformed cells. An example of direct sequencing of ELE/RET and RET/ELE transcripts at the fusion point is given in Fig. 2.

Novel Forms of ELE/RET Rearrangement

The importance of ELE/RET rearrangement in radiation-induced childhood carcinomas is further supported by the fact that, in addition to the common form of ELE/RET fusion, novel types of ELE/RET rearrangements are found in these tumors. Truncated forms were observed in four cases, and in three of these the downstream end of the fused ELE gene was shorter by a complete ELE exon (144 bp). This exon, which represents the 3′ end of the fused ELE fragment in the regular ELE/RET rearrangement, is missing in this particular truncated RET/PTC3 rearrangement. This observation is confirmed by the finding that the missing exon appears in the reciprocal transcript, thus extending its length by 144 bp. In another single case, a short truncation by 18 bp was observed in the ELE/RET transcript (Klugbauer et al. 1996, 1998a).

Breakpoint /Recombination Sites and RET Activation

The various types of ELE/RET rearrangements appear to be due to DNA strand breaks at different breakpoints in the genomic DNA. In order to elucidate the site and structure of the DNA at the breakpoints, genomic DNA was sequenced. These analyses revealed a spread of breakpoints in introns 4 and 5 and in exon 5 for the ELE gene (Klugbauer et al. 1996, 1998a; Bongarzone et al. 1997). For RET genomic DNA, the breakpoints were clustered in intron 11 (Smanik et al. 1995; Klugbauer et al. 1998a), except for one intraexonic breakpoint in RET exon 11, as reported by Pierotti's group (Fugazzola et al. 1996). At the breakpoints, both contributing germline sequences show a

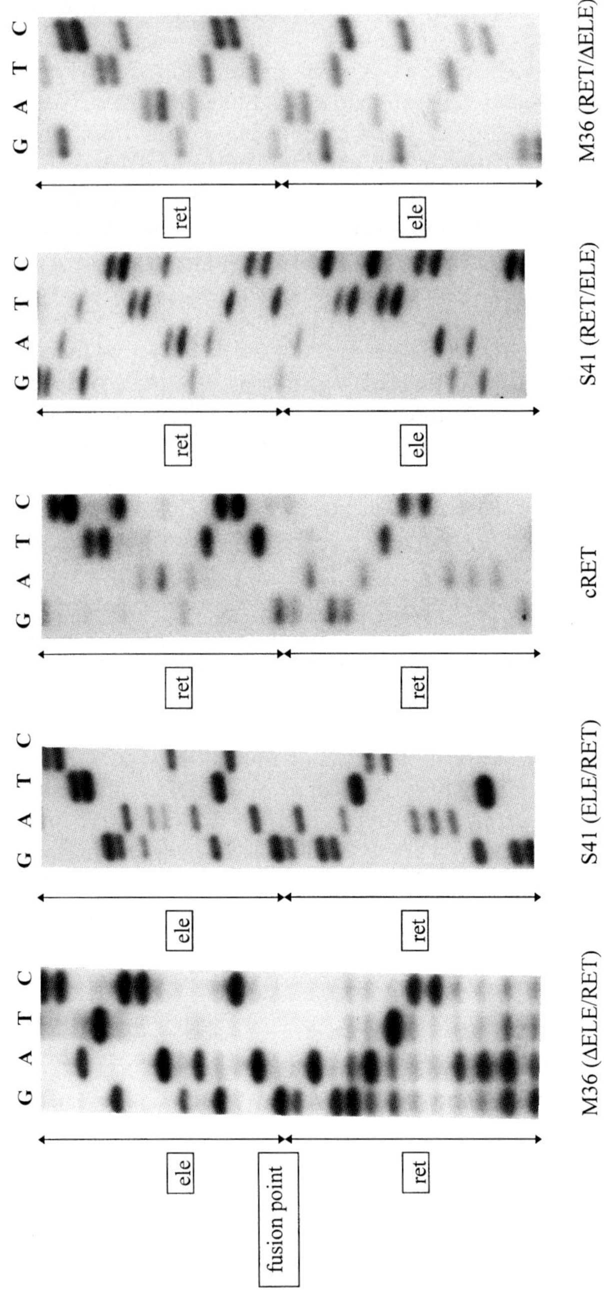

Fig. 2. Sequence analysis of the fusion point region of RET/PTC3 (tumor S41, i.e., RET/PTC3r1) and its truncated form (tumor M36, RET/ΔELE, i.e., RET/PTC3r2) in both normal and reciprocal transcripts. (From Klugbauer et al. 1996)

short nucleotide match, obviously a prerequisite for recombination (Smanik et al. 1995; Bongarzone et al. 1997; Klugbauer et al. 1998a).

It can be concluded from the site of recombination that, in all forms of ELE/RET rearrangement leading to thyroid carcinomas, the inclusion of a well-preserved ELE part at least 5' prime of intron 4 is required. With this portion of the ELE gene present in the fusion product, the actual length at the 3' end of the ELE fusion part differs considerably and appears to be irrelevant to the oncogenic potential of the fused gene. ELE-1 apparently contains a potential coiled-coil region of amino acid sequences upstream from the fusion point. This sequence and the structure appear to be essential for oligomerization of the fusion protein and thus for ligand-independent constitutive activation of the RET tyrosine kinase.

On the other hand, by the 5' fused ELE fragment, RET becomes devoid of its extracellular and transmembrane domains, leaving the cytoplasmic part, which exhibits tyrosine kinase activity, under the control of the ubiquitously expressed ELE1 gene. At the 5' part of the fused gene, at least exon 12 and the RET tyrosine kinase domain have to be preserved. Both, the 5' regulatory part of ELE and the 3' tyrosine kinase part of RET are obviously essential to trigger a thyrocyte in the transformed state. Ectopic, constitutive activation of an intracytoplasmic RET tyrosine kinase with putatively altered substrate specificity appears to be an essential prerequisite of radiation-induced papillary thyroid carcinomas in children after Chernobyl.

Novel Types of RET Rearrangement

In a few cases, we have found additional types of RET rearrangement in thyroid carcinomas in the radiation-exposed children from Belarus. In one of these patients, the RET tyrosine kinase domain was fused at its 5' end to a gene which we designated RET fused gene 5 (RFG5). Part of this gene had previously been reported to be fused to the RET gene after transfection of NIH 3T3 cells with DNA from a human sigmoid colon cancer and was called RET-II (Ishizaka et al. 1989), but the RET-II gene has not been detected in the colon tumor itself or in any other human tumor, suggesting that the RET-II rearrangement was an NIH 3T3 transfection artifact. However, we found this fused gene in rare thyroid carcinomas in children exposed to radioactive fallout after Chernobyl (Klugbauer et al. 1998b). Analysis of the whole cDNA sequence revealed coiled-coil regions that appear to be responsible for activation of the RET tyrosine kinase domain by dimerization of the upstream RFG5-fused gene. A hydrophobic domain is missing, indicating that the fusion protein could be cytoplasmic, as are the other oncogenic RET fusion proteins.

Conclusions

The basic principle in oncogenic activation of the RET tyrosine kinase by replacing the 5′ end of RET by a cytoplasmic fusion protein exhibiting dimerization potential is common to the majority of childhood papillary thyroid carcinomas that developed after Chernobyl. Under physiological conditions, RET tyrosine kinase is regulated by the unusually complex multicomponent interaction of GDNF, GDNFR-α, and RET at the cell surface membrane. If the essential part of RET, the tyrosine kinase domain, is activated by fusion to a protein that exhibits dimerization potential, the physiological safeguard is eliminated: RET becomes constitutively activated and thus oncogenic. Cytoplasmic translocation adds to this release from physiological inhibition by providing the chance to interact with new critical substrates.

Having found several rare RET-fused partners in RET activation among childhood papillary thyroid carcinomas after Chernobyl, it might be predicted that the high probability of radiation-induced double strand breaks in the thyroid of the exposed population will give rise to even more new rare gene fusion products in these tumors in the future. However, the probability of an ELE/RET recombination is obviously significantly higher than any other type of fusion leading to oncogenic activation. The fact that both genes are located on chromosome 10q11.2 in immediate vicinity to one another might enhance the probability of chromosomal inversion.

It is evident from the results of the present study and the data from the literature that RET rearrangement appears to be a critical molecular event in radiation-induced thyroid carcinogenesis in children. RET/PTC rearrangement exhibits a significantly higher prevalence in radiation-induced carcinomas than in spontaneous papillary thyroid carcinomas (Table 6). This was confirmed by a recent comparative study on tumors that developed in France either spontaneously, i.e., without a proven history of radiation, or after childhood therapeutic irradiation. RET rearrangement was significantly more frequent in tumors in irradiated patients than in spontaneous thyroid carcinomas (Bounacer et al. 1997). In this study, RET/PTC1 (i.e., H4/RET rearrangement) was 3.5 times more frequent than RET/PTC3 (i.e., ELE/RET fusions). This is in contrast to the high prevalence of the RET/PTC3 type of rearrangement found in our studies after Chernobyl (Klugbauer et al. 1995, 1996, 1998a; Rabes and Klugbauer 1997). Almost identical results obtained by three other groups (Ito et al. 1994; Fugazzola et al. 1995; Nikiforov et al. 1997) confirmed our findings. Compiling the available data on childhood thyroid carcinomas after Chernobyl, ELE/RET rearrangements are 3.5 times more frequent than H4/RET rearrangements (Table 6).

In additon to radiation, young age at exposure could also be a critical determinant for the preference of ELE/RET rearrangements. However, the recent studies from France do not support this idea. In patients with a childhood history of radiation, ELE/RET rearrangements were infrequent in thyroid carcinomas (Bounacer et al. 1997). The available data are summarized in Table 7. This is in agreement with results of a study on age-re-

Table 6. RET/PTC rearrangements in spontaneous and radiation-induced papillary thyroid tumors

Country	Spontaneous		Total (n)	Radiation-induced		Total (n)	Reference
	(n)	(%)		(n)	(%)		
Canada	3	5	60	–	–	–	Sugg et al. (1996)
France	8	11	70	–	–	–	Santoro et al. (1992)
France	2	10	19	–	–	–	Said et al. (1994)
United Kingdom	2	6	30	–	–	–	Wynford -Thomas (1993)
Italy	14	33	42	–	–	–	Santoro et al. (1994)
Italy	18	35	52	–	–	–	Bongarzone et al. (1994)
Japan	1	9	9	–	–	–	Ishizaka et al. (1991)
Japan	1	3	38	–	–	–	Wajjwalku et al. (1992)
Saudi Arabia	1	3	40	–	–	–	Zou et al. (1994)
USA	4	11	36	–	–	–	Jhiang et al. (1992)
USA	11	17	65	–	–	–	Santoro et al. (1992)
USA	11	65	17	–	–	–	Nikiforov et al. (1997)
Belarus	–	–	–	4	56	7	Ito et al. (1994)
Belarus	–	–	–	36	61	59	Klugbauer et al. (1995, 1996) Rabes and Klugbauer (1997)
Belarus	–	–	–	4	66	6	Fugazzola et al. (1995)
Belarus	–	–	–	29	76	38	Nikiforov et al. (1997)
France	3	15	20	16	84	19	Bounacer et al. (1997)
Total	79	15.8	500	89	69.0	129	

lated RET activation in thyroid carcinomas in Italy. Although Bongarzone et al. (1996) detected significantly more RET rearrangements in the age-group of 4–30 years than in older patients, RET rearrangements of the ELE/RET type were found in only one patient in children and adolescents up to the age of 19 years, in contrast to five patients with H4/RET or RIα/RET rearrangements in this group. This suggests that young age per se does not favor the RET/PTC3 type of rearrangement. Radiation history was not taken into account in this study.

It is possible that external irradiation leads to a type of RET rearrangement (RET/PTC1, i.e., H4/RET; in vitro: Ito et al. 1993b; in vivo: Bounacer et al. 1997) which is different from that induced by internal thyroid irradiation after the uptake of large amounts of radioactive iodine isotopes (RET/PTC3, i.e., ELE/RET, Klugbauer et al. 1995, 1996, 1998a; Fugazzola et al. 1995, Nikofov et al. 1997; Rabes and Klugbauer 1997). The probability of double strand breaks and of recombination processes depends on the dose. At the present time, definite conclusions about the role of several parameters (e.g., dose of irradiation, age, physiological stage of the thyroid gland, or hyperplastic processes after radiation-induced cell loss) in the induction and progression of thyroid carcinomas in children after Chernobyl are difficult to draw. It also has to be considered that an ELE/RET rearrangement might endow an affected cell with a more effective growth advantage than other types of RET rearrangement, thus leading to the very rapid development of thyroid carcinomas after Chernobyl.

Table 7. Prevalence of ELE/RET (PTC3) and H4/RET (PTC1) rearrangements in papillary thyroid carcinomas after the Chernobyl reactor accident (Belarus) and after external therapeutic radiation (France)

	Total RET rearranged tumors (n)	PTC1 tumors (n)	PTC3 tumors (n)	PTC3 tumors (%)	Reference
Belarus after Chernobyl (age at accident, 2–10 years)	9	2	7	77.8	Klugbauer et al. (1995, 1996)
Belarus after Chernobyl (age at accident, 1–8 years)	4	0	3	75.0	Fugazzola et al. (1995)
Belarus after Chernobyl (age at accident, 1–18 years)	36	8	23	63.9	Rabes and Klugbauer (1997)
Belarus after Chernobyl (age at surgery, 5–18 years	33	6	22	66.7	Nikiforov et al. (1997)
France (age at radiation therapy, 1–20 years)	12	10	2	16.7	Bounacer et al. (1997)
(age at radiation therapy, over 20 years)	6	4	2	33.3	

The present data suggest that the RET paradigm is an important tool in elucidating mechanisms of irradiation-induced thyroid carcinogenesis in children. A straight line linking a specific class of carcinogenic factors, a specific type of molecular genetic alteration, and a specific group of cancers – the ultimate goal of molecular genetic epidemiology – can at least tentatively be drawn in this cohort of children. All of them suffer from papillary thyroid carcinomas that developed rapidly after high-dose internal thyroid irradiation by uptake of iodine radionuclides. The majority of the tumors exhibit RET rearrangements, and although the ELE/RET type of rearrangement is not the only one, it appears to be a typical molecular alteration.

Acknowledgements. This work was supported by grants from the Dr.-Mildred-Scheel-Stiftung für Krebsforschung, the Wilhelm Sander-Stiftung, the Matthias-Lackas-Stiftung, and the K.L. Weigand'sche Stiftung to H.M.R. We are most grateful to Professor E. Lengfelder, Institute of Radiation Biology, Ludwig Maximilians University of Munich, Germany, and to Professor E. Demidchik, Chair of Oncology, Medical High School of Minsk, Belarus, for the excellent cooperation. Thanks are due to the Otto Hug Strahleninstitut and Christine Frenzel for support of this work.

References

Avantaggiato V, Dathan NA et al (1994) Developmental expression of the RET protooncogene. Cell Growth Diff 5:305–311

Balonov M, Jacob P et al (1996) Pathways, levels and trends of population exposure after the Chernobyl accident. In: Karaoglou A, Desmet G, Kelly GN et al (eds) The radiological consequences of the Chernobyl accident. EUR 16544 EN, Brussels, pp 235–249

Bartsch H, Hollstein M et al (1995) Screening for putative radon-specific p53 mutation hotspot in German uranium miners. Lancet 346:121

Baverstock K, Egloff B et al (1992) Thyroid cancer after Chernobyl. Nature 359:22

Bhatia K, Gutiérrez MI et al (1992) PCR detection of a neutral CGA/CGG dimorphism in exon 6 of the human p53 gene. Nucleic Acids Res 220:928

Bongarzone I, Monzini N et al (1993) Molecular characterization of a thyroid tumor-specific transforming sequence formed by the fusion of ret tyrosine kinase and the regulatory subunit RIα of cyclic AMP-dependent protein kinase A. Mol Cell Biol 13:358–366

Bongarzone I, Butti MG et al (1994) Frequent activation of ret protooncogene by fusion with a new activating gene in papillary thyroid carcinomas. Cancer Res 54:2979–2985

Bongarzone I, Fugazzola L et al (1996) Age-related activation of the tyrosine kinase receptor protooncogenes RET and NTRK1 in papillary thyroid carcinoma. J Clin Endocrinol Metabol 81:2006–2009

Bongarzone I, Butti MG et al (1997) Comparison of the breakpoint regions of ELE1 and RET genes involved in the generation of RET/PTC3 oncogene in sporadic and in radiation-associated papillary thyroid carcinomas. Genomics 42:252–259

Bounacer A, Wicker R et al (1997) High prevalence of activating ret proto-oncogene rearrangements, in thyroid tumors from patients who had received external radiation. Oncogene 15:1263–1273

Bressac B, Kew M et al (1991) Selective G to T mutations of p53 gene in hepato-cellular carcinoma from southern Africa. Nature 350:429–431

Demidchik EP, Drobyshevskaya IM et al (1996) Thyroid cancer in children in Belarus. In: Karaoglou A, Desmet G et al (eds) The radiological consequences of the Chernobyl accident. EUR 16544 EN, Brussels, pp 677–678

Dobashi Y, Sugimura H et al (1994) Stepwise participation of p53 gene mutation during dedifferentiation of human thyroid carcinomas. Diagn Mol Pathol 3:9–14

Durbec P, Marcos-Guierrez CV et al (1996) GDNF signalling through the Ret receptor tyrosine kinase. Nature 381:789–793

Fagin JA, Matsuo K et al (1993) High prevalence of mutations of the p53 gene in poorly differentiated human thyroid carcinomas. J Clin Invest 91:179–184

Favus MJ, Schneider AB et al (1976) Thyroid cancer occurring as a late consequence of head-and-neck irradiation. N Engl J Med 294:1019–1025

Fugazzola L, Pilotti S et al (1995) Oncogenic rearrangements of the RET proto-oncogene in papillary thyroid carcinomas from children exposed to the Chernobyl nuclear accident. Cancer Res 55:5617–5620

Fugazzola L, Pierotti MA (1996) Molecular and biochemical analysis of RET/PTC4, a novel oncogenic rearrangement between RET and ELE1 genes, in a post-Chernobyl papillary thyroid cancer. Oncogene 13:1093–1097

Furmanchuk AW, Averkin JI et al (1992) Pathomorphological findings in thyroid cancers of children from the Republic of Belarus: a study of 86 cases occurring between 1986 ('post-Chernobyl') and 1991. Histopathology 21:401–408

Goretzki P, Lyons J et al (1992) Mutational activation of ras and gsp oncogenes in differentiated thyroid cancer and their biological implication. World J Surg 16:576–582

Grieco M, Santoro M et al (1990) PTC is a novel rearranged form of the ret proto-oncogene and is frequently detected in vivo in human thyroid papillary carcinomas. Cell 60:557–563

Hancock SL, Cox RS et al (1991) Thyroid diseases after treatment of Hodgkin's disease. New Engl J Med 325:599–605

Hara H, Fulton N et al (1994) N-RAS mutation: an independent prognostic factor for aggressiveness of papillary thyroid carcinoma. Surgery 116:1010–1016

Harach HR, Williams ED (1995) Childhood thyroid cancer in England and Wales. Br J Cancer 72:777–783

Harris CC (1993) p53: at the crossroads of molecular carcinogenesis and risk assessment. Science 262:1980–1981

Hillebrandt S, Streffer C et al (1996) Mutations in the p53 tumour suppressor gene in thyroid tumours of children from areas contaminated by the Chernobyl accident. Int J Radiat Biol 69:39–45

Hsu IC, Metcalf RA et al (1991) Mutational hotspot in the p53 gene in human hepatocellular carciomas. Nature 350:427–428

Ishizaka Y, Ochiai M (1989) Activation of the ret II oncogene without a sequence encoding a transmembrane domain and transforming activity of two ret-II oncogene products differing in carboxy-termini due to alternative splicing. Oncogene 4:789–794

Ishizaka Y, Kobayashi S et al (1991) Detection of ret^{PTC}/PTC transcripts in thyroid adenomas and adenomatous goiter by an RT-PCR method. Oncogene 6:1667–1672

Ito T, Seyama T et al (1992) Unique association of p53 mutations with undifferentiated but not with differentiated carcinomas of the thyroid gland. Cancer Res 52:1369–1371

Ito T, Seyama T et al (1993a) Genetic alterations in thyroid tumor progression: association with p53 gene mutations. Jpn J Cancer Res 84:526–531

Ito T, Seyama T et al (1993b) In vitro irradiation is able to cause RET oncogene rearrangement. Cancer Res 53:2940–2943

Ito T, Seyama T et al (1994) Activated RET oncogene in thyroid cancers of children from areas contaminated by Chernobyl accident. Lancet 344:259

Jhiang S, Caruso DR et al (1992) Detection of the PTC/ret ^{tpc} oncogene in human thyroid cancers. Oncogene 7:1331–1337

Jhiang S, Smanik A et al (1994) Development of a single-step duplex RT-PCR detecting different forms of ret activation, and identification of the third form of in vivo ret activation in human papillary thyroid carcinoma. Cancer Lett 78:69–76

Jing S, Wen D et al (1996) GDNF-induced activation of the ret protein tyrosine kinase is mediated by GDNFR-a, a novel receptor for GDNF. Cell 85:1113–1124

Karga H, Lee JK et al (1991) RAS oncogene mutations in benign and malignant thyroid neoplasms J Clin Endocrinol Metabol 73:832–836

Kazakov VS, Demidchik EP (1992) Thyroid cancer after Chernobyl. Nature 359:21

Klugbauer S, Lengfelder E et al (1995) High prevalence of RET rearrangement in thyroid tumors of children from Belarus after the Chernobyl reactor accident. Oncogene 11: 2459–2467

Klugbauer S, Lengfelder E et al (1996) A new form of RET rearrangement in thyroid carcinomas of children after the Chernobyl reactor accident. Oncogene 13:1099–1102

Klugbauer S, Demidchik EP et al (1998a) Detection of a novel type of RET rearrangement (PTC5) in thyroid carcinomas after Chernobyl and analysis of the involved RET-fused gene RFG5. Cancer Res 58:198–203

Klugbauer S, Demidchik EP et al (1998b) Molecular analysis of new subtypes of ELE/RET rearrangements, their reciprocal transcripts and breakpoints in papillary thyroid carcinomas of children after Chernobyl. Oncogene 16:671–675

Lemoine NR, Mayall ES (1988) Activated RAS oncogenes in human thyroid cancers. Cancer Res 48:4459–4463

Lyons J, Landis C et al (1990) Two G protein oncogenes in human endocrine tumors. Science 249:655–659

Marsh DJ, Mulligan LM et al (1997) RET proto-oncogene mutations in multiple endocrine neoplasia type 2 and medullary thyroid carcinoma. Horm Res 47:168–178

Matsuo K, Friedman E et al (1993) The thyrotropin receptor is not an oncogene for thyroid tumors: structural studies of the TSH-R and the a-subunit of G_s in human thyroid neoplasmas. J Clin Endocrinol Metab 76:1446–1451

Minoletti F, Butti MG et al (1994)The two genes generating RET/PTC3 are localized in chromosomal band 10q11.2. Genes Chromosomes Cancer 11:51–57

Nakamura T, Yana I et al (1992) p53 gene mutations associated with anaplastic transformation of human thyroid carcinomas. Jpn J Cancer Res 83:1293–1298

Namba H, Rubin SA et al (1990) Point mutations of RAS oncogenes are an early event in thyroid tumorigenesis. Mol Endocrinol 4:1471–1479

Nikiforovy, Gnepp DR (1994) Pediatric thyroid cancer after the Chernobyl disaster. Cancer 74:748–766

Nikoforov YE, Nikiforova MN et al (1996) Prevalence of mutations of ras and p53 in benign and malignant thyroid tumors from children exposed to radiation after the Chernobyl nuclear accident. Oncogene 13:687–693

Nikoforov YE, Rowland JM et al (1997) Distinct pattern of ret oncogene rearrangements in morphological variants of radiation-induced and sporadic thyroid papillary carcinomas in children. Cancer Res 57:1690–1694

O'Sullivan C, Barton C et al (1991) Activating point mutations of the gsp oncogene in human thyroid adenomas. Mol Carcinog 4:345–349

Pacini F, Vorontsova T et al (1997) Post-Chernobyl thyroid carcinoma in Belarus children and adolescents: comparison with naturally occurring thyroid carcinoma in Italy and France. J Clin Endocrinol Metabol 82:3563–3569

Pierotti MA, Bongarzone I et al (1996) Cytogenetics and molecular genetics of carcinomas arising from thyroid epithelial follicular cells. Genes Chromosomes Cancer 16:1–14

Prentice RL, Kato H et al (1982) Radiation exposure and thyroid cancer incidence among Hiroshima and Nagasaki residents. Natl Cancer Inst Mongr 62:207–212

Rabes HM, Klugbauer S (1997) Strahleninduzierte Schilddrüsenkarzinome bei Kindern: Hohe Prävalenz von RET-Rearrangement. Verh Dtsch Ges Pathol 81:139–144

Ron E, Modan B et al (1989) Thyroid neoplasia following low-dose radiation in childhood. Radiat Res 120:516–531

Ron E, Lubin JH et al (1992) Thyroid cancer incidence. Nature 360:113

Ron E, Lubin JH et al (1995) Thyroid cancer after exposure to external radiation: a pooled analysis of seven studies. Radiat Res 141:259–277

Russo D, Arturi F et al (1995) Genetic alterations in thyroid hyperfunctioning adenomas. J Clin Endocrinol Metab 80:1347–1351

Said S, Schlumberger M et al (1994) Oncogenes and anti-oncogenes in human epithelial thyroid tumors. J Endocrinol Invest 17:371–379

Santoro M, Carlomagno F et al (1992) Ret oncogene activation in human thyroid neoplasms is restricted to the papillary cancer subtype. J Clin Invest 89:1517–1522

Santoro M, Dathan NA et al (1995) Molecular characterization of RET/PTC3; a novel rearranged version of the RET proto-oncogene in a human thyroid papillary carcinoma. Oncogene 9:509–516

Santoro M, Grieco M et al (1994) Molecular defects in thyroid carcinomas: role of the RET oncogene in thyroid neoplastic transformation. Eur J Endocrinol 133:513–522

Schneider AB, Ron E et al (1993) Dose-response relationships for radiation-induced thyroid cancer and thyroid nodules: evidence for the prolonged effects of radiation on the thyroid. J Clin Endocrin Metabol 77:362–369

Shi Y, Zou M et al (1991) High rates of RAS codon 61 mutation in thyroid tumors in an iodide-deficient area. Cancer Res 51:2690–2693

Shore RE (1992) Issues and epidemiological evidence regarding radiation-induced thyroid cancer. Radiat Res 131:98–111

Shore RE, Woodard E et al (1985) Thyroid tumors following thymus irradiation. J Natl Cancer Inst 6:1177–1184

Shore RE, Hildreth N et al (1993) Thyroid cancer among persons given X-ray treatment in infancy for an enlarged thymus gland. Am J Epidemiol 137:1068–1080

Smanik PA, Furminger TL et al (1995) Breakpoint characterization of the ret/PTC oncogene in human papillary thyroid carcinoma. Hum Mol Gen 4:2313–2318

Smida J, Zitzelsberger H et al (1997) p53 mutations in childhood thyroid tumours from Belarus and in thyroid tumours without radiation history. Int J Cancer 73:802–807

Sozzi G, Bongarzone I et al (1994) A t(10;17) translocation creates the RET/PTC2 chimeric transforming sequence in papillary thyroid carcinoma. Genes Chromosomes Cancer 9:244–250

Suarez HG, DuVillard JA et al (1990) Presence of mutations in all three RAS genes in human thyroid tumors. Oncogene 5:565–570

Suarez HG, DuVillard JA et al (1991) gsp mutations in human thyroid tumors. Oncogene 6:677–679

Suchy B, Waldmann V et al (1998) Absence of RAS and p53 mutations in thyroid carcinomas of children after Chernobyl in contast to adult thyroid tumours. Br J Cancer 77:952–955

Sugg SL, Zheng L et al (1996) ret/PTC-1, 2, and -3 oncogene rearrangements in human thyroid carcinomas: implications for metastatic potential? J Clin Endocrinol Metab 81:3360–3365

Takahashi M (1995) Oncogenic activation of the ret protooncogene in thyroid cancer Crit Rev Oncog 6:35–46

Takahashi M, Ritz J et al (1985) Activation of a novel human transforming gene, ret, by DNA rearrangement. Cell 42:581–588

Taylor JA, Watson MA et al (1994) p53 mutation hotspot in radon-associated lung cancer. Lancet 343:86–87

Thompson DE, Mabuchi K et al (1994) Cancer incidence in atomic bomb survivors. II. Solid tumors, 1958–1987. Radiat Res 137:S17–S67

Treanor JJS, Goodman L et al (1996) Characterization of a multicomponent receptor for GDNF. Nature 382:80–83

Trupp M, Arenas E et al (1996) Functional receptor for GDNF encoded by the c-ret proto-oncogene. Nature 381:785–789

Tsuzuki T, Takahashi M et al (1995) Spatial and temporal expression of the ret proto-oncogene product in embryonic, infant and adult rat tissues. Oncogene 10:191–198

Wajjwalku W, Nakamura S et al (1992) Low frequency of rearrangements of the ret and trk proto-oncogenes in Japanese thyroid papillary carcinomas. Jpn J Cancer Res 83:671–675

Waldmann V, Rabes HM (1997) Absence of $G_s\alpha$ gene mutations in childhood thyroid tumors after Chernobyl in contrast to sporadic adult thyroid neoplasia. Cancer Res 57:2358–2361.

Wright PA, Lemoine NR et al (1989) Papillary and follicular thyroid carcinomas show a different pattern of RAS oncogene mutation. Br J Cancer 60:576–577

Wynford-Thomas D (1993) Molecular basis of epithelial tumorigenesis: the thyroid model. Crit Rev Oncol 4:1–23

Wynford-Thomas D (1997) Origin and progression of thyroid epithelial tumours: cellular and molecular mechanisms. Horm Res 47:145–157

Yoshimoto K, Iwahana H et al (1993) Rare mutations of the $G_s\alpha$ subunit gene in human endocrine tumors. Cancer 72:1386–1393

Zou M, Shi Y et al (1993) p53 mutations in all stages of thyroid carcinomas. J Clin Endocrinol Metabol 77:1054–1058

Zou M, Shi Y et al (1994) Low rate of ret proto-oncogene activation (PTC/ret[ptc]) in papillary thyroid carcinomas from Saudi Arabia. Cancer 73:176–180

Thyroid Carcinomas in RET/PTC Transgenic Mice

S. M. Jhiang[1,2], J.-Y. Cho[1,2], T. L. Furminger[1,2], J. E. Sagartz[3], Q. Tong[1,2], C. C. Capen[3], and E. L. Mazzaferri[1,2]

[1] Department of Physiology, Ohio State University, Columbus, OH 43210, USA
[2] Department of Internal Medicine, Ohio State University, Columbus, OH 43210, USA
[3] Department of Veterinary Biosciences, Ohio State University, Columbus, OH 43210, USA

Abstract

The RET/PTC oncogene, a rearranged form of the RET proto-oncogene, has been found to be associated with human papillary thyroid carcinomas. To investigate whether RET/PTC causes papillary thyroid carcinoma, we generated a transgenic mouse model of papillary thyroid carcinoma with targeted expression of RET/PTC1 in the thyroid gland. Thyroid tumors in these RET/PTC1 transgenic mice are characterized by a slow growth rate, thyroid-stimulating hormone (TSH)-responsive tumor progression, and loss of radioiodide-concentrating activity despite continued expression of thyroglobulin (Tg). The time of tumor onset appears to be dependent on the expression level of RET/PTC1 in these transgenic mice. In high-copy RET/PTC1 transgenic mice, cellular abnormalities, including a slightly increased proliferation rate, aberrant follicle formation, and loss of radioiodide-concentrating activity, can be readily identified at embryological day 18. To identify which signaling pathway or pathways perturbed by RET/PTC1 are essential for RET/PTC1 to induce tumor development, we generated transgenic mice carrying a thyroid-targeted RET/PTC1 triple mutant, which contains tyrosine to phenylalanine mutations at tyrosine residues 294, 404, and 451. Initial characterization of the thyroid glands of these RET/PTC1 triple-mutant transgenic mice showed no change in follicular morphology or radioiodide-concentrating activity. This finding suggests that signaling pathways mediated by one or more of these three phosphotyrosine binding sites are essential for RET/PTC1 to induce thyroid tumor development. Finally, in order to investigate whether tumors induced by RET/PTC3 are more aggressive than those tumors induced by RET/PTC1, we also generated thyroid-targeted RET/PTC3 transgenic mice.

Recent Results in Cancer Research, Vol. 154
© Springer-Verlag Berlin · Heidelberg 1998

Introduction

The RET proto-oncogene (c-RET) encodes a receptor tyrosine kinase with an extracellular domain, a transmembrane domain, and a cytoplasmic tyrosine kinase domain (Itoh et al. 1989). The ligands of c-RET have been recently identified as glial cell line-derived neurotrophic factor and neuturin, for which c-RET serves as a signaling component for the corresponding receptor complex (Buj-Bello et al. 1997; Klein et al. 1997; Robertson and Mason 1997). The RET/PTC oncogenes, encoding chimeric oncoproteins with the cytoplasmic domain of c-RET fused to the N terminus of other genes, are frequently detected in human papillary thyroid carcinomas (Jhiang and Mazzaferri 1994). While the RET/PTC1 oncogene is the major form of RET rearrangement found in spontaneous papillary thyroid carcinoma, the RET/PTC3 oncogene is the most common form of RET rearrangement found in papillary thyroid carcinoma in children from areas contaminated by the Chernobyl accident (Klugbauer et al. 1995).

Tg-PTC1 Transgenic Mice

To investigate whether RET/PTC is a genetic lesion that leads to the development of papillary thyroid carcinoma, we generated a transgenic mouse model of papillary thyroid carcinoma with targeted expression of RET/PTC1 in the thyroid gland using the bovine thyroglobulin (Tg) promoter. Three transgenic founders were identified. However, due to reproductive problems with one of the three lines, most of our studies were focused on the other two transgenic lines, Tg-PTC1#1 (low-copy transgenic mice) and Tg-PTC1#42 (high-copy transgenic mice). All transgenic offspring from these two transgenic lines developed bilateral thyroid tumors with biological features remarkably similar to human papillary thyroid carcinomas. Our study indicates that RET/PTC is not only a biomarker associated with papillary thyroid carcinoma, but is also a specific genetic lesion that leads to the development of papillary thyroid carcinoma (Jhiang et al. 1996).

Histological and Cytological Features

All transgenic offspring from Tg-PTC1#42 and Tg-PTC1#1 transgenic lines developed bilateral thyroid carcinomas which were invasive into surrounding tissues and elicited a modest amount of fibrous stroma. These thyroid tumors contained a mixture of solid, cribriform, and follicular architecture, with a minor degree of papillary formation. Colloid formation was poor or absent. The nuclei were variable in size and irregularly shaped. Some of the nuclei were vesicular and occasionally formed nuclear grooves and pseudo-inclusions, which are distinctive cytological characteristics observed in human papillary thyroid carcinomas (Jhiang et al. 1996).

Thyroglobulin Expression, Radioiodide Uptake, and Thyroxine Suppression

In human thyroid tumors, continued expression of Tg enables physicians to measure patients' serum Tg levels to monitor for the presence of residual and/or recurrent thyroid cancers in patients who have undergone total thyroidectomy. Similarly, in Tg-PTC1 transgenic mice, Tg expression has been detected throughout tumor progression, from early stages to advanced tumors containing spindle cell populations (Cho et al., submitted). In agreement with the observation that most human thyroid tumors are presented as "cold nodules," radioiodide-trapping activity was lost in RET/PTC1-induced thyroid tumors (Cho et al., submitted). Thyroxine (T4) supplementation is often prescribed to patients who have unresectable or metastatic thyroid tumors in order to suppress the growth of residual neoplastic tissues. Likewise, thyroid tumor development and progression is markedly delayed in Tg-PTC1 transgenic mice by administration of exogenous T4 (Sagartz et al., submitted). Thyroid tumors from T4-treated transgenic mice had remarkably less cellularity and showed mostly distended follicles filled with colloid.

Tumor Onset

To investigate whether RET/PTC1 requires additional genetic lesions to induce thyroid tumor development in Tg-PTC1 transgenic mice, the time of tumor onset was determined in both Tg-PTC1#42 and Tg-PTC1#1 transgenic mice (Cho et al., submitted). Tg-PTC1#42 transgenic mice developed bilateral thyroid carcinomas, originating from the central portion of each lobe of the thyroid glands by as early as 4 days of age. However, Tg-PTC1#1 transgenic mice had bilateral thyroid carcinomas at 21 days of age. Taken together, the time of tumor onset appears to be dependent on the expression level of RET/PTC1 in Tg-PTC1 transgenic mice. In the case of Tg-PTC1#42 transgenic mice, where RET/PTC1 was expressed at a very high level in thyroid follicular cells with a high intrinsic proliferation rate, additional genetic lesions appear to be less essential for RET/PTC1 to induce thyroid tumor development.

Cellular Abnormalities Preceding Tumor Development

To understand the molecular and cellular mechanisms underlying thyroid tumor development in Tg-PTC1 transgenic mice, cellular abnormalities preceding tumor development were investigated (Cho et al., submitted). A slightly increased proliferation rate, distorted morphology of thyroid follicles, and loss of radioiodide-trapping activity can be readily identified in Tg-PTC1#42 transgenic mice at embryological day 18. The early onset of these distinctive cellular changes most likely results from the signaling pathways activated by RET/PTC1 and not from secondary abnormalities associated with cellular transformation.

Tg-PTC1 (Y294F, Y404F, Y454F) Transgenic Mice

We and others have shown that RET/PTC oncoproteins form constitutive dimers and that constitutive activation of the RET/PTC tyrosine kinase is essential for RET/PTC transforming activity (Tong et al. 1997). It is generally believed that tyrosine kinase activation leads to phosphorylation of its own tyrosine residues and that the resulting phosphotyrosine residues serve as docking sites to recruit signaling proteins to pass on the signaling cascades. The cytoplasmic domain of c-RET in RET/PTC oncoproteins have 16 tyrosine residues, and the long isoform of c-RET has two extra tyrosine residues at the C terminus (Itoh et al. 1989). Among these tyrosine residues, pY294, pY404, and pY451 of RET/PTC1 were identified as the docking sites for Grb7/Grb10, phospholipase C (PLC)-γ, and Shc/Enigma, respectively (Arighi et al. 1997; Borrello et al. 1994, 1996; Durick et al. 1996; Pandey et al. 1996). To investigate whether signaling pathways mediated by these three phosphotyrosine residues are essential for RET/PTC1 to induce thyroid tumor development in vivo, we generated transgenic mice with thyroid-targeted expression of a RET/PTC1 triple mutant, carrying tyrosine to phenylalanine mutations at tyrosine residues 294, 404, and 451.

Initial characterization of the thyroid glands of these RET/PTC1 triple-mutant transgenic mice showed no change in thyroid follicle morphology or radioiodide-concentrating activity, compared to nontransgenic littermates (Furminger et al., manuscript in preparation). The RET/PTC1 triple mutant is expressed in the thyroid glands of the corresponding transgenic mice as demonstrated by reverse-transcription polymerase chain reaction (RT-PCR). This finding suggests that signaling pathways mediated by one or a combination of pY294, pY404, and/or pY451 are essential for RET/PTC1 to induce thyroid tumor development.

Tg-PTC3 Transgenic Mice

A dramatic increase in thyroid cancer has been reported in children who were exposed to radiation from the Chernobyl nuclear reactor explosion. It has been reported that these thyroid tumors are more aggressive than those thyroid tumors occurring in the general population. About 60% of these Chernobyl-related thyroid tumors contain RET rearrangements, with the predominant form of RET/PTC oncogene being RET/PTC3 (Klugbauer et al. 1995). To investigate whether tumors induced by RET/PTC3 are more aggressive than those tumors induced by RET/PTC1, we also generated transgenic mice with thyroid-targeted expression of RET/PTC3.

The thyroid glands of the RET/PTC3 transgenic mice showed only subtle morphological changes, such as coalescing follicles at 3 weeks of age. However, the radioiodide-trapping activity was significantly reduced in the thyroid glands of 1-month-old RET/PTC3 transgenic mice that showed no thyroid tumor formation. RET/PTC3 is expressed in the thyroid glands of these transgenic mice, as demonstrated by RT-PCR. However, the expression level of RET/PTC3 in the corresponding transgenic mice is much lower than that of RET/PTC1 in Tg-PTC1#42 transgenic mice, as demonstrated by western blot analysis. Therefore, the temptation to conclude that RET/PTC3 is a weaker tumor inducer than RET/PTC1 awaits proof that the expression level of RET/PTC3 in these transgenic mice is comparable to that of RET/PTC1 in Tg-PTC1#1 low-copy transgenic mice.

Concluding Remarks

We developed a transgenic mouse model of papillary thyroid carcinoma with targeted expression of RET/PTC1 in the thyroid gland. Despite differences between tumors in transgenic mice and human papillary thyroid carcinomas in terms of temporal expression profiles and the mechanisms regulating RET/PTC1 expression, thyroid tumors in these transgenic mice show remarkable similarities to human papillary thyroid carcinomas in many aspects. Based on our studies, it appears that thyroid tumor development and progression in Tg-PTC transgenic mice is primarily determined by the expression levels of RET/PTC. Signaling pathways perturbed by RET/PTC in thyroid follicular cells could conceivably be interrupted by other factors if RET/PTC expression occurs at a low level. Therefore, we hypothesize that both the intensity and duration of RET/PTC activation in proliferating thyroid follicular cells are essential to confer thyroid tumor development both in transgenic mice and in humans.

References

Arighi F, Alberti L, Torriti F, Ghizzoni S, Rizzetti MG, Pelicci G, Pasini B, Bongarzone I, Piutti C, Pierotti MA, Borrello MG (1997) Identification of Shc docking site on Ret tyrosine kinase. Oncogene 14:773–782

Borrello MG, Pelicci G, Arighi E, De Filippis L, Greco A, Bongarzone I, Rizzetti M, Pelicci PG, Pierotti MA (1994) The oncogenic versions of the Ret and trk tyrosine kinases bind Shc and Grb2 adapter proteins. Oncogene 9:1661–1668

Borrello MG, Alberti L, Arighi E, Bongarzone I, Battistini C, Bardelli A, Pasini B, Piutti C, Rizzetti MG, Mondellini P, Radice MT, Pierotti MA (1996) The full oncogenic activity of Ret/ptc2 depends on tyrosine 539, a docking site for phospholipase Cγ. Mol Cell Biol 16:2151–2163

Buj-Bello A, Adu J, Pinon LGP, Horton A, Thompson J, Rosenthal A, Chinchetru M, Buchman VL, Davies AM (1997) Neuturin responsiveness requires a GPI-linked receptor and RET receptor tyrosine kinase. Nature 387:721–724

Cho J-Y, Sagartz JE, Capen CC, Mazzaferri EL, Jhiang SM (1998) Cellular abnormalities preceding tumor development in thyroid-targeted RET/PTC1 transgenic mice. Oncogene (submitted)

Durick K, Wu R, Gill GN, Taylor SS (1996) Mitogenic signaling by Ret/ptc2 requires association with Enigma via a LIM domain. J Biol Chem 271:12691-12694

Itoh F, Ishizaka Y, Tahira T, Ikeda I, Imai K, Yachi A, Sugimura T, Nagao M (1989) Recent studies on the ret proto-oncogene. Tumor Res 24:1–13

Jhiang SM, Mazzaferri EL (1994) The ret/PTC oncogene in papillary thyroid carcinoma. J Lab Clin Med 123:331–337

Jhiang SM, Sagartz JE, Tong Q, Parker-Thornburg J, Capen CC, Cho J-Y, Xing S, Ledent C (1996) Targeted expression of the RET/PTC1 oncogene induces papillary thyroid carcinoma and congenital hypothyroidism in transgenic mice. Endocrinology 137:375–378

Klein RD, Sherman D, Ho W, Stone D, Bennett GL, Moffat B, Vandlen R, Simmons L, Gu Q, Hongo J, Devaux B, Poulsen K, Armanini M, Nozaki C, Asai N, Goddard A, Phillips H, Henderson CE, Takahashi M, Rosenthal A (1997) A GPI-linked protein that interacts with RET to form a candidate neuturin receptor. Nature 387:717–721

Klugbauer S, Lengfelder E, Demidchik EP, Rabes HM (1995) High prevalence of RET rearrangement in thyroid tumors of children from Belarus after the Chernobyl reactor accident. Oncogene 11:2459–2467

Pandey A, Liu X, Dixon JE, Di Fiore PP, Dixit VM (1996) Direct association between the Ret receptor tyrosine kinase and the Src homology 2-containing adapter protein Grb7. J Biol Chem 271:10607–10610

Robertson K, Mason I (1997) The GDNF-RET signalling partnership Trends Genet 13:1–3

Sagartz JE, Jhiang SM, Tong Q, Capen CC (1998) Thyroxine supresses the development and progression of thyroid carcinomas in transgenic mice with targeted expression of the ret/PTC1 oncogene. Am J Pathol (submitted)

Tong Q, Xing S, Jhiang SM (1997) Leucine zipper mediated dimerization is essential for the PTC1 oncogenic activity. J Biol Chem 272:9043–9047

Signal Transduction by the Receptor Tyrosine Kinase Ret

D. H. J. van Weering and J. L. Bos

Laboratory for Physiological Chemistry, Utrecht University, P.O. Box 80042,
3508 TA Utrecht, The Netherlands

Abstract

Ret is the receptor for glial cell line-derived neurotrophic factor (GDNF) and
neurturin (NTN). Defects in this receptor underlie several genetic syndromes. The receptor is a transmembrane tyrosine kinase which transduces
Ret-mediated signaling to a variety of signaling pathways, most notably the
Ras signlaing pathway and the phosphatidylinositol-3 kinase pathway. These
pathways are activated through the interaction of adaptor proteins to tyrosine phosphorylated receptor. The ultimate biological effects, depending on
the cell type, include morphological changes in the cytoskeleton, cell scattering, proliferation, and differentiation.

Introduction

Receptor tyrosine kinases are transmembrane proteins which are present in
the plasma membrane. They consist of an extracellular ligand-binding domain and an intracellular tyrosine kinase domain and are activated by binding to their specific ligands. Ligands can induce receptor dimerization, because they are either dimers or monomers containing two different domains
for binding of two receptor molecules at the same time (Lemmon and Schlessinger 1994). Dimerization of these receptors leads to activation of the tyrosine kinase and receptor autophosphorylation (Ullrich and Schlessinger 1990;
Heldin 1995). After receptor activation, several cytoplasmic proteins become
activated due to tyrosine phosphorylation, translocation, or allosteric activation. This activation subsequently results in the activation of elements
further downstream. Since various proteins interact with the active receptor,
a variety of signaling pathways is also activated. Figure 1 shows the most important players of three signaling pathways induced by activated receptor tyrosine kinases, namely the Ras pathway, the phosphatidyl inositol-3 kinase
(PI3K)-actin cytoskeleton pathway, and the PI3K-protein kinase B (PKB)
pathway. For the sake of clarity, this scheme is by no means complete with
respect to all possible interactions and involved proteins. The Ras-extracellu-

Recent Results in Cancer Research, Vol. 154
© Springer-Verlag Berlin · Heidelberg 1998

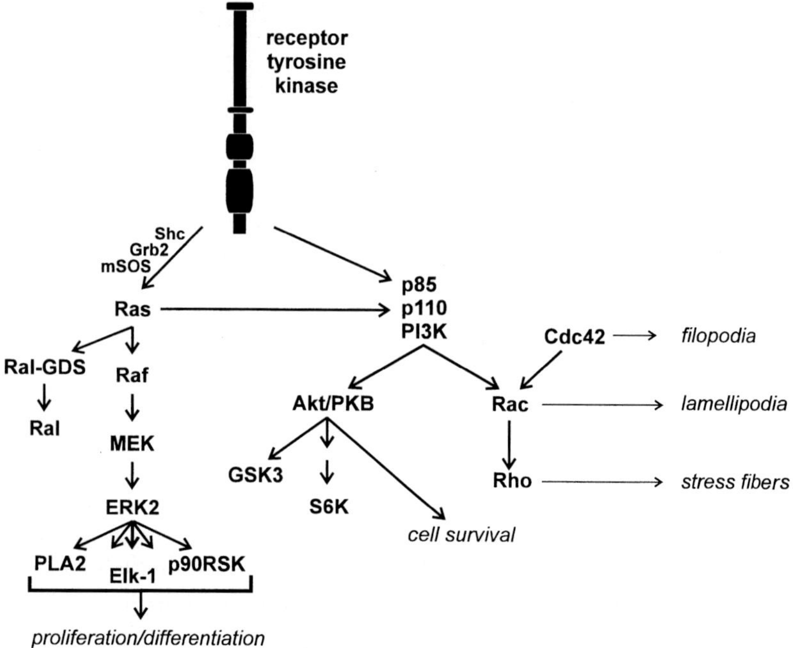

Fig. 1. Three main signal transduction pathways activated by most receptor tyrosine kinases

lar signal-regulated kinase 2 (ERK2) pathway is involved in changes in gene transcription, resulting in cellular proliferation or differentiation. The actin cytoskeleton is involved in diverse cellular processes, e.g. cell division, cellular shape change, cellular migration, and axon outgrowth. A key role in the rearrangement of the actin cytoskeleton is played by PI3K and members of the Rho family of GTPases, including Cdc42, Rac, and Rho. The PI3K-PKB pathway is also involved in regulation of gene expression via S6K, but also in regulation of other signaling pathways involving glycogen, synthase kinase 3 (GSK3) or β-catenin (Avruch et al. 1994; Bos 1995; Symons 1996). Recently, a novel signaling pathway downstream from Ras has been identified which involves Ral guanine nucleotide exchange factors and the small GTPase Ral (Feig et al. 1996).

Ret is a member of the family of receptor tyrosine kinases. In order to understand the function of Ret not only in normal development, but also in diseases such as multiple endocrine neoplasia type 2 (MEN2) and Hirschsprung's disease, it is important to know which signaling pathways are activated by Ret. To study Ret signal transduction, different approaches have been used with respect to stimulation of the tyrosine kinase activity of Ret. Because the ligands of Ret, glial cell line-derived neurotrophic factor (GDNF), and neurturin (NTN) have only recently been identified, very few papers have appeared in which GDNF was used to study Ret signal transduction. For most studies, constitutively active Ret mutants such as the Ret/PTC oncogenes or full-length Ret harboring the activating MEN2A and MEN2B point mutations were used. Alternatively, a chimeric receptor consisting of the human epithelial growth factor (EGF) receptor ligand binding domain fused to the intracellular domain of Ret (HERRet) was introduced into cells. Stimulation of this chimeric receptor with EGF results in Ret tyrosine kinase activity, which can therefore be used to study Ret signal transduction.

First, Ret-binding proteins will be discussed, followed by an overview of the role of tyrosine residues in protein binding to Ret. Next, signal transduction by constitutively active mutants of Ret will be addressed, followed by results from studies with the HERRet chimeric receptor. Finally, we will consider GDNF signaling.

Ret-Binding Proteins

In order to understand more about the signal transduction events involved in the effects of Ret tyrosine kinase activation in the cell, several groups have investigated which signaling molecules bind to constitutively active Ret and to EGF-stimulated HERRet. The results of these studies are summarized in Table 1.

Grb2 is an adaptor protein consisting of SH2 and SH3 domains. Grb2 binding to active Ret could only be shown in vitro for the p51 isoform of Ret, which contains a Grb2-SH2 binding consensus sequence (Y^*XNX). No association was observed with the p9 or p43 isoforms, which lack this sequence (Pandey et al. 1995; Durick et al. 1990). Another adaptor molecule is Shc. Shc-binding to Ret has been shown using constitutively active mutants of Ret [Borrello et al. 1994; Asai et al. 1996). Shc binding to receptor tyrosine kinases is mediated by the PTB domain in Shc, which recognizes the consensus sequence $(L)xNPxY^*$ (Bork and Margolis 1995; van der Geer et al. 1995). Although no sequence exactly matching the consensus is present in Ret, it has recently been shown that Shc proteins bind to tyrosine residue 1062 ($IeNklY^*$) in active Ret (Asai et al. 1996). A third adaptor molecule, Grb10, which also binds to active Ret, is a member of the Grb7 family of SH2 domain-containing adaptor proteins. The central domain of the adaptor molecule is similar to a *Caenorhabditis* gene that contains a pleckstrin homology (PH) domain and may be crucial for migration of a subset of *C. elegans* neuronal cells. Although Grb10 was originally identified in a screen for SH2-containing proteins using the C terminus of the EGF receptor, it binds with much higher affinity to activated Ret. The role of Grb10 in Ret signaling is currently unknown (Pandey et al. 1995; Durick et al. 1996; Doi et al. 1995).

Enigma is a recently identified protein with unknown function. It interacts with Ret via a LIM domain. Cysteine-rich LIM domains recognize tyrosine-containing tight-turn structures in proteins, but do not require phosphorylation of the tyrosine residue for binding (Wu and Gill 1994). Indeed, Enigma

Table 1. Ret-binding proteins as determined by in vitro and in vivo studies

Protein	Ret-PTC (p51 form)	HERRet (p9 form)
In vitro binding[a]		
GST-Grb2-SH2	+[c]	–[d]
GST-Shc-SH2	+[c]	ND
Grb10 (yeast-2-hybrid)	+[d]	ND
GST-Grb10	ND	+[d]
Enigma (yeast-2-hybrid)	+[d]	ND
GST-Enigma-LIM	ND	+[d]
PLCγ (yeast-2-hybrid)	+[d]	ND
GST-PLCγ-SH2	ND	+[d]
GST-Src-SH2	ND	+[d]
In vivo binding[b]		
Grb2	+/–[c]	–[f]
Shc	+[c]	–[f]
Grb10	ND	+[g]
RasGAP	ND	+[h]
PI3K	ND	–[h]
PLCγ	+[e]	+[h]

PLC, phospholipase C; ND, not determined; GST, glutathione-S transferase.
[a] Assayed by binding of the GST fusion proteins to active Ret in cell lysates.
[b] Assayed by co-immunoprecipitation of endogenous or transfected proteins
  together with active Ret from cell lysates.
[c] Borrello et al. 1994.
[d] Durrick et al. 1996.
[e] Borrello et al. 1996.
[f] van Weering et al. 1995.
[g] Pandey et al. 1995.
[h] Santoro et al. 1994.

binds to both the inactive and the active Ret tyrosine kinase domain (Durick et al. 1996). The importance of Enigma binding to Ret remains to be established, since in the initial report mutation of tyrosine residue 1062 abrogated Enigma binding and also the transforming activity of Ret. Now that is known that tyrosine 1062 is also the binding site for Shc, the importance of the interaction between Enigma and Ret may be questioned. Finally, phospolipase C (PLC)γ can bind to the tyrosine kinase domain of active Ret. PLCγ is involved in the activation of protein kinase C (PKC) and in the release of calcium from intracellular stores.

Binding of most of the above-mentioned proteins to the activated Ret tyrosine kinase domain requires phosphorylation of tyrosine residues in the receptor to function as docking sites for SH2 or PTB domains in the associating molecules. The first column of Table 2, shows which tyrosines are phosphorylated in constitutively active Ret. To determine which tyrosines are necessary for binding to certain proteins, specific tyrosine residues have been

Table 2. Tyrosine residues in the intracellular domain of Ret with details on thyrosine phosphorylation, mutational analysis, and binding proteins

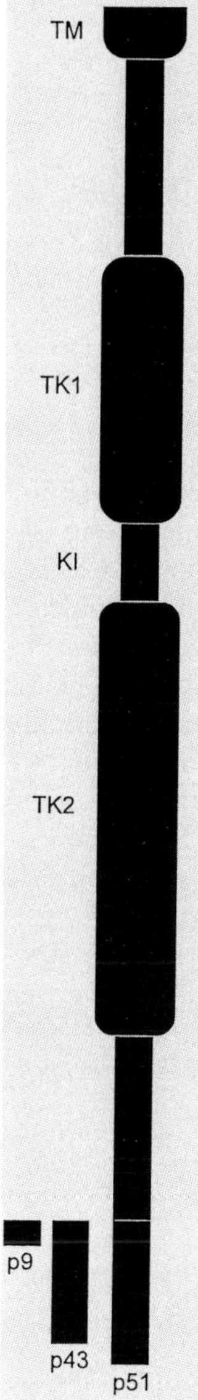

	Tyrosine phosphorylation		Y-F mutant; effect on BRDU inc.	Y-F mutant; effect on transforming activity		Binding protein
	MEN2A	MEN2B	*ret*/PTC2	MEN2A	MEN2B	
–Y660	–	–	ND	ND	ND	ND
–Y687	+	+/–	ND	ND	ND	ND
–Y752	ND	ND	ND	ND	ND	ND
–Y791	ND	ND	ND	ND	ND	ND
_/Y806	ND	ND	ND	ND	ND	ND
¬\Y809	ND	ND	ND	ND	ND	ND
–Y826	+	+	↓	ND	ND	ND
–Y864	ND	ND	ND	–	↓	ND
_/Y900	ND		↓	–	–	ND
¬\Y905	ND	ND	–	↓↓↓	–	Grb10
–Y928	ND	ND	ND	–	–	ND
–Y952	ND	ND	–	–	↓	NMD
–Y981	Nd	ND	↓↓↓	ND	ND	ND
–Y1015	+	+	ND	ND	ND	PLCγ
–Y1029	+	+	ND	ND	ND	ND
–Y1062	+	+	↓↓↓	ND	ND	Enigma/Shc
_/Y1090	–	–	ND	ND	ND	ND
¬\Y1096	+	+/–	–	ND	ND	Grb2

ND, not determined; MEN, multiple endocrine neoplasia; BrdU, bromodeoxyurdiine; PLC, phospholipase C; TM, transmembrane region; TK, fyrosine kinase domain; KI, kinase insert domain.

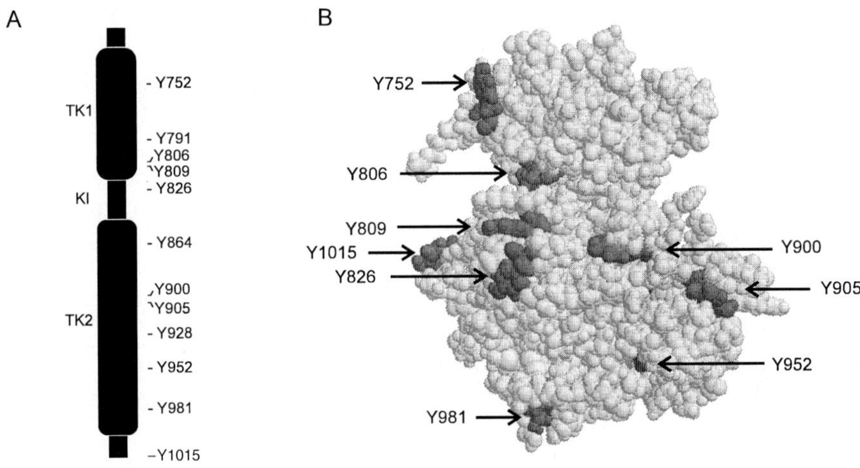

Fig. 2A, B. Position of tyrosine residues in **A** the amino acid sequence, and **B** in a three dimensional computer model of a part of the Ret tyrosine kinase domain

mutated to phenylalanine residues, which are resistant to phosphorylation. This method helps to determine which receptor-binding proteins are involved in the cellular responses after activation of Ret. Thus far, the binding sites for Grb10, PLCγ, Enigma, Shc, and Grb2 have been identified (Table 2). In order to select other tyrosine residues that are potentially interesting for mutational analysis, a model of the tyrosine kinase domain of Ret was made. The model is based on the three-dimensional structure of the kinase domain of the human insulin receptor. In this model, the three dimensional structure of the insulin receptor is retained, but the relative positions of the Ret amino acid residues have been calculated by computer after alignment of the two sequences. In Fig. 2, the position of all tyrosine residues exposed at the surface of the model are indicated. It is striking that all the exposed tyrosine residues are exposed on one side of the molecule. In agreement with this computer model, the binding sites for Grb10 (Y905) and PLCγ (Y1015) are well exposed at the surface of the molecule. Other known binding sites for signaling molecules are not included in this model since they are present outside the kinase domain of Ret.

Signaling by Constitutively Active Mutants of Ret

The first results on Ret signal transduction were obtained using cells transfected with constitutively active Ret mutants. Transfection of NIH3T3 fibroblasts with constitutively active mutants of Ret results in oncogenic transformation of the cells, as judged by focus formation in confluent monolayers, tumor formation in nude mice, and anchorage-independent growth in soft agar (Durick et al. 1995, 1996; Borrello et al. 1996; Iwashita et al. 1996; Liu et al 1996). Transforming activity of the Ret tyrosine kinase domain in the context of a fusion protein is comparable with that of the *erb*B2 kinase domain in the same context, but is approximately 100-fold higher than the transforming activity of the EGF receptor kinase domain (Romano et al. 1994). The transforming activity of Ret is cell type specific. Expression of the active Ret/PTC mutants in the neuronal cell line PC12 results in expression of immediate early and late genes implicated in neuronal differentiation of the cells, showing that active Ret induces neuronal differentiation of PC12 cells (Califano et al. 1995). In addition, Ret/PTC expression in Xenopus oocytes results in germinal vesicle breakdown (GVBD), a phenomenon involved in maturation of the oocyte (Grieco et al. 1995). These effects are mediated by endogenous Ras since inhibition of Ras, with a dominant negative mutant or with neutralizing antibodies blocked these differentiation events (Califano et al. 1995; Grieco et al. 1995).

Figure 2 shows the role of the individual tyrosine residues in Ret with respect to the transforming activity of Ret/PTC mutants. Mutation of both tyrosine 826 and tyrosine 900 to phenylalanine reduces the mitogenic activity of Ret/PTC2, and tyrosine 981 or 1062 is essential for the mitogenic activity of Ret/PTC2 (Durick et al. 1995, 1996). The role of PLCγ in the transforming activity by Ret/PTC is not clear. According to Durick et al. (1996), mutation of the binding site of PLCγ (Y1015) does not reduce transforming activity, while Borrello et al. (1996) claim that PLCγ binding and activation is essential for transforming activity.

A major drawback of the use of constitutively active mutants for studying signal transduction is that early signaling events cannot be investigated. Moreover, feedback mechanisms may have downregulated certain responses, which therefore remain unobserved. Thus an inducible system is more informative with respect to early events in Ret signal transduction.

HERRet-Induced Signal Transduction

In order to study early Ret signal transduction in the absence of a known ligand, Santoro et al. (1994) used a chimeric receptor consisting of the extracellular and transmembrane domain of the human EGF receptor fused to the tyrosine kinase domain of Ret (HERRet), stably transfected into NR6 fibroblasts which lack endogenous EGF receptors. EGF-induced stimulation of Ret tyrosine kinase activity in these cells results in HERRet tyrosine phosphorylation and in weak activation of PLCγ, as measured by PLCγ tyrosine phosphorylation and the production of inositol phosphates. PI3K activation was not detected in either co-immunoprecipitations or in vitro kinase assays. In these cells, HERRet stimulation also leads to activation of Ras. However, this Ras activity is not followed by ERK2 activation as would be expected (Santoro et al. 1994).

Since Ret is normally not expressed in fibroblasts, the unexpected signaling events observed in these cells might be due to the cell type rather than to the receptor. In order to test this, we stably transfected the EGF receptor-negative neuroepithelioma cell line SK-N-MC with the same HERRet chimeric receptor (yielding the SKF5 cells). Stimulation of HERRet in these cells resulted in Shc phosphorylation, Shc-Grb2-mSos complex formation, and activation of Ras. In contrast to fibroblasts, HERRet-induced activation of Ras in SKF5 cells was followed by ERK2 activation. ERK2 activation is dependent on Ras, since expression of a dominant negative mutant of Ras completely blocked ERK2 activation (van Weering et al. 1995). A possible explanation for the discrepancy between these two cell systems might be found at the level of Raf-1. In the fibroblast cell line, no MEK-1-phosphorylating activity is stimulated in response to Ret activity, while in SKF5 cells both Raf-1 and B-Raf are activated (D. H. J. van Weering and J. L. Bos, unpublished results).

Ret activation also leads to signal transduction towards PI3K-mediated events. First, Ret activation leads to the activation of PKB. Second, stimulation of SKF5 cells results in rapid formation of lamellipodia at the plasma membrane (van Weering and Bos 1997). Activation of PKB and formation of lamellipodia is mediated by PI3K, since the specific inhibitors wortmannin and LY294002 completely block Ret-induced PKB activation and lamellipodia formation. Ret-induced lamellipodia formation, but not PKB activation, is mediated by Rac, as determined by transient transfection assays using constitutively active and dominant negative mutants of this GTPase. The GTPases Rho and Cdc42 are not involved in lamellipodia formation. Ras is not necessary for Ret-induced signaling events, since in SKF5 cells expressing dominant negative Ras^{asn17}, Ret activation still leads to PKB activation and lamellipodia formation. However, transfection of constitutively active Ras into these cells does induce PKB activation and lamellipodia formation, and these signaling events are also mediated by PI3K (van Weering et al., submitted). Induction of PI3K-mediated events by constitutively active Ras has also been observed in fibroblasts, where constitutively active Ras activates PI3K via a direct interaction between Ras and the 110-kDa subunit of PI3K (Rodgriguez-Viciana et al. 1994, 1996). However, stimulation of SKF5 cells with basis fibroblast growth factor (bFGF) only weakly induced PI3K and PKB activation and did not induce lamellipodia formation, while bFGF strongly induces endogenous Ras activation (van Weering et al., submitted for publication).

The function of the Ret-induced lamellipodia is not exactly known, but since lamellipodia are involved in neurite outgrowth, which is also dependent on PI3K and GTPases of the Rho family, these lamellipodia might possibly represent early events in neuritogenesis. However, long-term stimulation of SKF5 cells does not result in neurite formation. Instead, over a time period of 4–6 h, the cells lose their intracellular contact and start to migrate away from each other (scattering) (van Puijenbroek et al. 1997). A process similar to scattering also occurs when immature neuroblasts in a developing embryo leave the neural tube to become neural crest cells (Newgreen and Gibbins 1982). Scattering of SKF5 cells may therefore be regarded as a form of differentiation of the cells. That lamellipodia formation is not required for scattering can be concluded from the fact that stimulation of SKF5 cells with bFGF does not result in lamellipodia formation, but does result in cell scattering. Platelet-derived growth factor (PDGF) stimulation has the opposite effect. This growth factor induces lamellipodia formation but not scattering (van Puijenbroek et al. 1997). It is therefore likely that lamellipodia formation and scattering are two independent processes that are both induced by Ret tyrosine kinase activity. Signaling events responsible for the scattering response most likely involve a prolonged activation of ERK2. Both bFGF and Ret induce prolonged ERK2 activation and scattering, while PDGF induces only transient ERK2 activation and no scattering (van Puijenbroek et al. 1997). If scattering is regarded as cellular differentiation, this system is analogous to the PC12 system in which EGF induces transient ERK2 activation followed by proliferation of the cells, while nerve growth factor (NGF) induces prolonged ERK2 activation and differentiation of the cells (Marshall 1995).

GDNF and NTN-Induced Signal Transduction

Because GDNF and NTN have only recently been identified as the ligands for Ret (Jing et al. 1996; Kotzbauer et al. 1996; Treanor et al. 1996), relatively little is known about GDNF- or NTN-induced Ret signal transduction. Both GDNF and NTN stimulate Ret tyrosine kinase activity via the (glycophosphatidyl inositol (GPI)-linked proteins GDNFR-α and NTNR-α (Jing et al. 1996; Treanor et al. 1996; Kotzbauer et al. 1996; Klein et al. 1997; Buj-Bello et al. 1997). With respect to signal transduction, GDNF induces Ret-dependent mesoderm induction in Xenopus embryos, which is thought to be mediated by ERK2 (Durbec et al. 1996; Umbhauer et al. 1995). Indeed, stimulation of SK-N-MC cells stably expressing full-length Ret (SKP2) with GDNF results in ERK2 activation. Although there is only a small increase in guanosine triphosphate (GTP)-bound Ras in the cells in response to GDNF stimulation, ERK2 activation is completely inhibited in the presence of a dominant negative mutant of Ras (van Weering and Bos 1997). These results are in agreement with the data we obtained with HERRet in the SKF5 cell line, which also show that Ret-induced ERK2 activation is mediated by Ras (van Weering et al. 1995). Another important effect of GDNF is that Ret-expressing neuroblasts, but not neuroblasts from Ret knockout mice, show axon outgrowth in response to GDNF stimulation (Durbec et al. 1996). Essential during axonogenesis is the formation of lamellipodia at the growth cone of the axon. Axon elongation is inhibited by cytochalasin D, which prevents actin polymerization, and by wortmannin, which inhibits PI3K activity (Kimura et al. 1994; Forscher and Smith 1988; Bentley and Toroian-Raymond 1986). In SKP2 cells, GDNF induces lamellipodia formation, and these lamellipodia are also dependent on PI3K activity. These results suggest that GDNF induces early events in neuritogenesis in this cell line (van Weering and Bos 1997).

Acknowledgments. This work was supported by the Foundation for Chemical Research (SON) with financial support from the Netherlands Organization for Scientific Research (NWO).

References

Asai N, Murakami H, Iwashita T, Takahashi M (1996) A mutation at tyrosine 1062 in MEN2A-RET and MEN2B-Ret impairs their transforming activity and association with Shc adaptor proteins. J Biol Chem 271:17644–17649

Avruch J, Zhang XF, Kyriakis JM (1994) Raf meets Ras: completing the framework of a signal transduction pathway. Trends Biochem Sci 19:279–283

Bentley D, Toroian-Raymond A (1986) Disoriented pathfinding by pioneer neurone growth cones deprived of filopodia by cytochalasin treatment. Nature 323:712–715

Bork P, Margolis B: A phosphotyrosine interaction domain. Cell 80:693–694

Borrello MG, Pelicci G, Arighi E, De Filippis L, Greco A, Bongarzone I, Rizzetti MG, Pelicci PG, Pierotti MA (1994) The oncogenic versions of the Ret and Trk tyrosine kinases bind Shc and Grb2 adaptor proteins. Oncogene 9:1661–1668

Borrello MG, Alberti L, Arighi E, Bongarzone I, Battistini C, Bardelli A, Pasini B, Piutti C, Rizzetti MG, Mondellini P, Radice MT, Pierotti MA (1996) The full oncogenic activity of Ret/ptc2 depends on tyrosine 539, a docking site for phospholipase C-gamma. Mol Cell Biol 16:2151–2163

Bos JL (1995) A target for phosphoinositide 3-kinase: Akt/PKB. Trends Biochem Sci 20:441–442

Buj-Bello A, Adu J, Pinon LG, Horton A, Thompson J, Rosenthal A, Chinchetru M, Buchman VL, Davies AM (1997) Neurturin responsiveness requires a GPI-linked receptor and the Ret receptor tyrosine kinase. Nature 387:721–724

Califano D, Monaco C, De Vita G, D'Alessio A, Dathan NA, Possenti R, Vecchio G, Fusco A, Santoro M, de Franciscis V (1995) Activated RET/PTC oncogene elicts immediate early and delayed response genes in PC12 cells. Oncogene 11:107–112

Durbec PL, Marcos-Gutierrez CV, Kilkenny C, Grigoriou M, Wartiowaara K, Suvanto P, Smith D, Ponder BAJ, Costantini F, Saarma M, Sariola H, Pachnis V (1996) GDNF signalling through the Ret receptor tyrosine kinase. Nature 381:789–793

Durick K, Yao VJ, Borrello MG, Bongarzone I, Pierotti MA, Taylor SS (1995) Tyrosines outside the kinase core and dimerization are required for the mitogenic activity of RET/ptc2. J Biol Chem 270:24642–24645

Durick K, Wu R-Y, Gill GN, Taylor SS (1996) Mitogenic signaling by Ret/ptc2 requires association with Enigma via a LIM domain. J Biol Chem 271:12691–12694

Feig LA, Urano T, Cantor S (1996) Evidence for a Ras/Ral signaling cascade. Trends Biochem Sci 21:438–441

Forscher P, Smith SJ (1988) Actions of cytochalasins on the organization of actin filaments and microtubules in a neuronal growth cone. J Cell Biol 107:1505–1516

Grieco D, Santoro M, Dathan NA, Fusco A (1995) Activated RET oncogene products induce maturation of Xenopus oocytes. Oncogene 11:113–117

Heldin CH (1995) Dimerization of cell surface receptors in signal transduction. Cell 80:213–223

Iwashita T, Asai N, Murakami H, Matsuyama M, Takahashi M (1996) Identification of tyrosine residues that are essential for transforming activity of the ret proto-oncogene with MEN2A or MEN2B mutations. Oncogene 12:481–487

Jing S, Wen D, Yu Y, Holst PL, Luo Y, Fang M, Tamir R, Antonio L, Hu Z, Cupples R, Louis J-C, Hu S, Altrock BW, Fox GM (1996) GDNF-induced activation of the Ret protein tyrosine kinase is mediated by GDNFR-alpha, a novel receptor for GDNF. Cell 85:1113–1124

Kimura K, Hattori S, Kabuyama Y, Shizawa Y, Takayanagi J, Nakamura S, Toki S, Matsuda Y, Onodera K, Fukui Y (1994) Neurite outgrowth of PC12 cells is suppressed by wortmannin, a specific inhibitor of phosphatidylinositol 3-kinase. J Biol Chem 269:18961–18967

Klein RD, Sherman D, Ho WH, Stone D, Bennett GL, Moffat B, Vandlen R, Simmons L, Gu Q, Hongo JA, Devaux B, Poulsen K, Armanini M, Nozaki C, Asai N, Goddard A, Phillips H, Henderson CE, Takahashi M, Rosenthal A (1997) A GPI-linked protein that interacts with Ret to form a candidate neurturin receptor. Nature 387:717–721

Kotzbauer PT, Lampe PA, Heuckeroth RO, Golden JP, Creedon DJ, Johnson EM Jr, Milbrandt J (1996) Neurturin, a relative of glial-cell-line-derived neurotrophic factor. Nature 384:467–470

Lemmon MA, Schlessinger J (1994) Regulation of signal transduction and signal diversity by receptor oligomerization. Trends Biochem Sci 19:459–463

Liu X, Vega QC, Decker RA, Pandey A, Worby CA, Dixon JE (1996) Oncogenic Ret receptors display different autophosphorylation sites and substrate binding specificities. J Biol Chem 271:5309–5312

Marshall CJ (1995) Specificity of receptor tyrosine kinase signaling: transient versus sustained extracellular signal-regulated kinase activation. Cell 80:179-185

Newgreen D, Gibbins I (1982) Factors controlling the time of onset of the migration of neural crest cells in the fowl embryo. Cell Tissue Res 224:145–160

Ooi J, Yajnik V, Immanuel D, Gordon M, Moskow JJ, Buchberg AM, Margolis B (1995) The cloning of Grb10 reveals a new family of SH2 domain proteins. Oncogene 10:1621–1630

Pandey A, Duan H, Di Fiore PP, Dixit VM (1995) The Ret receptor protein tyrosine kinase associates with the SH2-containing adapter protein Grb10. J Biol Chem 270:21461–21463

Rodriguez-Viciana P, Warne PH, Dhand R, Vanhaesebroeck B, Gout I, Fry MJ, Waterfield MD, Downward J (1994) Phosphatidylinositol-3-OH kinase as a direct target of Ras. Nature 370:527–532

Rodriguez-Viciana P, Warne PH, Vanhaesebroeck B, Waterfield MD, Downward J (1996) Activation of phosphoinsitide 3-kinase by interaction with Ras and by point mutation. EMBO J 15:2442–2451

Romano A, Wong WT, Santoro M, Wirth PJ, Thorgeirsson SS, Di Fiore PP (1994) The high transforming potency of erbB-2 and ret is associated with phosphorylation of paxillin and a 23 kDa protein. Oncogene 9:2923–2933

Santoro M, Wong WT, Aroca P, Santos E, Matoskova B, Grieco M, Fusco A, Di Fiore PP (1994) An epidermal growth factor receptor/ret chimera generates mitogenic and transforming signals: evidence for a ret-specific signaling pathway. Mol Cell Biol 14:663–675

Symons M (1996) Rho family GTPases: the cytoskeleton and beyond. Trends Biochem Sci 21:178–181

Treanor JJS, Goodman L, De Sauvage F, Stone DM, Poulsen KT, Beck CD, Gray C, Armanini MP, Pollock RA, Hefti F, Phillips HS, Goddard A, Moore MW, Buj Bello A, Davies AM, Asai N, Takahashi M, Vandlen R, Henderson CE, Rosenthal A (1996) Characterization of a multicomponent receptor for GDNF. Nature 382:80–83

Ullrich A, Schlessinger J (1990) Signal transduction by receptors with tyrosine kinase activity. Cell 61:203–212

Umbhauer M, Marshall CJ, Mason CS, Old RW, Smith JC (1995) Mesoderm induction in Xenopus caused by activation of MAP kinase. Nature 376:58–62

van der Geer P, Wiley S, Ka-Man Lai V, Olivier JP, Gish GD, Stephens R, Kaplan D, Shoelson S, Pawson T (1995) A conserved amino-terminal Shc domain binds to phosphotyrosine motifs in activated receptors and phosphopeptides. Curr Biol 5:404–412

van Puijenbroek AAFL, van Weering DHJ, van den Brink CE, Bos JL, van der Saag PT, de Laat SW, den Hertog J (1997) Cell scattering of SK-N-MC neuroepithelioma cells in response to Ret and FGF receptor tyrosine kinase activation is correlated with sustained ERK2 activation. Oncogene 14:1147-1158

van Weering DHJ, Medema JP, van Puijenbroek A, Burgering BMT, Baas PD, Bos JL (1995) Ret receptor tyrosine kinase activates extracellular signal-regulated kinase 2 in SK-N-MC cells. Oncogene 11:2207–2214

van Weering DHJ, Bos JL (1997) Glial cell line-derived neurotrophic factor induces Ret-mediated lamellipodia formation. J Biol Chem 272:249–254

Wu RY, Gill GN (1994) LIM domain recognition of a tyrosine-containing tight turn. J Biol Chem 269:25085–25090

VI. Population Genetics of Cancer Susceptibility

Complex Traits on the Map

J. Ott[1,2] and P. Lucek[2]

[1] Laboratory of Statistical Genetics, Rockefeller University,
  1230 York Avenue, New York, NY 10021, USA
[2] Department of Genetics and Development, Columbia University,
  701 West 168th Street, New York, NY 10032, USA

Abstract

The lod score method for localizing mendelian disease genes in human genetics is reviewed. Current ways of applying this technique to hypothesized genes underlying complex traits are discussed. In contrast to these parametric methods, allele-sharing methods using affected sib pairs are reviewed. Based on such allele-sharing data, a particular type of analysis is outlined which can identify sets of disease loci. This method makes use of pattern-recognition techniques as implemented in artificial neural networks (ANNs).

Introduction

Mendelian diseases, i.e., traits with a known, simple mode of inheritance (single recessive or dominant gene), are rather infrequent. One of the most frequent mendelian traits is cystic fibrosis. Among Caucasians, it has an incidence of 1:2000. In contrast, common heritable diseases generally follow unknown modes of inheritance. For example, schizophrenia has a population frequency of 1% and clearly has a genetic component; heritability (proportion of phenotypic variance due to genetic causes) accounts for at least 74%, yet the mode of inheritance is unclear. Presumably, multiple (perhaps interacting) loci are responsible for susceptibility to schizophrenia. Such diseases are called complex traits, and many cancers also fall into this category.

To determine the degree by which genetic factors play a role in the etiology of a complex trait, a common approach is to compare the recurrence risk for a monozygotic (MZ) twin K_{MZ} with that for a dizygotic (DZ) twin K_{DZ}. If K_{MZ} is much larger than K_{DZ}, this indicates the presence of underlying genes. How many such genes are involved has been investigated as follows (Risch 1990): The strength or effect size of a gene may be measured in terms of the degree by which it raises the recurrence risk for an offspring, K_O or a sibling K_S over that for a random person, which is the population prevalence K. The corresponding ratios $\lambda_O = K_O/K$ or $\lambda_S = K_S/K$ are then taken as measures for the genetic influence of a gene. With decreasing degree of

Recent Results in Cancer Research, Vol. 154
© Springer-Verlag Berlin · Heidelberg 1998

relationship, the corresponding λ values tend to decrease as well. The rate of drop-off is indicative of the number of genes involved in a trait (Risch 1990). While this is an appealing method, results of this and other segregation analysis techniques tend to be very approximate. Another, possibly more reliable approach, if feasible, is to look at animal models. As an example, results of planned crosses involving the nonobese diabetic (NOD) mouse have shown a minimum of nine loci to be responsible for diabetes in these animals (Risch et al. 1993). These diabetes genes tend to interact epistatically to produce disease susceptibility, and some of them act in a protective manner. These results lead to the conclusion that a similar number of genes are responsible for diabetes in humans.

To elucidate the mode of action of such genes, the current "genetic" approach (positional cloning) is to first localize a disease gene on the human gene map by genetic linkage analysis (Ott 1991; Weeks and Lathrop 1995). The next step is to characterize (clone) the gene by molecular genetics techniques. Further research is then directed toward functional analysis of the gene. This chapter is concerned with the first step of localizing disease genes on the human gene map. Brief introductions for parametric and nonparametric linkage analysis are given, followed by an outline on recent novel developments for the search of disease genes by pattern recognition techniques.

Lod Score Method for Mendelian Diseases

Genetic linkage analysis is based on the biological phenomenon of crossing-over. In meiosis, every two homologous chromosomes pair up. One arm of one homologue crosses over one arm of the other homologue, and a reciprocal exchange takes place (Fig. 1). Of the four gametic products of meiosis,

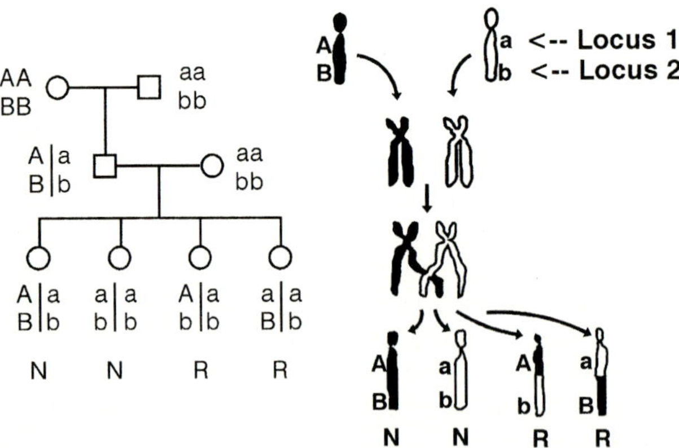

Fig. 1. Crossover in one pair of homologous chromosomes during meiosis (*right*) and corresponding interpretation of marker genotypes observed in family (*left*). *R*, recombination; *N*, nonrecombination

two show the effect of the crossover, while the other two are unaffected by it. In suitable families, for two genes on either side of the crossover point, a gamete containing the crossover point will appear as a so-called recombinant offspring, while a gamete lacking a crossover point will be seen as a nonrecombinant offspring. The proportion of recombinant offspring is referred to as the recombination fraction θ. The salient feature in all this is that crossovers take place randomly along a chromosome. For pairs of gene loci close together, crossovers rarely occur between them. Thus a small recombination fraction is indicative of close proximity of two loci. On the other hand, for loci far apart on a chromosome or located on different chromosomes, the recombination fraction is $\theta = 0.50$. Loci with a θ value significantly smaller than 0.50 are said to be genetically linked.

It is only in very special situations such as that shown in Fig. 1 that recombinant and nonrecombinant offspring can unambiguously be identified. Generally, missing observations, incomplete penetrance, and other complicating factors cloud our view of underlying genotypes. For example, for women susceptible to breast cancer (BRCA1 gene), the trait is not expressed at birth but only later in life (Claus et al. 1991; Hall et al. 1990), and there is also a difference of roughly 10 years in mean onset ages between genetic and nongenetic cases (Mérette and King 1992). Thus the recombination fraction must generally be estimated by the *maximum likelihood method*. The likelihood $L(\theta)$ is the probability of occurrence of the data (in our case, observations on family members) and depends on various parameters such as gene frequencies and the recombination fraction between a hypothesized disease locus and a genetic marker locus. $L(\theta)$ assumes different values depending on given values of θ. The likelihood by itself is less interesting than the likelihood ratio $L(\theta)/L(\frac{1}{2})$, whose logarithm $Z(\theta) = \log_{10}[L(\theta)L(\frac{1}{2})]$ is the so-called lod score (Morton 1955). The value of θ that maximizes the lod score is taken as the best estimate of the recombination fraction. With a given disease inheritance model and assumed parameter values, the lod score is generally computed for some set of family data with the aid of a computer program. Well-known linkage programs are LINKAGE (Lathrop et al. 1984), Mendel (Lange et al. 1988), and Genehunter (Kruglyak et al. 1996; Kong and Cox 1997).

Localizing a hypothetical disease gene on the human gene map amounts to estimating recombination fractions between disease locus and each of the markers on the map and testing whether an estimated value of θ is significantly smaller than 0.50, which represents absence of linkage. Traditionally, significance is said to be established when the maximum lod score over all families attains a value of at least 3 (Morton 1955). In a genome-wide search, as often carried out today, somewhat higher critical limits are called for (Lander and Kruglyak 1995).

Lod scores and Complex Traits

As the mode of inheritance of complex traits is unknown, it is not obvious how the lod score method should be applied to such traits, i.e., what inheritance model should be specified for analysis purposes. Often, researchers estimate a mendelian model that is as dose to "reality" as possible by setting disease allele frequency and penetrances in such a way that the inheritance model predicts appropriate population prevalence and sib recurrence risk of the disease. More frequently, multiple inheritance models are tried in the analysis (Weeks et al. 1990; Curtis and Sham 1995), which necessitates some form of correction for multiple testing (Ott 1991).

Because of these difficulties, the lod score method is often abandoned for complex traits. Instead, nonparametric methods are employed that do not require specification of disease inheritance models. Below, a very common type of such methods is described.

Complex Traits – Allele-Sharing Methods

In so-called affected sib pair (ASP) methods, all calculations are done for marker genotypes and no assumptions are made regarding disease inheritance. The only connection with disease is that attention is focused on siblings affected with the trait under study.

Assume a marker locus with consecutively numbered alleles, two parents with genotypes *1/2* and *3/4*, and two affected offspring. If marker inheritance is random (no connection with disease), parent *1* transmits alleles *1* and *2* with equal frequencies to each of the two offspring. In other words, the two offspring either do or do not share an allele received from this parent, where these two cases occur with equal frequencies. However, if parent 1 carries a disease susceptibility allele at a locus tightly linked with the marker under study, then the disease allele is in coupling with one or the other of the two marker alleles. In that case, two affected offspring tend to share an allele from parent 1 more often than expected by chance. In other words, for a given parent, the average number of alleles shared by the two sibs is equal to 0.50 without linkage and tends to exceed 0.50 with linkage. For both parents considered jointly, the two offspring either share 0, one, or two alleles with an average of one under no linkage. Testing for linkage amounts to determining whether the observed number of alleles shared over many ASPs is significantly higher than expected by chance. Well-known applications of such ASP methods include genome screens carried out to localize diabetes susceptibility genes (Davies et al. 1994; Hashimoto et al. 1994).

While it is in principle possible to carry out ASP analyses by hand for one marker at a time, more efficient methods consider all markers on a chromosome jointly. Powerful approaches for such analyses have been developed and implemented in computer programs (Kruglyak et al. 1996; information on the ASPEX program is available at URL ftp://lahmed.stanford.edu/pub/aspex/

index.html). A successful application of such a method to inflammatory bowel disease has recently been described (Hugot et al. 1996), with a commentary carrying the same title as this chapter (Ott 1996).

Multilocus Allele-Sharing Methods with Neural Networks

Essentially all currently available methods, including the multipoint ASP methods, either implicitly or explicitly work under the assumption of a single disease locus. However, for complex traits, it is generally believed that multiple, possibly interacting loci confer susceptibility rather than a single disease locus. We have therefore begun to develop pattern recognition techniques with the aim of identifying *sets* of marker loci that jointly show deviations from random allele sharing. Some of the markers may act only as modifiers for others. For example, allele sharing may be increased at marker 17 only when allele sharing is elevated at marker 99. If there are interactions among disease loci, pattern recognition techniques will be able to recognize these interactions and will therefore be more powerful than conventional ASP methods.

Pattern recognition techniques are often used to predict an outcome (e.g., disease diagnosis) on the basis of observed predictor variables. This is achieved by monitoring observations with known predictor variables and outcomes. Linear discriminant analysis may then be applied to determine the set of predictor variables that best predict outcome. For allele-sharing data in ASPs, we have turned to a particular type of pattern recognition technique called *artificial neural network* (ANN), which can be shown to be able to carry out nonlinear discriminant analysis (Bishop 1995). The network architecture we are using is a feed-forward ANN with three neuronal layers (input, hidden, and output).

Here, only a brief nontechnical description can be given; a more detailed account has been provided elsewhere (P. Lucek et al., manuscript submitted). ANNs were originally developed as simple models for the way nerve cells transmit impulses in the brain. In ANNs, neurons are modeled as nodes that are arranged in layers. A given node potentially receives impulses from all nodes in the layer preceding it and potentially sends an impulse ("fires") to each node in the layer following it. Whether a node fires is determined by the sum of all impulses received and some threshold function. Based on multiple observations at the input nodes and predetermined values of the output nodes, ANNs "learn" how best to connect input and output nodes via pathways through hidden nodes. The "strengths" of connections among pairs of nodes in adjacent layers are called weights, and iteratively estimating these weights is referred to as training a network. A common training (learning) algorithm is the back-propagation method. Initially, weights have some assumed starting values, which are modified and optimized in the course of learning. These weights are analogous to the coefficients associated with predictor variables in discriminant or multiple regression analysis. ANNs may be seen to carry out simple calculations in a highly parallel manner, which enables them to do tasks for which other methods are unsatisfactory.

Our allele-sharing observations have a very simple structure: For each parent, at any marker, an ASP shows sharing ($x=1$) or no sharing ($x=-1$) or provides no information ($x=0$). Thus, for all markers studied on the genome, observations form an array (a matrix) of x values with m rows (markers) and n columns (parents). The ANN has m input nodes, a hidden layer with a smaller number of nodes, and an output layer with two nodes O_1 and O_2. We "train" the network (estimate the weights) with both observed allele-sharing data and data randomly generated on the computer. The rationale is that ASP data contain "signal" (disease loci) and "noise" (random allele sharing at markers not linked with disease loci), while randomly generated data only contain "noise." Correspondingly, training of the ASP data is done with output nodes set to $O_1=O_2=1$, while for randomly generated data we have $O_1=0$ and $O_2=1$. We then differentiate between weights to the two output nodes, O_1-O_2 ("signal + noise"–"noise"="signal"), and compute a compound contribution value, C_i, $i=1\ldots m$, for each marker locus.

Application of our methods to published allele-sharing data for a genome screen of diabetes genes (Davies et al. 1994) showed that the ANN recognizes all markers found by conventional methods. In addition, it points to markers not implicated in the original study. In particular, one of the genes (IDDM4) implicated in diabetes was seen in the original genome screen only after sib pairs were subdivided into two groups, those that showed allele sharing at HLA for both parents and those that did not, which indicates an interaction between IDDM4 and a diabetes gene (IDDM1) at the HLA region. In contrast, the neural network recognized IDDM4 without subdividing data.

Our neural network approach to gene mapping appears promising for various complex traits, including cancer genes. Data types other than affected sib pairs, where recognizing patterns among observations is important, may also be suitable for analysis by neural nets. For example, many cancers are homozygous for a marker, while the individual is heterozygous. This loss of heterozygosity (LOH) is a well-known method for identifying cancer genes. In a genomic survey for LOH, neural nets may be able to pick out patterns of interactions among cancer-causing genes that would otherwise be difficult to recognize.

Acknowledgements. Research leading to the development of neural network approaches for complex traits has been generously supported by grant MH44292 from the U.S. National Institute of Mental Health (NIMH) and by grant 5T32AM07367 (Medical Scientist Training Program) from the U.S. National Institute of Health (NIH).

References

Bishop CM (1995) Neural networks for pattern recognition. Clarendon, Oxford
Claus EB, Risch N, Thompson WD (1991) Genetic analysis of breast cancer in the cancer and steroid hormone study. Am J Hum Genet 48:232–242

Curtis D, Sham PC (1995) Model-free linkage analysis using likelihoods. Am J Hum Genet 57:703–716

Davies JL, Kawaguchi Y, Bennett ST, Copeman JB, Cordell HJ, Pritchard LE, Reed PW, Gough SCL, Jenkins SC, Palmer SM, Balfour KM, Rowe BR, Farrall M, Barnett AH, Bain SC, Todd JA (1994)A genome-wide search for human type 1 diabetes susceptibility genes. Nature 371:130–136

Hall JM, Lee MK, Morrow J, Newman B, Anderson L, Huey B, King MC (1990) Linkage analysis of early onset familial breast cancer to chromosome 17q21. Science 250:1684–1689

Hashimoto L, Habita C, Beressi JP, Delepine M, Besse C, Cambon-Thomson A, Deschamps I, Rotter JI, Djoulah S, James MR, Froguel P, Weissenbach J, Lathrop GM, Julier C (1994) Genetic mapping of a susceptibility locus for insulin-dependent diabetes mellitus on chromosome 11q. Nature 71:161–164

Hugot J-P, Laurent-Puig P, Gower-Rousseau C, Olson JM, Lee JC, Beaugerie L, Naom I, Dupas J-L, Van Gossum A, Orholm M, Bonaiti-Pellie C, Weissenbach J, Mathew CG, Lennard-Jones JE, Cortot A, Colombel J-F, Thomas G (1996) Mapping of a susceptibility locus for Crohn's disease on chromosome 16. Nature 379:821–823

Kong A, Cox NJ (1997) Allele-sharing models: LOD scores and accurate linkage tests. Am J Hum Genet 61:1179–1188

Kruglyak L, Daly MJ, Reeve-Daly MP, Lander ES (1996) Parametric and nonparametric linkage analysis: a unified multipoint approach. Am J Hum Genet 58:1347–1363

Lander E, Kruglyak L (1995) Genetic dissection of complex traits: guidelines for interpreting and reporting linkage results. Nature [Genet] 11:241–247

Lange K, Weeks D, Boehnke M (1988) Programs for pedigree analysis: MENDEL, FISHER, and dGENE. Genet Epidemiol 5:471–472

Lathrop GM, Lalouel JM, Julier C, Ott J (1984) Strategies for multilocus linkage analysis in humans. Proc Natl Acad Sci USA 81:3443–3446

Mérette C, King M-C, Ott J (1992) Heterogeneity analysis of breast cancer families by using age at onset as a covariate. Am J Hum Genet 50:515–519

Morton NE (1955) Sequential tests for the detection of linkage. Am J Hum Genet 7:277–318

Ott J (1991) Analysis of human genetic linkage. Johns Hopkins University Press, Baltimore

Ott J (1996) Complex traits on the map. Nature 379:772–773

Risch N (1990) Linkage strategies for genetically complex traits. I. Multilocus models. Am J Hum Genet 46:222–228

Risch N, Ghosh S, Todd JA (1993) Statistical evaluation of multiple-locus linkage data in experimental species and its relevance to human studies: application to nonobese diabetic (NOD) mouse and human insulin-dependent diabetes mellitus (IDDM). Am J Hum Genet 53:702–714

Weeks DE, Lathrop GM (1995) Polygenic disease: methods for mapping complex disease traits. Trends Genet 11:513–519

Weeks DE, Lehner T, Squires-Wheeler E, Kaufmann C, Ott J (1990) Measuring the inflation of the lod score due to its maximization over model parameter values in human linkage analysis. Genet Epidemiol 7:237–243

Genetic Mapping of Cancer Susceptibility/Resistance Loci in the Mouse

G. Manenti, L. De Gregorio, M. Gariboldi, F. S. Falvella, N. Zanesi, M. A. Pierotti, and T. A. Dragani

Division of Experimental Oncology A, Istituto Nazionale Tumori, Via G. Venezian 1, 20133 Milan, Italy

Abstract

Genetic linkage experiments using crosses between mouse inbred strains with an inherited predisposition and resistance to lung cancer make it possible to investigate the genetics of the complex inheritance of susceptibility and resistance to lung cancer. We have previously mapped a major locus (pulmonary adenoma susceptibility 1, *Pas1*) affecting inherited predisposition to lung cancer in mice onto chromosome 6, near *Kras2*. Appropriate crosses that include *Pas1/*$^+$ mice provide a model system for identifying loci that can modify the lung cancer predisposition phenotype caused by *Pas1*. Using this approach, we mapped the pulmonary adenoma resistance 1 (*Par1*) locus on to mouse chromosome 11; this locus selectively inhibits lung tumor development in *Pas1/*$^+$ animals and therefore behaves like a modulator gene of *Pas1*. More recently, we have mapped lung tumor modifier loci specifically affecting the initiation and progression of lung cancer. Thus experimental models provide an essential tool for the mapping of lung cancer susceptibility/resistance genes and for the subsequent cloning of candidate genes.

Background

Exposure to environmental carcinogens, in particular to cigarette smoke, represents a major risk factor for lung cancer (Loeb et al. 1984; IARC 1986). However, genetic factors may also play a role in lung cancer risk, as evidenced by the fact that not all heavy smokers develop lung cancer, and neoplasms may also occur in the lungs of nonsmokers. Several studies have indicated an excess risk of lung cancer in relatives of lung cancer patients and suggested that inheritance of an autosomal locus influences the risk and age of onset of this disease (Sellers et al. 1992). However, lung cancer pedigrees are rare, indicating a possible polygenic nature of inherited predisposition (Law 1990; Amos et al. 1992; Dragani et al. 1995).

Recent Results in Cancer Research, Vol. 154
© Springer-Verlag Berlin · Heidelberg 1998

Mouse inbred strains with an inherited predisposition or resistance to lung cancer provide an important tool for investigating the genetics of this complex disease (Malkinson 1989; Dragani et al. 1995). Analysis of the genetics of lung tumors started at the turn of the century, when inbred strains of mice with different incidences of lung tumor were first produced. As early as 1926, Lynch suggested that dominant factors might be involved in the inheritance of susceptibility to lung tumors in mice. Later, different studies indicated that mouse strains genetically susceptible to the development of spontaneous lung tumors are also particularly susceptible to lung tumorigenesis induced by chemical carcinogens. However, susceptibility to pulmonary tumorigenesis is not a discrete genetic trait, but rather is expressed in various degrees (Andervont 1939; Heston 1940; Lynch 1940; Shimkin 1940). Heston (1942) stated that a variable number of genetic factors are present among both susceptible strains and resistant ones. More recently, genetic linkage studies have confirmed a polygenic model for lung tumor susceptibility.

The *Pas1* Locus in Mice and Humans

In an (A/J×C3H/He)F2 cross, we have previously mapped the major locus affecting inherited predisposition to lung cancer in mice (pulmonary adenoma susceptibility 1, *Pas1*) onto the mouse chromosome 6, near *Kras2*. A/J mice are susceptible to lung tumors and carry a *Pas1/$^+$* allele (Gariboldi et al., 1993). Two subsequent reports in laboratory mice (*Mus musculus musculus*) and one other study from our laboratory in interspecific mice confirmed both the chromosomal location and the strong contribution of *Pas1* to lung tumor development and identified additional minor loci (Devereux et al. 1994; Festing et al. 1994; Manenti et al. 1995). Recently, we have found that, in addition to the A/J strain, the SWR/J and the BALB/c strains also carry the Pas1/$^+$ allele (Manenti et al. 1997b).

The *Pas1* location around *Kras2* is intriguing and may indicate that the A/J-derived allele of *Kras2* is the factor conferring predisposition to lung cancer. Indeed, somatic mutations frequently occur at the *Kras2* gene in both spontaneous and chemically induced lung tumors (for a review, see Dragani et al. 1995). Furthermore, several studies have reported a very good association between polymorphisms (a 37-bp duplication and several specific base changes) in the second intron of the *Kras2* gene and the susceptibility to develop lung tumors in different inbred or recombinant inbred (RI) strains (Ryan et al. 1987; Malkinson 1991; Chen et al. 1994). We found that, based on these polymorphisms, *M. spretus* should be classified as a susceptible strain. In fact, the *M. spretus Kras2* has only one copy of the 37-bp sequence and shows those polymorphisms at nucleotides 288 and 296 that have been suggested to be typical features of susceptible or high–intermediate strains. However, the *M. spretus* strain shares *Kras2* polymorphisms specific to susceptible strains but not the *Pas1* locus, as excluded by linkage analysis. The close association between the *Kras2* polymorphisms and *Pas1* in *M. musculus* mice, together with the lack of this association in *M. spretus*, may be explained in terms of evolutionary distance. Indeed, *Kras2* and *Pas1* may be closely associated but distinct, and the phylogenetic distance between *M. spretus* and *M. musculus* mice may account for the rare recombination between the genomic structure of *Kras2* intron 2 and *Pas1* (Manenti et al. 1995).

Genetic linkage studies in lung cancer pedigrees and in affected sib pairs would allow unambiguous mapping of the human lung cancer susceptibility gene or genes, but familial clusters of lung cancer are rare, and the poor prognosis of the disease prevents the collection of blood samples in eligible families. The mapping near *Kras2* of a major locus affecting inherited predisposition to lung cancer in mice (*Pas1*; Gariboldi et al. 1993) prompted us to test the possible association of KRAS2 polymorphisms with risk and prognosis of lung adenocarcinoma in humans.

In the Italian population, we carried out a linkage disequilibrium study by genotyping lung adenocarcinoma patients and healthy blood donor subjects for three genetic markers located in the putative region of interest: PTHLH (12p11.2), KRAS2 (12p12.1), and CDKN1B (12p13). Homozygosity of the A2 allele at a *RsaI* polymorphism of KRAS2 proto-oncogene and the presence of allele 2 at a VNTR polymorphism in the PTHLH gene, respectively, showed borderline statistically significant associations with low and high lung cancer risk. Furthermore, the same alleles were significantly associated with a better and poorer tumor prognosis, respectively. In contrast, no association was found for the most telomeric marker, the CDKN1B gene (Manenti et al. 1997 a).

Linkage disequilibrium studies with genetic markers located close to a disease gene have been successful in high-resolution mapping of genes responsible for rare diseases in isolated populations, with the disease gene most probably originating from a few founders. However, the power of this approach is expected to be much lower for common diseases and for studies in heterogeneous populations. Indeed, lung cancer is a common rather than a rare disease, and the Italian population is not an isolated population. Therefore, our results, although preliminary and deserving confirmation in other populations, may provide evidence for the existence of the human PAS1 gene on chromosome 12p11.2–12.1. Similarly, the results also suggest that the mouse model of inherited predisposition to lung tumorigenesis is predictive of a human genetic mechanism of susceptibility to lung cancer.

The *Pas1* Locus

Appropriate crosses that include *Pas1/*[+] mice provide a model system for identifying loci that can modify the lung cancer predisposition phenotype caused by *Pas1*. In an interspecific cross between the A/J and the *M. spretus* strains (termed ASB), approximately 50% of the ASB mice developed lung tumors (Manenti et al. 1995). This is compatible with the presence of one highly penetrant major susceptibility gene deriving from the A/J strain (*Pas1*). However, lung tumor susceptibility was as much as 14-fold lower in the ASB population than in susceptible control (A/J×C57BL/6J)F1 mice (Manenti et al. 1995). This result suggested the existence of one or more *M. spretus*-derived loci that strongly reduced the expressivity of *Pas1* in ASB mice. Indeed, linkage analysis in male and female groups indicated that a genomic region of chromosome 11 was significantly associated with the expressivity of lung tumor susceptibility. Interval mapping analysis showed that the highest lod score occurred at the *Rara* locus. We named the lung tumor resistance locus *Par1* (pulmonary adenoma resistance 1). *Par1* selectively inhibits lung tumor development in $Pas1/^+$ animals and therefore behaves, like a modulator gene of *Pas1* (Manenti et al. 1996).

The lod score peak was located on the region of chromosome 11 that contains the retinoic acid receptor (*Rara*) gene (Manenti et al. 1996). Retinoids and retinoid receptors are known to regulate the proliferative and differentiating capacities of various mammalian cell types, including lung epithelial cells (Ahn et al. 1995; Seewaldt et al. 1995; Chytil 1996). Retinoids are also used in a variety of chemopreventive and chemotherapeutic settings. Indeed, chemoprevention of oral, skin, and head and neck cancers has been reported, as well as the therapy of acute promyelocytic leukemia or of squamous cell carcinoma of the cervix and the skin (for reviews, see Benner et al. 1995; Lotan 1996). The *Rara* gene could therefore be considered, an obvious candidate gene for *Par1*. We analyzed the loss of heterozygosity, nucleotide sequence comparison, gene expression, and biochemical activity of the *Rara* gene from the *M. spretus* ($Par1/^+$) and A/J ($Par1/^-$) mouse strains. The two *Rara* alleles were distinguished by two amino acid variations, but showed similar biochemical activity and expression levels, leading to *Rara* gene being ruled out as a candidate *Par1* gene (Gariboldi et al. 1998).

The mapping of a genetic locus conferring dominant resistance to lung cancer opens important perspectives for the near future. The tumor resistance loci may represent a new special category of genetic modifiers of cancer. Once the relative genes are cloned, it will be possible to study the biochemical mechanisms of inherited resistance to cancer. Eventually, it could be possible to devise new therapeutic strategies for cancer, based on the biochemistry of these genes, that would imply the use of our own natural molecules. Thus the putative anticancer effects of tumor resistance loci would in principle not be conditioned by adverse side effects, as in the case of the therapeutic drugs now available for cancer patients.

Acknowledgements. This work was partially funded by grants from Finalised Project CNR "ACRO" and from the Associazione and Fondazione Italiana Ricerca Cancro (AIRC and FIRC), Italy.

References

Ahn MJ, Langenfeld J, Moasser MM et al (1995) Growth suppression of transformed human bronchial epithelial cells by all-trans-retinoic acid occurs through specific retinoid receptors. Oncogene 11:2357–2364

Amos CI, Caporaso NE, Weston A (1992) Host factors in lung cancer risk: a review of interdisciplinary studies. Cancer Epidemiol Biomarkers Prev 1:505–513

Andervont HB (1939). Pulmonary tumors in mice. VI. Time of appearance of tumors induced in strain A mice following injection of 1,2,5,6-dibenzanthracene. Public Health Rep (Wash) 54:1512–1519

Benner SE, Lippman SM, Hong WK (1995) Current status of retinoid chemoprevention of lung cancer. Oncology 9:205–210

Chen B, Johanson L, Wiest JS et al (1994) The second intron of the K-*ras* gene contains regulatory elements associated with mouse lung tumor susceptibility. Proc Natl Acad Sci USA 91:1589–1593

Chytil F. (1996). Retinoids in lung development. FASEB J 10:986–992

Devereux TR, Wiseman RW, Kaplan N et al (1994) Assignment of a locus for mouse lung tumor susceptibility to proximal chromosome 19. Mamm Genome 5:749–755

Dragani TA, Manenti G, Pierotti MA (1995) Genetics of murine lung tumors. Adv Cancer Res 67:83–112

Festing MFW, Yang A, Malkinson AM (1994) At least four genes and sex are associated with susceptibility to urethane-induced pulmonary adenomas in mice. Genet Res 64:99–106

Gariboldi M, Manenti G, Canzian F et al (1993) A major susceptibility locus to murine lung carcinogenesis maps on chromosome 6. Nature [Genet] 3:132–136

Gariboldi M, Vivat V, De Gregorio L et al (1988) Analysis of *Rara* gene as a candidate for pulmonary adenoma resistance 1 (*Par1*). Mol Carcinog 21:13–16

Heston WE (1940) Lung tumors and heredity. I. The susceptibility of four inbred strains of mice and their hybrids to pulmonary tumors induced by subcutaneous injection. J Natl Cancer Inst 1:105–111

Heston WE (1942) Genetic analysis of susceptibility to induced pulmonary tumors in mice. J Natl Cancer Inst 3:69–78

International Agency for Research on Cancer (1986) Tobacco smoking. IARC Monogr Eval Carcinog Risks Chem Hum 38:35–394

Law MR (1990) Genetic predisposition to lung cancer. Br J Cancer 61:195–206

Loeb LA, Ernster VL, Warner KE et al (1984) Smoking and lung cancer: an overview. Cancer Res 44:5940–5958

Lotan R (1996) Retinoids in cancer chemoprevention. FASEB J 10:1031–1039

Lynch CJ (1926) Studies on the relation between tumor susceptibility and heredity. III. Spontaneous tumors of the lung in mice. J Exp Med 43:339–355

Lynch CJ (1940) Influence of heredity and environment upon number of tumor nodules occurring in lungs of mice. Proc Soc Exp Biol Med 43:186–189

Malkinson AM (1989) The genetic basis of susceptibility to lung tumors in mice. Toxicology 54:241–271

Malkinson AM (1991) Genetic studies on lung tumor susceptibility and histogenesis in mice. Environ Health Perspect 93:149–159

Manenti G, Falvella FS, Gariboldi M et al (1995) Different susceptibility to lung tumorigenesis in mice with an identical *Kras2* intron 2. Genomics 29:438–444

Manenti G, Gariboldi M, Elango R et al (1996) Genetic mapping of a pulmonary adenoma resistance locus (*Par1*) in mouse. Nature [Genet] 12:455–457

Manenti G, De Gregorio L, Pilotti S et al (1997a) Association of chromosome 12p genetic polymorphisms with lung adenocarcinoma risk and prognosis. Carcinogenesis 18:1917–1920

Manenti G, Gariboldi M, Fiorino A et al (1997b) *Pas1* is a common lung cancer susceptibility locus in three mouse strains. Mamm Genome 8:801–809

Ryan J, Barker PE, Nesbitt MN et al (1987) *KRAS2* as a genetic marker for lung tumor susceptibility in inbred mice. J Natl Cancer Inst 79:1351–1357

Seewaldt VL, Johnson BS, Parker MB et al (1995) Expression of retinoic acid receptor beta mediates retinoic acid-induced growth arrest and apoptosis in breast cancer cells. Cell Growth Diff 6:1077–1088

Sellers TA, Potter JD, Bailey-Wilson JE et al (1992) Lung cancer detection and prevention: evidence for an interaction between smoking and genetic predisposition. Cancer Res 52:2694s–2697s

Shimkin MB (1940) Induced pulmonary tumors in mice. I. Susceptibility of seven strains of mice to the action of intravenously injected methylcholanthrene. Arch Pathol 29:229–238

Cancer Epidemiology in Migrant Populations

M. McCredie[1,2]

[1] Department of Preventive and Social Medicine, University of Otago,
Dunedin, New Zealand
[2] Cancer Epidemiology Research Unit, New South Wales Cancer Council,
Sydney, Australia

Abstract

Migrant studies have taken advantage of the wide geographical variation in
cancer risk. Cancer rates in migrants, obtained from routinely collected incidence or mortality statistics, are compared with those in the host country
and in the country of origin; the rate of change with time since migration
(or age at migration) and in subsequent generations is assessed; and the
results are interpreted in the light of differences in socio-economic status
and the degree of cultural assimilation. Rapid changes in cancer risk following migration imply that life-style or evvironmental factors are of overriding
importance in aetiology. The susceptibility of fair-skinned races to ultraviolet
(UV)-associated skin cancers is an example of racial differences based on inherited factors, but the long-term excess or deficit of other cancers in migrants has not yet been atributed definitively to genetic rather than persisting life-style factors. Are there racial differences in metabolism, DNA repair
mechanisms or altered expression of oncogenes or tumour suppressor genes?
Several genetic polymorphisms affecting the metabolism of known occupational carcinogens or hormonal factors do vary by race. While classical
epidemiology has shown that the environment predominates in determining
cancer incidence, molecular epidemiology has identified several examples of
genetically determined differences between races.

Introduction

Migrant studies have taken advantage of the large geographical variation in
cancer risk (Parkin et al. 1977), the term 'geographical' covering a variety of
circumstances including racial, cultural and economic as well as physical
(Muir 1973). Differences in environmental exposures and host susceptibility
are possible explanations for these disparate cancer rates, while the influence
of social class and of the health system in the relevant country (upon which
the diagnosis and reporting of cancers depend) also has to be kept in mind.

Recent Results in Cancer Research, Vol. 154
© Springer-Verlag Berlin · Heidelberg 1998

Investigations of migrant populations may be used to assess the relative importance of environmental and genetic influences in cancer aetiology and to gain insight into the time relationships between environmental exposures and appearance of cancer. Cancer risks may be compared between populations of similar genetic background but living in different physical, social and cultural environments and between populations of different genetic backgrounds living in the same geographical environment (Parkin and Khlat 1996; Thomas and Karagas 1996).

Cancer rates in migrants, obtained from routinely collected incidence or mortality statistics, are compared with those in the host country and in the country of origin, the rate of change with time since migration (or age at migration) and between different generations of migrants (Parkin and Iscovich 1997) is assessed; and the results are interpreted in the light of possible differences in socio-economic status and the degree of cultural assimilation. The major contribution of the earliest formal migrant studies, which were of Japanese (Locke and King 1980) and Chinese (King and Haenszel 1977) migrants to the United States, was to demonstrate that for most cancer sites the risk changed towards that of the host country over time and from one generation to the next. This was irrespective of whether a particular cancer was common or rare in the country of origin.

Migrant studies must be interpreted with caution, as migrants are self-selected and not representative of the population in their country of birth. They may come from particular regions within that country or from specific social or religious groups with distinctive cancer patterns and are likely to be healthier in order to undertake the journey and to pass the medical examination often required by the host country. Migrants generally travel from a poorer to a more industrialized country.

Rapid changes in cancer risk following migration imply that life-style or environmental factors are important in aetiology and that either the relevant agents act late in carcinogenesis (e.g. aspects of diet in respect of large bowel cancer; McMichael et al. 1980) or the introduction of preventive strategies at this stage is effective (e.g. for cancer of cervix; Parkin et al. 1990). However, if the change was slow so that the rate in the migrants remained closer to that in the country of birth, either the migrants retained in their environment factors which modify cancer progression (e.g. southern European migrants with respect to large bowel cancer; McMichael and Giles 1988) or exposures early in life (i.e. at an early stage in carcinogenesis) were more relevant. Epidemiology alone cannot distinguish between the effects of genetic susceptibility from those of persisting cultural influences.

Cancers classified by Thomas and Karagas (1996) as being partly related to a diet rich in animal products (e.g. colon, breast, ovary, prostate, testis) are more common in industrialised countries, being generally linked with a higher standard of living. For these, migrant rates generally increase, except when it is predominantly those of high social class who emigrate. Smoking-related cancers (e.g. lung, larynx, bladder, pancreas) also tend to be more common in migrants than in their country of origin, but here comparisons are less informative, partly because the findings reinforce what is already known about smoking habits. They may, however, be used to identify possible protective factors, e.g. in male Greek migrants to Australia, whose lung cancer rate is lower than expected (McCredie et al. 1990 a) from their prevalence of smoking (McMichael and Giles 1988). Cancers related to contamination of food by carcinogens (e.g. liver, stomach) and those with a probable infectious aetiology (e.g. cervix, liver, nasopharynx), tend to become less common in migrants than in their countries of origin (Thomas and Karagas 1996).

Examples from Routinely Collected Incidence or Mortality Data

The United States, Israel, Australia and Britain, each with large immigrant populations, have been fruitful sources of investigation. Breast cancer rates are somewhat higher in migrants to the United States from Mexico, Puerto Rico, China and Japan than in the country of origin. However, even in their US-born descendants, rates are only half that in the US-born white population (Thomas and Karagas 1996). This is in contrast to the pattern seen in migrants from European countries, whose breast cancer rates generally approach that of US-born white women. In Australia, where information on time since migration is available, breast cancer mortality rates in European migrants increase with the number of years spent in Australia, until after 17 years they are generally at least as high as those in the Australia-born population (Armstrong et al. 1983).

Rates of colon cancer, as for breast cancer, are low in the countries of origin and somewhat higher in migrants from Latin America, China or Japan. However, rates for their US-born descendants more closely approached those of the US-born whites than did rates of breast cancer (Thomas and Karagas 1996). Rates for male European migrants are slightly greater than the rate for US-born whites, while those for female European migrants are more variable but generally similar to that for US-born white women (Thomas and Karagas 1996). Male southern European migrants to Australia had almost the same rates as the Australian-born after 17 years, but rates for female European migrants tended to remain somewhat lower than that for the Australia-born population (Armstrong et al. 1983). This implies that the life-style of the female migrants (probably aspects of diet; McMichael and Giles 1988) changed more slowly than that of their male counterparts. In Israel, there was a marked increase in rates of colon cancer over time both in the migrants and in the Israel-born population (Parkin et al. 1990). When this was taken into account, there was no change in risk of colon cancer, relative to that in the Israel-born population, with increasing duration of residence in Israel for migrants from Europe or America, Western Asia or North Africa, the risk remaining significantly low in the latter.

For stomach cancer, mortality rates were lower in migrants to the United States than in their countries of origin but consistently higher than the rates for US-born whites (Thomas and Karagas 1996). The residual excess in rates was not related to the level of risk in the country of origin. In the offspring of Asian migrants rates fell further but, except in the Chinese, some residual excess risk persisted. Among migrants to Australia, stomach cancer rates declined with the passage of time in Australia, but a small residual excess remained 17 years after migration (Armstrong et al. 1983). A similar excess persisted among migrants to Israel 30 years after migration (Parkin et al. 1990). Dietary factors (smoked, cured, salted or pickled products) have been implicated in the aetiology of stomach cancer, and constituents of fresh fruits and vegetables may be protective (Nomura 1996). The decline in rates of stomach cancer in first-generation migrants provides evidence that exposures in adult life are of aetiological importance.

With Australia's majority of fair-skinned people, high levels of ultraviolet (UV) radiation and past propensity for sunbathing, it is not surprising that its rates of skin cancer, including melanoma, are the highest in the world. Compared with the Australia-born population, migrants from all countries except New Zealand have significantly lower incidence rates of melanoma (McCredie et al. 1990b). Moreover, the risk of dying from melanoma among migrants to Australia from the British Isles and from Central and Eastern Europe was substantially higher if migration had occurred at an early age (Khlat et al. 1992). In the olive-skinned southern Europeans, this effect was not seen. In Israel, the darker-skinned migrants from North Africa and Western Asia have markedly lower rates of melanoma than the Israel-born population even 30 years after migration (Parkin et al. 1990). Although there was an increasing trend in melanoma rates in European and American migrants with time since migration, rates remained 40% below those of the Israel-born population 30 years after migration. The evidence suggests that it is exposure early in life that contributes most to the genesis of melanoma in fair-skinned people.

Examples from Case-Control Studies

Additional information obtained from individuals can enhance knowledge gained from data at the population level. In a case-control study of breast cancer risk in Asian Americans, women who had a single move from East Asia to the United States had a risk of breast cancer which was the same in those who migrated during childhood or early adolescence (<16 years), early reproductive life (16–25 years) or at a later age (26–35 years) (Ziegler et al. 1993). However, the risk was lower among women who migrated after the age of 35. A similar (and interrelated) pattern was seen for duration of residence in the United States. The risk of breast cancer rose during the period 8–14 years of residence but not thereafter. Among Asian American women born in the United States, there was a steadily increasing risk according to whether the mother and one or both grandmothers had been born in the United States. The place of birth of fathers or grandfathers did not influence the risk. Whether the migrants came from an urban or rural environment in Asia also contributed to the picture, with those migrating from urban centres in East Asia having a 40% lower risk of breast cancer than Asian American women born in the United States, while those from rural regions had an even lower risk. These observations point to cultural influences having a much stronger effect than genetic factors in the aetiology of breast cancer.

By contrast, in a case-control study of squamous cell carcinoma of the oesophagus, the risk was higher in African Americans than in US-born whites in each category of alcohol and tobacco consumption (Brown et al. 1994). As the excess of oesophageal cancer in African Americans could not be explained simply by exposure to these known risk factors, a strong genetic influence or some unidentified risk factor is postulated.

Genetic Factors Varying by Race

The susceptibility of fair-skinned races to UV-associated skin cancers is an obvious example of racial differences based on inherited factors. Can the persisting excess or deficit of other cancers in migrants many years after migration be explained by genetic factors rather than by life-style? Are there racial differences in metabolism, or DNA repair mechanisms or altered expression of oncogenes or tumour suppressor genes? Certainly several genetic polymorphisms affecting the metabolism of known occupational carcinogens do vary by race, e.g. CYP1A1 and CYP2D6; for polycyclic aromatic hydrocarbons (Zahm and Fraumeni 1995).

An example of the interaction of environmental and genetic factors is provided by bladder cancer, generally caused by environmental exposure to aromatic amines which are activated by N-hydroxylation and detoxified by N-acetylation or conjugation with glutathione. N-Acetyltransferase is coded by a single gene with two major alleles. Individuals homozygous for the slow acetylator allele display the slow acetylator phenotype, inactivating carcinogenic (and other) aromatic amines more slowly than rapid acetylators. This implies a higher risk of bladder cancer among slow metabolizers. Glutathione S-transferase M1 (GSTM1) is part of a family of enzymes that detoxify reactive chemical entities by promoting their conjugation to glutathione. *GSTM1* is polymorphic in humans with inherited homozygous deficiency being associated with no GSTM1 enzymic activity. 3- and 4-amino-biphenyl (3-ABP, 4-ABP) are aromatic amines present in tobacco smoke. Adducts of these compounds with haemoglobin can be used as biomarkers of the internal dosage of the N-hydroxylated metabolites of 3- and 4-ABP.

Male bladder cancer rates are higher in US-born whites, intermediate in African Americans and lower in Asian Americans (Parkin et al. 1997), although their smoking habits are known to be comparable (Yu et al. 1994). Acetylator status was assessed and the levels of 3- and 4-ABP-haemoglobin adducts measured in 133 Los Angeles men who were either lifetime non-smokers or current smokers; among the latter, there was a reasonably wide range of number of cigarettes smoked per day (Yu et all. 1994). The proportion of slow acetylators was highest in the US-born whites, intermediate in the African Americans and lowest in the Asian Americans. The geometric mean level of 3- and 4-ABP-haemoglobin adducts followed the same pattern, indicating that slow acetylators were exposed to higher levels of activated 3- and 4-ABP in vivo compared with rapid acetylators. There were higher mean levels of adducts in cigarette smokers compared with non-smokers, the levels increasing with the number of cigarettes smoked per day. There were also higher mean levels of adducts in slow acetylators independent of race or of level of smoking. When the *GSTM1* genotype (null versus non-null) was considered together with acetylation phenotype, whites had less than one half the prevalence of the 'protective' profile (rapid acetylator, *GSTM1* non-null) relative to African and Asian Americans (Yu et al. 1995). Thus we have an example in which genetically determined levels of activity of two enzymes appear to contribute substantially to racial susceptibility to one important cancer.

An example of another aspect of metabolism known to vary between races is seen within the prostate, where the conversion of testosterone to dihydroxytestosterone by the enzyme 5-*a*-reductase controls cell division. Since cell proliferation is an important influence in human carcinogenesis, racial variation in the secretion or metabolism of testosterone may be responsible for the worldwide variation in prostate cancer risk. A series of studies has measured two serum markers of 5-*a*-reductase activity ($3a,17\beta$-androstanediol glucuronide and androsterone glucuronide; Ross et al. 1992), a polymorphic marker in the SRD5A2 gene (Reichardt et al. 1995), which encodes the type II steroid 5-*a*-reductase, and the highly polymorphic androgen receptor (AR) (Coetzee and Ross 1994), which is required to translate the androgen response.

Incidence rates of prostate cancer vary widely in African Americans, US-born whites and Japanese (Parkin et al. 1997). Measures of circulating testosterone, sex hormone-binding globulin, two serum markers of 5-*a*-reductase activity (Ross et al. 1992), the CAG repeat in the *AR* gene (Coetzee and Ross 1994) and the V89L missense substitution in the SRD5A2 gene (Reichardt et al. 1995) all parallel the pattern seen for prostate cancer; in addition the TA repeat in the SRD5A2 gene was found only in African Americans (Reichardt et al. 1995). On this evidence, it is not unreasonable to postulate that the racial differences in prostate cancer are largely accounted for by inherited metabolic factors.

It is not yet known to what extent similar mechanisms might operate for other cancers. Polymorphic metabolism may help to explain the residual low risk of breast cancer in the offspring of Japanese migrants, the higher rates of myeloma and cancers of the oesophagus and pancreas in African Americans, and the high rate of lung cancer (especially adenocarcinoma) in Chinese women (Parkin et al. 1997; McCredie et al. 1990b), who have a low prevalence of smoking (Maclennan et al. 1977).

With regard to inherited mutations in 'single' genes (e.g. BRCA1), there are as yet few data on population prevalence and penetrance, and we do not know whether there are significant racial differences. However, 'single' genes are likely to account for only a small minority of cancers (Caporaso and Goldstein 1995).

The Earliest Migrants to Australasia

There appears to be a contrasting pattern of cancer incidence in the people who first migrated to Australia, the Aborigines, and the Maori who ante-dated European settlement in New Zealand. The Aborigines, who now comprise only 1%–2% of the Australian population, were separated from the rest of the world from the time of their arrival perhaps 40,000 years ago and lived as hunters and gatherers until white colonisation 200 years ago. However, there appear to be no differences in cancer incidence between aboriginal and white Australians, which cannot be explained purely by socio-economic or life-style factors. Maori people, who came to New Zealand only about 1000 years ago and were followed by Europeans some 150 years ago, now comprise 13% of the population. As well as showing an excess of cancers associated with a lower standard of living, Maori show some clear-cut differences (Smith et al. 1985). For example, women who have at least half Maori ancestry have a moderate excess risk of breast cancer, despite their reproductive risk factor profile generally being more favourable than that of white New Zealanders (M. McCredie et al., manuscript in preparation). As Maori are on the whole well integrated into New Zealand life, genetic factors may be responsible.

While classical epidemiology has shown that the environment is the predominant factor in determining cancer incidence, molecular epidemiology has identified several examples of genetically determined differences between races and there are likely to be more.

References

Armstrong BK, Woodings TL, Stenhouse NS, McCall MG (1983) Mortality from cancer in migrants to Australia – 1962 to 1971. University of Western Australia, Nedlands

Brown LM, Hoover RN, Greenberg RS, Schoenberg JB, Schwartz AG, Swanson GM, Liff JM, Silverman DT, Hayes RB, Pottern LM (1994) Are racial differences in squamous esophageal cancer explained by alcohol and tobacco use? J Natl Cancer Inst 86:1340–1345

Caporaso N, Goldstein A (1995) Cancer genes: single and susceptibility: exposing the difference. Pharmacogenetics 5:59–63

Coetzee GA, Ross RK (1994) Re: Prostate cancer and the androgen receptor. J Natl Cancer Inst 86:872–873

Khlat M, Vail A, Parkin DM, Green A (1992) Mortality from melanoma in migrants to Australia: variation by age at arrival and duration of stay. Am J Epidemiol 135:1103–1113

King H, Haenszel W (1973) Cancer mortality among foreign- and native-born Chinese in the United States. J Chronic Dis 26:623–646

Locke FB, King H (1980) Cancer mortality among Japanese in the United States. J Natl Cancer Inst 65:1149–1156

Maclennan R, da Costa J, Day NE, Law CH, Ng YK, Shanmugaratnam K (1977) Risk factors for lung cancer in Singapore Chinese, a population with high incidence rates. Int J Cancer 20:854–860

McCredie M, Coates MS, Ford JM (1990a) Cancer incidence in European migrants to New South Wales. Ann Oncol 1:219–225

McCredie M, Coates MS, Ford JM (1990b) Cancer incidence in migrants to New South Wales. Int J Cancer 46:228–232

McMichael AJ, Giles GG (1988) Cancer in migrants to Australia: extending the descriptive epidemiological data. Cancer Res 48:751–756

McMichael AJ, McCall MG, Hartshorne JM, Woodings TL (1980) Patterns of gastrointestinal cancer in European migrants to Australia: the role of dietary change. Int J Cancer 25:431–437

Muir CS (1973) Geographical differences in cancer patterns. IARC Sci Publ 7:1–13

Nomura A (1996) Stomach cancer. In: Schottenfeld D, Fraumeni JF Jr (eds) Cancer epidemiology and prevention, 2nd edn. Oxford University Press, New York, pp 707–724

Parkin DM, Iscovich J (1997) Risk of cancer in migrants and their descendants in Israel: II. Carcinomas and germ-cell tumours. Int J Cancer 70:654–660

Parkin DM, Khlat M (1996) Studies of cancer in migrants: rationale and methodology. Eur J Cancer 32A:761–771

Parkin DM, Steinitz R, Khlat M, Kaldor J, Katz L, Young J (1990) Cancer in Jewish migrants to Israel. Int J Cancer 45:614–621

Parkin DM, Whelan SL, Ferlay J, Raymond L, Young J (eds) (1997) Cancer incidence in five continents, vol 7. IARC Sci Publ 143

Reichardt JKV, Makridakis N, Henderson BE, Yu MC, Pike MC, Ross RK (1995) Genetic variability of the human SRD5A2 gene: implications for prostate cancer risk. Cancer Res 55:3973–3975

Ross RK, Bernstein L, Lobo RA, Shimizu H, Stanczyk FZ, Pike MC, Henderson BE (1992) 5-Alpha-reductase activity and risk of prostate cancer among Japanese and US white and black males. Lancet 339:887–889

Smith AH, Pearce NE, Joseph JG (1985) Major colorectal cancer aetiological hypotheses do not explain mortality trends among Maori and non-Maori New Zealanders. Int J Epidemiol 14:79–85

Thomas DB, Karagas MR (1996) Migrant studies. In Schottenfeld D, Fraumeni JF Jr (eds) Cancer epidemiology and prevention, 2nd edn. Oxford University Press, New York, pp 236–254

Yu MC, Skipper PL, Taghizadeh K, Tannenbaum SR, Chan KK, Henderson BE, Ross RK (1994) Acetylator phenotype, aminobiphenyl-hemoglobin adduct levels, and bladder cancer risk in white, black, and Asian men in Los Angeles, California. J Natl Cancer Inst 86:712–716

Yu MC, Ross RK, Chan KK, Henderson BE, Skipper PL, Tannenbaum SR, Coetzee GA (1995) Glutathione S-transferase M1 genotype affects aminobiphenyl-hemoglobin adduct levels in white, black, and Asian smokers and nonsmokers. Cancer Epidemiol Biomarkers Prev 4:861–864

Zahm SH, Fraumeni JF Jr (1995) Racial, ethnic, and gender variations in cancer risk: considerations for future research. Environ Health Perspect 103:283–286

Ziegler RG, Hoover RN, Pike MC, Hildeheim A, Nomura AMY, West DW, Wu-Williams AH, Kolonel LN, Horn-Ross PL, Rosenthal JF, Hyer MB (1993) Migration patterns and breast cancer risk in Asian-American women. J Natl Cancer Inst 85:1819–1827

Molecular Epidemiology of Hereditary Nonpolyposis Colorectal Cancer in Finland

L. A. Aaltonen

Department of Medical Genetics, Haartman Institute, P.O. Box 21,
00014 University of Helsinki, Finland

Abstract

The population frequency of germline mutations predisposing to hereditary nonpolyposis colorectal cancer (HNPCC) is unknown. Several epidemiological studies have addressed the problem, and estimates on the proportion of the total colorectal cancer burden accounted for by HNPCC have varied between 0.5% and 13%. In the absence of any clinical diagnostic hallmarks, the definition of HNPCC is based on family history. The problem in defining the syndrome is reflected in the wide range of frequency estimates. The molecular background of HNPCC has recently been clarified. Defects in a total of five different mismatch repair genes have been associated with the syndrome. Tumors associated with HNPCC display microsatellite instability (or replication error, RER). RER analysis followed by germline mutation analysis in the mismatch repair genes allows molecular diagnosis in a proportion of HNPCC patients. These diagnostic methods are likely to contribute to our understanding of the epidemiology of HNPCC. In Finland, the centralized health care system, population history, and recent advances in molecular genetic research have together created tools to evaluate the molecular epidemiology of HNPCC in the country.

Introduction

The epidemiology of HNPCC has been studied extensively. Many efforts have been made to define the proportion of the total colorectal cancer burden accounted for by HPNCC. Unlike the hereditary intestinal polyposis syndromes, HNPCC lacks clinical diagnostic hallmarks, and the diagnosis is thus based on family history. The so-called Amsterdam criteria for HNPCC include the following:
1. At least three relatives should have histologically verified colorectal cancer; one of them should be a first-degree relative of the other two.
2. At least two successive generations should be affected.

Recent Results in Cancer Research, Vol. 154
© Springer-Verlag Berlin · Heidelberg 1998

3. In one of the relatives colorectal cancer should be diagnosed under 50 years of age. In addition, the different polyposis syndromes have to be excluded (Vasen et al. 1991).

While these criteria have been very useful in defining the syndrome for research purposes, the lack of specific clinical features and laboratory analyses have hampered epidemiological studies on HNPCC.

Studies to estimate the frequency of HNPCC have typically included a set of unselected colorectal cancer patients, whose family histories have then been scrutinized. Such studies have failed to give consistent results on the frequency of the syndrome, and the results vary from 0.5% to 13% (Aaltonen et al. 1994; Houlston et al. 1992). Recently, the molecular background of the disease has in part been revealed. Germline mutations of five DNA mismatch repair gene – MSH2, MLH 1, PMS1, PMS2, and MSH6 (GTBP) – have been associated with HNPCC (Bronner et al. 1994; Fishel et al. 1993; Leach et al. 1993; Miyaki et al. 1997; Nicolaides et al. 1994; Papadopoulos et al. 1994). Furthermore , it has been shown that tumors derived from HNPCC patients display microsatellite instability, also referred to as the replication error (RER) phenomenon. This can be easily demonstrated by genotyping tumor tissue DNA with microsatellite markers. Tumor tissue DNA displays alleles that are not present in normal tissue DNA. This phenomenon is present in approximately 10%–15% of all colorectal cancers (Aaltonen et al. 1993; Ionov et al. 1993; Thibodeau et al. 1993), but only a subset of the patients have HNPCC. The usefulness of RER testing in the detection of HNPCC is thus still to be clarified.

Tools for Molecular Genetic Research

Many successful studies on hereditary diseases have been conducted in Finland. The success of this kind of research work has been due to several factors. First, Finland has a centralized health care system. People from one geographical area usually attend their local health centers and hospitals, and patient records can be obtained for research purposes from the units of the public health care provided that the authorization of the appropriate officials has been obtained. Second, Finland has a long history of population registration. The Finnish Population Register Center is a computerized unit which holds information on all individuals living in Finland. Every individual has a unique social security number, and the register can identify the first-degree relatives of an individual. Constructing pedigrees with the Population Register information can thus be performed automatically. Pedigrees can often be traced back for centuries with the help of church records, which have the status of an official population registry and have turned out to be very accurate. Third, the data of the Finnish Cancer Registry is an important tool for cancer research. The registry is population based, has a legal status, and has been functioning since 1953. All cancer cases that come to the attention of physicians are reported to the registry. The data set is almost complete and includes information on tumor site, histology, stage and age of the patient at diagnosis. The registry is based on social security numers (Kyllönen et al. 1987; Teppo et al. 1994). Thus pedigrees constructed in the Population Registry can be automatically linked to the Cancer Registry files, and pedigrees depicting family history of cancer can be drawn. Cross-linking two registries, as described above, is a very potential tool, and discussion about the ethical implications of such procedures should be conducted. In the case of cross-linking the Cancer Registry data with the Population Registry data, the conclusion has been that such a procedure can be performed for research purposes and after authorization by the appropriate officials. Fourth, the unique population history of the Finns has laid the foundation for effective identification of genes underlying hereditary diseases. Although Finland has been inhabited for thousands of years, the population is hypothesized to have expanded from a small number to the present 5 million within the last 2000 years. During this time, there has been little immigration. Thus same hereditary diseases are rarer in Finns than in other European populations, and some are more frequent. Examples of the former are cystic fibrosis and phenylketonuria. The more frequent diseases comprise many rare recessive disorders as well as some dominant traits. The genetic homogeneity of the population greatly facilitates disease gene identification studies. The background of a hereditary disease is likely to be more homogenous in this population, whereas similar studies in more mixed populations could be hampered by a mixed molecular background, genetic heterogeneity, and different mutations in a homogenous disease (de la Chapelle 1993). The use of linkage disequilibrium in mapping disease genes in Finns is a good example of the advantages of the population structure for the molecular studies (Hästbacka et al. 1992). Homogenous populations greatly facilitate not only studies on mendelian disease genes, but also identification of genes underlying multifactorial diseases.

HNPCC Mutations in the Finnish Population

After the MSH2 (chromosome 2p) and MLH1 (chromosome 3p) gene loci had been identified (Lindblom et al. 1993; Peltomäki et al. 1993), linkage studies were performed in Finnish HNPCC families. While little evidence of linkage to 2p was obtained, multiple families displayed close linkage to 3p markers. Interestingly, many of the families (11 out of 18 studied) turned out to have a shared ancestry and/or shared 3p marker haplotype (Nyström-Lahti et al. 1994). This indicated that a single ancestral founder mutation might underlie a large proportion of the Finnish HNPCC cases. Sequence analysis of the newly identified MLH1 gene revealed a deletion of exon 16 at the cDNA level, which turned out to be due to a 3.5-kb genomic deletion comprising both this exon and the intronic sequence (referred as mutation I). This deletion was perhaps promoted by an Alu-mediated recombination

(Nyström-Lahti et al. 1995). Most families segregating this mutation originated from Eastern Finland. Another relatively frequent MLH1 mutation, destroying the splice acceptor site of exon 6 (referred as mutation II), was also detected. At present, more than 50 families with either MSH2 or MLH1 mutations have been identified, and the majority of these segregate mutation I or mutation II.

The age of the two founder mutations was subsequently studied by analyzing the extent of the conserved haplotype, and it was concluded that mutation I was introduced to the Finnish population 16–43 generations (400–1075 years) ago. Mutation II was estimated to be five to 21 generations (125–525 years) old. These estimates were in agreement with genealogical data, suggesting a common ancestor born 500 and 300 years ago, respectively (Moisio et al. 1996).

To determine the population frequency of MSH2 and MLH1 mutations, a prospective multicenter study was launched. In this work, normal and tumor tissue is prospectively collected, after informed consent, from hundreds of colorectal cancer patients. Nine central hospitals covering South-Eastern Finland are participating in the study. The tumors are analyzed for RER using multiple microsatellite markers. The RER-positive cases are then scrutinized for mutations in the MLH1 and MSH2 mismatch repair genes by genomic sequencing. However, regardless of their RER status, all samples are analyzed for the founder mutation 1 (easy to test, cannot be detected by sequencing). Preliminary results indicate that the proportion of all colorectal cancers accounted for by HNPCC (as defined by germline mutations in the MSH2 and MLH1 genes) is smaller than estimated in many previous epidemiological studies. The results of the study suggest that routine molecular screening of colorectal cancer patients for HNPCC is not warranted with the present methods. The family histories of all patients are scrutinized with the help of the Population Registry and Cancer Registry. Patients frequently have a first-degree relative with colorectal or endometrial cancer. It is likely that MLH1 and MSH2 are not the only major genes predisposing to familial nonpolyposis colorectal cancer. In the Jewish population, a mutation in the APC gene that confers an increased risk for colorectal cancer without polyposis has been identified (Laken et al. 1997). It is likely that examples of other colorectal cancer susceptibility genes will be identified in the future. Thus the absence of MSH2 and MLH1 mutations should not affect clinical screening of a family with colon cancer if the family history indicates that such screening is necessary.

It is important to diagnose HNPCC families. A recent 10-year study conducted in Finland showed that clinical screening programs could significantly reduce the incidence of colorectal cancer in the screening group as compared with the control group and completely prevented colorectal cancer-related deaths (Järvinen et al. 1995). The psychosocial effects of the molecular diagnosis of HNPCC must be carefully monitored, and genetic testing must always be accompanied by appropriate counseling. However, the rationale of such testing in HNPCC is clear, and if patients wish to participate in the clinical cancer screening programs offered, they are likely to benefit in view of reduced cancer morbidity and mortality. It should be emphasized that clinical screening must be made available to patients regardless of their willingness to take predictive genetic testing.

References

Aaltonen LA, Peltomäki P, Leach F, Sistonen P, Pylkkänen L, Mecklin J-P, Järvinen H, Powell S, Jen J, Hamilton S, Petersen G, Kinzler K, Vogelstein B, de la Chapelle A (1993) Clues to the pathogenesis of familial colorectal cancer. Science 260:812–816

Aaltonen LA, Sankila R, Mecklin J-P, Järvinen H, Pukkala E, Peltomäki P, de la Chapelle A (1994) A novel approach to estimate the proportion of hereditary non-polyposis colorectal cancer of total colorectal cancer burden. Cancer Detect Prev 18:57–63

Bronner CE, Baker SM, Morrison PT, Warren G, Smith LG, Lescoe MK, Kane M, Earabino C, Lipford J, Lindblom A, Tannergård P, Bollag RJ, Godwin AR, Ward DC, Nordensjöld M, Fishel R, Kolodner R, Liskay M (1994) Mutation in the DNA mismatch repair gene homologue hMLH1 is associated with hereditary non-polyposis colon cancer. Nature 368:258–261

De la Chapelle A (1993) Disease gene mapping in isolated human populations: the example of Finland. J Med Genet 30:857–865

Fishel R, Lescoe MK, Rao MRS, Copeland NG, Jenkins NA, Garber J, Kane M, Kolodner R (1993) The human mutator gene homolog MSH2 and its association with hereditary nonpolyposis colorectal cancer. Cell 75:1027–1038

Hästbacka J, de la Chapelle A, Kaitila I, Sistonen P, Weaver A, Lander E (1992) Linkage disequilibrium mapping in isolated founder populations: diastrophic dysplasia in Finland. Nature [Genet] 2:204–211

Houlston RS, Collins A, Slack J, Morton NE (1992) Dominant genes for colorectal cancer are not rare. Ann Hum Genet 56:99–103

Ionov Y, Peinado MA, Malkhosyan S, Shibata D, Perucho M (1993) Ubiquitous somatic mutations in simple repeated sequences reveal a new mechanism for colonic carcinogenesis. Nature 363:558–561

Järvinen HJ, Mecklin J-P, Sistonen P (1995) Screening reduces colorectal cancer rate in families with hereditary nonpolyposis colorectal cancer. Gastroenterology 108:1405–1411.

Kyllönen J, Teppo L, Lehtonen M (1987) Completeness and accuracy of registration of colorectal cancer in Finland. Ann Chir Gynaecol 76:185–190

Laken SJ, Petersen GM, Gruber SB, Oddoux C, Ostrer H, Giardiello FM, Hamilton SR, Hampel H, Markowitz A, Klimstra D, Jhanwar S, Winawer S, Offit K, Luce MC, Kinzler KW, Vogelstein B (1997) Familial colorectal cancer in Ashkenazim due to a hypermutable tract in APC. Nature Genet 17:79–83

Lindblom A, Tannergård P, Werelius B, Nordenskjöld M (1993) Genetic mapping of a second locus predisposing to hereditary non-polyposis colon cancer. Nature [Genet] 5:279–282

Leach FS, Nicolaides NC, Papadopoulos N, Liu B, Jen J, Parsons R, Peltomäki P, Sistonen P, Aaltonen LA, Nyström-Lahti M, Guan X-Y, Fournier REK, Todd S, Lewis T, Leach RJ, Naylor SL, Weissenbach J, Mecklin J-P, Järvinen H, Petersen GM, Hamilton SR, Green J, Jass J, Watson P, Lynch HT, Trent JM, de la Chapelle A, Kinzler KW, Vogelstein B (1993) Mutations of a mutS homolog in hereditary nonpolyposis colorectal cancer. Cell 75:1215–1225

Miyaki M, Konishi M, Tanaka K, Kikuchi-Yanoshita R, Muraoka M, Yasuno M, Igan T, Koike M, Chiba M, Mori T (1997) Germline mutation of MSH6 as the cause of hereditary nonpolyposis colorectal cancer Nature [Genet] 17:271–272

Moisio A-L, Sistonen P, Weissenbach J, de la Chapelle A, Peltomäki P (1996) Age and origin of two common MLH1 mutations predisposing to hereditary colon cancer. Am J Hum Genet 59:1243–1251

Nicolaides NC, Papadopoulos N, Liu B, Wei YF, Carter KC, Ruben SM, Rosen CA, Haseltine WA, Fleischmann RD, Fraser CM, Adams MD, Venter JC, Dunlop MG, Hamilton SR, Petersen GM, de la Chapelle A, Vogelstein B, Kinzler K (1994) Mutations of two PMS homologues in hereditary nonpolyposis colon cancer. Nature 371:75–80

Nyström-Lahti M, Sistonen P, Mecklin J-P, Pylkkänen L, Aaltonen L, Järvinen H, Weissenbach J, de la Chapelle A, Peltomäki P (1994) Close linkage to chromosome 3p and conservation of ancestral founding haplotype in hereditary nonpolyposis colorectal cancer families. Proc Natl Acad Sci USA 91:6054–6058

Nyström-Lahti M, Kristo P, Nicolaides NC, Chang S-Y, Aaltonen LA, Moisio AL, Järvinen HJ, Mecklin J-P, Kinzler KW, Vogelstein B, de la Chapelle A, Peltomäki P (1995) Founding mutations and Alu-mediated recombination in hereditary colon cancer. Nature 1:1203–1206

Papadopoulos N, Nicolaides NC, Wei Y-F, Ruben SM, Carter KC, Rosen CA, Haseltine WA, Fleichmann RD, Fraser CM, Adams MD, Venter JC, Hamilton SR, Petersen GM, Watson P, Lynch HT, Peltomäki P, Mecklin J-P, de la Chapelle A, Kinzler KW, Vogelstein B (1994) Mutation of a mutL homolog is associated with hereditary colon cancer. Science 263:1625–1629

Peltomäki P, Aaltonen LA, Sistonen P, Pylkkänen L, Mecklin J-P, Järvinen H, Green J, Jass J, Weber J, Leach F, Petersen G, Hamilton S, de la Chapelle A, Vogelstein BA (1993) Genetic mapping of a locus predisposing to human colorectal cancer. Science 260:810–812

Teppo L, Pukkala E, Lehtonen M (1994) Data quality and quality control of a population-based cancer registry. Acta Oncol 33:365–369

Thibodeau SN, Bren G, Schaid D (1993) Microsatellite instability in cancer of the proximal colon. Science 260:816–819

Vasen HFA, Mecklin J-P, Meera Khan P, Lynch HT (1991) The international collaborative group on hereditary non-polyposis colorectal cancer (ICG-HNPCC). Dis Colon Rectum 34:424–425

VII. Virus and Cancer:
The HBV/HCV Paradigm

The PreS2 Activators of the Hepatitis B Virus: Activators of Tumour Promoter Pathways

E. Hildt[1] and P. H. Hofschneider[2]

[1] Institute of Experimental Surgery, Technical University of Munich,
Ismaninger Strasse 22, 81675 Munich, Germany
[2] Max Planck Institute of Biochemistry, Department of Viral Research,
Am Klopferspitz 18 a, 80636 Martinsried, Germany

Abstract

In addition to causing acute and chronic hepatitis, hepatitis B virus (HBV) is considered to be a major cliological factor in the development of human hepatocellular carcinoma (HCC). Epidemiological studies have demonstrated an approximately 10-fold increase in the relative risk of HCC among HBV carried compared to noncarriers. Almost all HBV-associated HCCs studied so far harbor chromosomally integrated HBV DNA. Integrated viral DNA can encode two types of transcriptional activators, the HBx protein and the PreS2 activators [the large surface proteins (LHBs) and truncated middle surface proteins (MHBs)]. The activator function of the PreS2 activators is based on the cytoplasmic orientation of the PreS2 domain. The PreS2 domain is PKC-dependent phosphorylated. Moreover, the PreS2 domain binds of PKCα/β and triggers a PKC-dependent activation of the c-Raf-1/MAP2-kinase signal transduction cascade, resulting in an activation of transcription factors such as AP-1 and NF-kB. Furthermore, by activation of this signaling cascade, the PreS2 activators cause an increased proliferation rate of hepatocytes. According to the two-step model of carcinogenesis (initiation/promotion), the PreS2 activators could exert a tumour-promoter-like function by activation of the PKC/c-Raf-1/MAP2-kinase signaling cascade: cells harboring critical mutations (initiation) may be positively selected (promotion). Such a multistep process may account for the long latency period in HCC development, but it also leads to the hypothesis that each tumor reflects an individual case.

Introduction

About 15% of all tumours in humans worldwide are associated with viruses (Parkin et al. 1984). Viruses can therefore be considered to be the most oncogenic agents. In addition to causing acute and chronic hepatitis, the human hepatitis B virus (HBV) is considered to be a major etiological factor in the development of human hepatocellular carcinoma (HCC) (for a review,

Recent Results in Cancer Research, Vol. 154
© Springer-Verlag Berlin · Heidelberg 1998

see Buendia 1992). HBV is considered to be causative in the development of tumours in about 30% of all virus-associated tumours. At present, more than 200 million people are chronically infected, and every year 2 million die as a result of the infection, 700 000 of whom die of HBV-associated HCC (Szmuness 1978). Epidemiological studies demonstrated an approximately 100-fold increase in the relative risk of HCC among HBV carriers compared to non-carriers (Beasley et al. 1981; Beasley 1988). Almost all HBV-associated HCCs studied so far harbour chromosomally integrated HBV DNA. The long latency period between infection and the development of HCC cannot be explained by common mechanisms of viral oncogenesis; accordingly, HBV harbours no classical oncogene. HBV DNA does not integrate at specific sites of the host genome. Thus a common *cis*-effect onto flanking cellular genes can be ruled out as a general mechanism of HBV-associated carcinogenesis.

Integrated HBV DNA can encode for two types of transcriptional activators: the HBx (Twu and Schloemer 1987; Wollersheim et al. 1988; Zahm et al. 1988) and the PreS2 activators LHBs (large hepatitis B virus surface protein) and MHBs[t] (C-terminally truncated middle surface proteins) (Caselmann et al. 1990; Kekulé et al. 1990; Hildt et al. 1996b). The HBx activators have been extensively described (for reviews, see Kekulé 1994; Caselmann 1996; Hildt et al. 1996c), whereas the structure and the transcriptional activator mechanism of the family of the PreS2 activators has not yet been very well characterized. Since new results on the PreS2 activators have recently been obtained, we will focus on a putative role of the PreS2 activators in the process of HBV-associated hepatocarcinogenesis.

Genomic Organization of the Hepadnaviridae

Hepadnaviridae are subdivided into mammalian and avian-hepadnaviruses. The mammalian hepadnaviruses include HBV, which can also infect chimpanzees, woodchuck hepatitis virus (WHV) and the ground squirrel hepatitis B virus (GSHV). The duck hepatitis B virus (DHBV) and the heron hepatitis B virus belong to the avian-hepadnaviruses. The hepadnaviridae share the following features:
- An only partially double-stranded genomic DNA comprising a complete coding strand (negative strand) and an incomplete non-coding strand (positive strand).
- An RNA-dependent DNA polymerase contained in the nucleocapsid of the virion.
- Replication through a pre-genomic RNA template, which relates the hepadnaviruses to the retroviruses.
- A high degree of species and organ specificity.

The hepadnadiruses are the smallest known DNA viruses. The partially double-stranded DNA genome is about 3 kb in size, and in the case of HBV it is 3.2 kb. The viral genome uses all three reading frames and contains at least four different open reading frames coding for the viral polymerase, the Hbc and HBe antigen, the HBx activator and the preS/S gene encoding the three surface antigens (for details, see Ganem 1991; Caselmann, 1996). The preS/S gene consists of a single open reading frame, which is divided into the preS1, the preS2 and the S region by three in-frame ATG codons. By alternate translational initiation at each of the three AUG codons, the large (LHBs; PreS1+PreS2+S), the middle (MHBs; PreS2+S) or the small (SHBs; S) surface protein can be synthesized, all of which can be glycosylated at amino acid 146 of the S region. MHBs can also be glycosylated at amino acid 4 of the PreS2 region and can therefore be detected in three forms: p30 (representing the unglycosylated protein), gp33 (representing the monoglycosylated form) and gp36 (representing the biglycosylated protein) (Stibbe and Gerlich 1983). MHBs harbours three hydrophobic regions serving as transmembrane regions. MHBs is therefore synthesized as an integral membrane protein, which is secreted after modifications in the endothelial reticulum (ER) and Golgi complex. MHBs is not directly essential for the assembly of the viral particle. Surprisingly, LHBs is not glycosylated in the PreS2 region. Recent reports demonstrated that, in the case of LHBs, the PreS1/PreS2 domains are not co-translationally translocated across the ER membrane, resulting in a cytoplasmic orientation, since the transmembrane region I (according to the structure of SHBs and MHBs) is not used (Bruss et al. 1994; Ostapchuk et al. 1994). The transmembrane region II, however, is translocated. During viral assembly, a fraction of the PreS1/PreS2 domain is post-translationally translocated across the membrane, resulting in a localization on the viral surface of the PreS1/PreS2 domain. In contrast to MHBs, the LHBs protein expressed in the absence of MHBs and SHBs is not secreted (Chisari et al. 1986, 1989) and becomes intracellularly enriched. In the case of strong overexpression, intracellular accumulation of LHBs can result in the development of ground glass hepatocytes.

In chronic infection, single or multiple copies of the HBV DNA can be integrated into the host genome. This apparently occurs before the later development of HCC. Almost all HBV-associated HCCs harbour integrated HBV DNA. The integrated HBV DNA in the tumours is usually rearranged and partially deleted. Each tumour is monoclonal with respect to the HBV integrate, and the tumours have individual integration patterns. As a common feature of many HBV integrates isolated from HCCs, destruction of the open reading frames coding for the viral polymerase and the Hbc antigen can be observed, resulting in a replication-incompetent HBV genome. The open reading frame of the S region and, in about 60% of cases the open reading frame of the HBx activator remain intact; in the case of the S open reading frame, however, truncation of the 3' end can frequently be observed (Yamamoto et al. 1993; Schlüter et al. 1994). From these 3' end truncated preS/S genes, C-terminally truncated MHBs (MHBs[t]) can be expressed.

The presence and functionality of the MHBs[t] activator was first observed by analysis of the subcloned unique 5.6-kb integrate of the human hepatoma cell line huH4 (Kekulé et al. 1990) and then in HCC tissue comprising a

2.0 kb integrate (Caselmann et al. 1990). Deletions of 3′-terminal sequences of the sequences coding for the surface antigen which could result in expression of the MHBs[t] activators can be observed in one third of the integrates derived from HBV-associated HCCs (Yamamoto et al. 1993; Schlüter et al. 1994).

Structural Characterization of the PreS2 Activators MHBs[t] and LHBs

Initial detailed analysis of subcloned viral HBV DNA revealed that the transcriptional activator function of MHBs[t] is generated by 3′ truncations within a considerably extended area of the preS2/S gene (Lauer et al. 1992, Natoli et al. 1992). It was shown that generation of the transcriptional activator function requires deletion of the sequences encoding the hydrophobic region III, corresponding to the 70 C-terminal amino acids of full-length MHBs (Fig. 1b). The transcriptional activator function of MHBs[t] does not require the PreS1 region (Kekulé et al. 1990). In co-transfection experiments, stepwise deletions and mutagenesis demonstrated that a frameshift at $nt_{HBV}129$, corresponding to amino acid 47, abolishes the activator function, whereas truncation at $nt_{HBV}221$, corresponding to amino acid 76, generates a functional MHBs[t] activator (Lauer et al. 1992). This fragment corresponds to the truncated preS2/S[t] originally isolated from the human hepatoma cell line

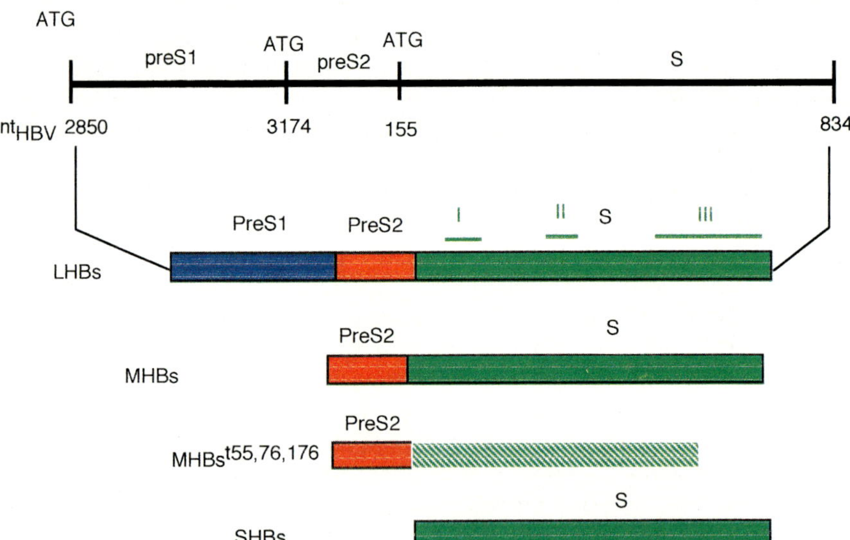

Fig. 1. Genomic organization of the surface antigen. Structure of the preS/S gene (subtype ayw) and representation of the large, middle and small three surface proteins LHBs, MHBs and SHBs, respectively. The structure of the functional MHBs[t] activators is given. The *hatched box* indicates the range which can be deleted for generation of functional MHBs[t] activators. *I, II* and *III* mark the position of the transmembrane regions. *HBV,* hepatitis B virus

huH4. Based on these data, MHBs^{t76} was considered to be a minimal transcriptional activator, and a TAO region (*trans*-activity on) was defined as encompassing deletions within nt$_{HBV}$573-221, corresponding to MHBs$^{t194-76}$ (Lauer et al. 1992).

In order to gain better insight into the mechanism of MHBs^t-dependent transcriptional activation, a preliminary analysis of the subcellular localization of MHBs^t was performed using the MHBs^{t167} activator (Meyer et al. 1992a). An ER localization was suggested in this study. A more detailed analysis based on immunofluorescence and various cell fractionation experiments revealed that MHBs^{t76} is indeed an ER-localized activator (Hildt et al. 1993). Moreover, this study demonstrated that, in contrast to full-length MHBs, MHBs^{t76}, is retained at the ER and does not enter the Golgi complex and therefore is not secreted.

On the basis of these observations, it was speculated that intracellular retention per se causes the functional difference between the structure protein MHBs and the transcriptional activator MHBs^t (Meyer et al. 1992a). It was hypothesized that the intracellular retention causes ER overloading and subsequent generation of radicals. At first glance, this appears to be a possible mechanism, especially for the observed MHBs^t -dependent activation of nuclear factor (NF)-κB (Meyer et al. 1992; Lauer et al. 1994; Pahl and Bäuerle 1994). However, in a comparative study, it was shown that retention of full-length MHBs in the ER by fusion of the ER retention signal KDEL to its C terminus is not sufficient for the activation of NF-κB or the generation of any transcriptional activator function (Hildt et al. 1995).

The real reason for the functional difference between the full-length structural protein MHBs and the activator protein MHBs^t was revealed by the observation that MHBs^{t76} derived from Sf9 cells (Hildt et al. 1993) or HepG2 cells (Hildt et al. 1995, 1996a) is unglycosylated, although the glycosylation site at Asn-4 is still present. Based on this finding, it was speculated that, in all functional MHBs^t activators, the glycosylation site at amino acid 4 of the PreS2 domain is inaccessible to the glycosyltransferases, which are located in the lumen of the ER-Golgi network. Proteolytic digestion of microsomal vesicles derived from MHBs or MHBs^{t76} producing Sf9 cells revealed that the PreS2 domain is only accessible for the proteases in the case of MHBs^{t76}. This shows that, in the case of MHBs^{t76}, the PreS2 domain faces the cytoplasm (corresponding to the outside of the microsomal vesicles), whereas in the case of full-length MHBs the PreS2 domain leads into the lumen of the ER (Hildt et al. 1995). This topological difference not only causes the functional difference between MHBs and MHBs^t, but it also seems to explain the intracellular retention. It has been shown that only properly folded proteins are secreted (Hurtley and Helenius 1989). The inverted membrane topology (Fig. 2) of the PreS2 domain at MHBs^t with respect to MHBs represents an obvious misfolding and can therefore be considered to cause the intracellular retention.

The cytoplasmic orientation of the PreS2 domain was found to be a prerequisite for transcriptional activation; on the other hand, in the case of MHBs^{t76}, which was thus far considered to be a minimal transcriptional acti-

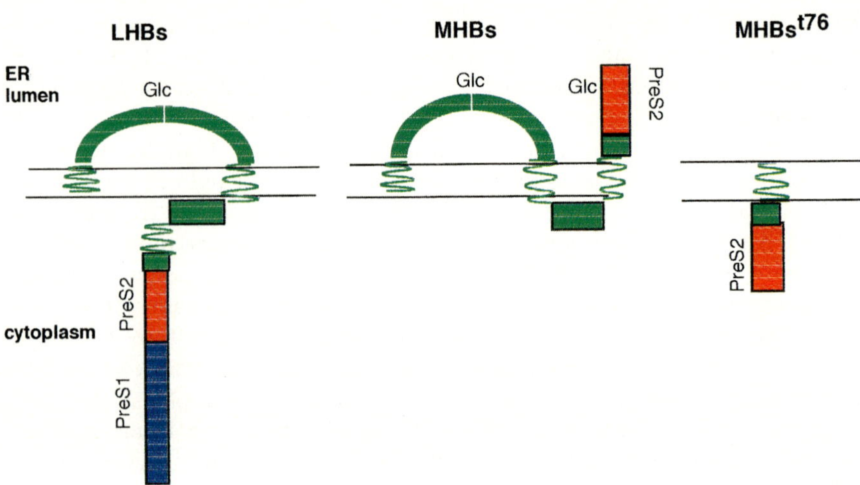

Fig. 2. Transmembrane topology of LHBs, MHBs and MHBs^t. The luminal and cytoplasmic sides of the endoplasmic reticulum (*ER*) membrane are indicated. In MHBs, the PreS2 region faces the lumen of the ER; in MHBs^t and LHBs, the PreS2 region projects into the cytoplasm

vator, the hydrophobic transmembrane region encompassing amino acids 63–76 is buried in the ER membrane, and interaction with cytosolic binding partners can thus be ruled out. It was therefore investigated whether the insertion of MHBs^t proteins into the ER membrane is essential for their functionality. MHBs^t proteins lacking all three transmembrane regions were found to be functional transcriptional activators as well (Hildt et al. 1995). As demonstrated by immunofluorescence and cell fractionation, they are not associated with the ER membrane and therefore homogeneously distributed all over the cytoplasm and the nucleus (Hildt et al. 1995). Based on these observations, two subtypes of MHBs^t activators can be distinguished: (1) the ER-localized subtype (i.e. MHBs^t76) and (2) the non-ER-localized subtype (i.e. MHBs^t63). Both subtypes have in common the fact that, in contrast to full-length MHBs, the PreS2 domain is exposed to the cytoplasm. In cotransfection experiments stepwise deletion revealed that the minimal transcriptional activator unit is located between amino acids 6 and 52 of the PreS2 domain (Hildt et al. 1995). This is in accordance with the previously described data, which demonstrated that a frameshift mutation at $nt_{HBV}129$, corresponding to amino acid 47, abolishes the transcriptional activator function (Lauer et al. 1992).

Since functional MHBs^t activators were found to be unglycosylated, highly purified MHBs^t activators could be isolated not only from eukaryotic expression systems (Sf9 cells, HepG2, CCL13 cells; Hildt et al. 1993, 1995, 1996a), but also from an *Escherichia coli* system (Hildt et al. 1993, 1995). The functionality of these MHBs^t proteins isolated from different sources was shown by electric field-mediated transfer into reporter cell lines (Hildt et al. 1993,

1995, 1996a). Various deletion and point mutants isolated from the bacterial expression system were used for physicochemical analysis by circular dichroism (CD) spectroscopy and gel filtration. The gel filtration experiments demonstrated that MHBs[t] proteins form stable dimers. By mutagenesis and subsequent CD spectroscopic analysis of the mutated fragments, it was found that dimerization is mediated by an amphipathic α-helix within the PreS2 domain (aa 41–52). The integrity of the α-helix is a prerequisite for both the transcriptional activator function and the dimerization.

A detailed analysis of highly purified MHBs[t76] derived from eukaryotic expression systems by two-dimensional gel electrophoresis, electrospray mass spectrometry and metabolic labelling using ^{32}P-ortho-phosphate revealed that, in contrast to full-length MHBs, both subtypes of the MHBs[t] proteins are phosphoproteins (Hildt et al. 1996a, 1998; Urban et al. 1997). For both subtypes, the phosphorylation site was mapped to a Ser/Thr cluster at amino acids 27–31. Destruction of the phosphorylation site abolished the transcriptional activator function.

Identification of LHBs as a Transcriptional Activator

The cytoplasmic orientation of the PreS2 domain was shown to cause the transcriptional activator function of MHBs[t]. Recent reports demonstrated that, during protein biosynthesis of LHBs, a fraction of the PreS1/PreS2 domain faces the cytoplasm (Bruss et al. 1994; Ostapchuk et al. 1994). An analysis of the transcriptional activator potential of LHBs revealed that, like MHBs[t] proteins, it is indeed a transcriptional activator (Hildt et al. 1996b). The activator function of LHBs is not affected by the co-expression of SHBs and MHBs. An analysis of the mechanism of LHBs-dependent transcriptional activation revealed that MHBs[t] and LHBs share the same mechanism for transcriptional activation (Hildt et al. 1996b; also see below), since in both cases the cytoplasmic orientation of the PreS2 domain is a prerequisite for the transcriptional activator function. On the basis of these observations, LHBs and the MHBs[t] activators have been included in the family of PreS2 activators. Most importantly, however, in contrast to the coding sequences for MHBs[t], which are only generated during the integration process, the sequence encoding LHBs is constitutively present in the viral genome. It is therefore tempting to speculate on the role of the activator function of LHBs during viral replication, i.e. LHBs could trigger activation of the other viral promoters. An elevated LHBs to SHBs ratio causes intracellular retention of LHBs. This intracellularly retained LHBs could exert a transcriptional activator effect, resulting in enhanced SHBs synthesis and ensuring the proper ratio of LHBs to SHBs for the assembly of the viral particle. This hypothesis is supported by the recent observation that, in the case of DHBV, which lacks an HBx homologous protein, the PreS/S protein also shows transcriptional activator function (Rothmann et al. submitted).

Mechanism of PreS2 Activator-Dependent Transcriptional Activation

Since LHBs- and MHBs[t]-dependent transcriptional activation is based on the cytoplasmic orientation of the PreS2 domain, and since in a recent report it was shown that LHBs- and MHBs[t]-dependent transcriptional activation is mediated by the same pathways (Hildt et al. 1996b, 1998), the MHBs[t]-dependent transcriptional activation here is considered to be paradigmatic for all PreS2 activators. The PreS2-dependent activation is pleiotropic and shows no tissue specificity. A wide variety of different target sequences was found to be activated by the MHBs[t] proteins (Table 1). MHBs[t] binds directly neither to DNA nor to DNA-binding proteins. MHBs[t] activators exert their effects through the activation of various non-related transcription factors such as AP-1, AP-2 and NF-κB (see Table 1). From this it can be concluded that MHBs[t] interferes with one or more early steps of signal transduction.

By various experimental approaches protein kinase C (PKC)-α and PKC-β were identified as cellular binding partners of the PreS2 domain (Hildt et al. 1998). Moreover, MHBs[t] was found to be a novel activator of PKC-α/β. The MHBs[t]-dependent activation of PKC is independent of diacylglycerol (DAG), but requires the presence of Ca^{2+}. MHBs[t] therefore represents a novel type of PKC activator. Inhibition of PKC or its depletion demonstrated that its acti-

Table 1. Overview of the promoters and minimal promoter elements activated by MHBs[t]

Target sequences	Transcription factor	References
Cellular promoters		
c-myc/P2	AP-1	Kekulé et al. 1990; Lauer et al. 1994; Natoli et al. 1992
c-Ha-ras	SP-1	Meyer et al. 1992b
c-fos	SRF	Natoli et al. 1992; Lauer et al. 1994
α_1-Antitrypsin		Meyer et al. 1992b
Interleukin-6	MRF	Meyer et al. 1992b
Viral Promoter/enhancer		
HBV enhancer I		Meyer 1992b
RSV-LTR		Lauer et al. 1994
SV40 early promoter/enhancer		Kekulé et al. 1990; Caselmann et al. 1990
HSV TK-promoter		Meyer et al. 1992b
HIV1-LTR	NFκB	Meyer et al. 1992a
HTLV1-LTR		Meyer et al. 1992a
Synthetic minimal promoters		
AP-1	AP-1	Hildt et al. 1993
AP-2	AP-2	Lauer et al. 1994
NF-κB	NFκB	Natoli et al. 1992; Meyer et al. 1992
SP-1	SP-1	Meyer et al. 1992b
SRE	SRF	Natoli et al. 1992
TRE		

HBV, hepatitis B virus; HSV, herpes simplex virus; HIV, human immunodeficiency virus; HTLC, human T-lymphotrophic virus; NF, nuclear factor; RSV, Rous sarcoma virus; LTR, long terminal repeat; SRE, serum response element; SRF, serum response factor; TRE, TPA responsive element.

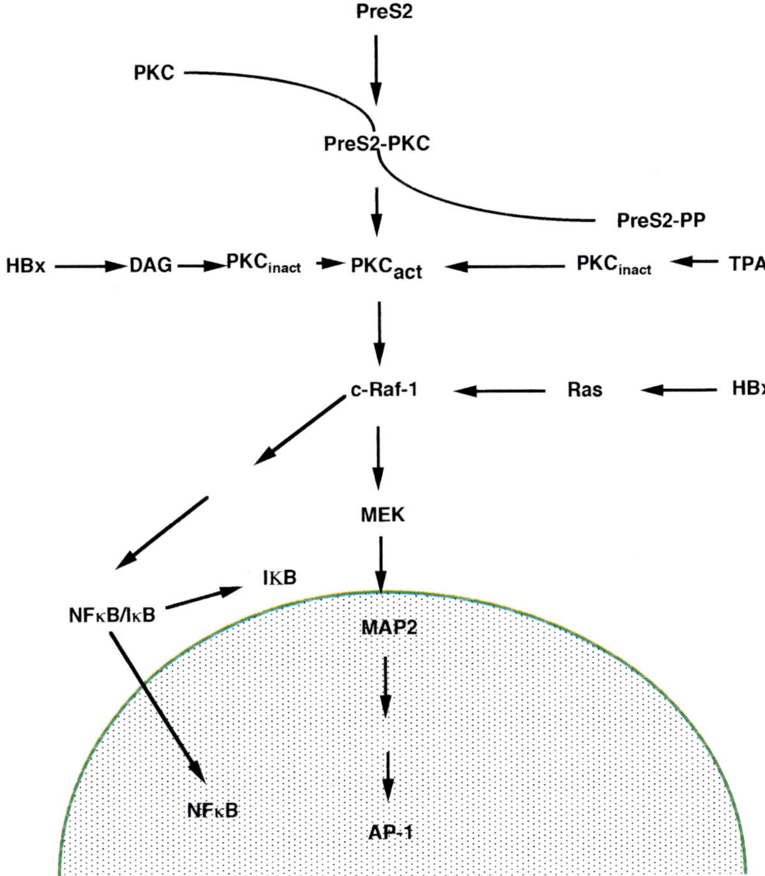

Fig. 3. Signaling pathways triggered by the PreS2 activators. The figure summarizes the work of different groups described in the text and is based on the results obtained from transient or stable cell culture expression systems and from the analysis of transgenic mice producing LHBs or MHBs[t76]. *PKC*, protein kinase C; *NF*, nuclear factor; *TPA*, tetradecanoyl phorbol myristate

vation is a prerequisite for MHBs[t]-dependent induction of AP-1 or NF-κB. The MHBs[t]-dependent activation of PKC is transduced into the nucleus by the c-Raf-1/MAP2 kinase signal transduction pathway. Co-expression of a transdominant negative mutant of c-Raf-1 kinase demonstrated that the functionality of c-Raf-1 kinase is essential for both the MHBs[t] activation of AP-1 and the activation of NF-κB (Hildt et al. 1998). In contrast to HBx (Benn and Schneider 1994, 1995), the activation of c-Raf-1 kinase in MHBs[t]-producing cells does not require the functionality of Ras.

The following model is suggested to describe PreS2-dependent transcriptional activation: the PreS2 domain is a binding partner of PKC; interaction between PreS2 and PKC causes DAG-independent activation of PKC and phosphorylation of the PreS2 domain. The activation of PKC is independent of Ras via the c-Raf-1/MAP2 kinase signal transduction pathway transduced into the nucleus (Fig. 3).

These data are in conflict with a previous model of MHBs^t-dependent transcriptional activation. Based on the ER localization of MHBs^{t167}, it was speculated that the intracellular retention of MHBs^{t167} could generate reactive oxygen intermediate (ROI), which subsequently trigger the activation of NF-κB. This concept seemed to be supported by the observation that radical scavengers such as *N*-acetyl-L-cysteine (NAC) or pyrolidine dithiocarbamate (PDTC) reduce the MHBs^{t167}-dependent activation of NF-κB (Meyer et al. 1992a). This model, however, is in conflict with several new sets of data. The intracellular retention of full-length MHBs (see above) does not cause an induction of NF-κB (Hildt et al. 1995). Non-membrane-associated MHBs^t proteins such as MHBs^{t55} show no difference compared to the membrane-associated MHBs^t proteins with respect to their NF-κB-inducing potential. The activation of NF-κB by MHBs^{t76} or MHBs^{t55} is not reduced by the presence of NAC in the culture fluid. The MHBs^{t76}-dependent activation of c-Raf-1 kinase or of MAP2 kinase, which in principle can both be activated by ROI (Stevenson et al. 1994), is not affected by the presence of NAC. Finally, in stable cell lines or in the livers of transgenic mice producing MHBs^{t76}, no increase in the level of dityrosine (a marker for the presence of radicals) was observed.

The conflicting results with respect to the different effects of NAC in the case of MHBs^{t167} and of MHBs^{t76} can be attributed to a significant difference in the amino acid composition of MHBs^{t76} and MHBs^{t167}. MHBs^{t167} harbours several Cys residues, whereas MHBs^{t76} has none. These Cys residues allow co-translational and post-translational interference with NAC (Weiss et al. 1996). It can therefore, be assumed that the observed effects of NAC on the activator function in the case of MHBs^{t167} models are caused by NAC-protein interactions and not by a reduction of the ROI level.

Transgenic Mouse Models

A variety of transgenic mice producing the HBV surface proteins dependent on different promoters were generated (for an overview, see Chisari 1995, 1996). Transgenic mice which strongly overproduce LHBs in the liver were produced (Chisari et al. 1986, 1989). In these mice, the expression of the transgene was driven under the control of a strong, liver-specific albumin promoter. Due to its overproduction, LHBs is not secreted and accumulates in the cell, resulting in ground glass hepatocytes. This overloading causes a situation analogous to a storage disease and results in permanent inflammation and radical formation with subsequent DNA damage and cellular stress. Until recently, the development of tumours in these mice was considered to be a consequence of overloading and of the resulting stress and inflammation. In the light of recent data showing that LHBs has a transcriptional activator function, the relevance of the transcriptional activation for the development of tumours under these conditions needs to be re-examined.

In a recent report, a synergy between tumor growth factor (TGF)-a and hepatitis B surface antigen (HBsAg) in hepatocellular proliferation and carcinogenesis was observed (Jakubczak et al. 1997). The double transgenic mice (TGF-a and HBsAg) developed HCCs within 8 months.

In contrast to LHBs, the MHBs[t] activators are only produced in very small amounts. Transgenic mice which only overproduce MHBs[t76] in the liver were therefore generated to allow an investigation of the effects caused by the activator function in the absence of nonspecific effects due to overproduction (E. Hildt et al. manuscript in preparation). The transgene which encodes MHBs[t76] was fused to the sequence coding for an amino-terminal hexa-histag to allow affinity purification under denaturing conditions. The transgene was expressed under the control of the liver- specific albumin promoter and the β-globin intron. The ploy A site was taken from SV40. The expression of the transgene in these mice was shown by immunofluoresence and by western blotting after enrichment by affinity chromatography. Determination of JNK2 (stress-activated protein kinase, SAP kinase) activity and of the level of various heat shock proteins demonstrated the absence of stress conditions in these animals in contrast to the LHBs animals. Transgenic mice producing MHBs[t76] are therefore a good tool for analysing the effects of PreS2-dependent activation in the absence of stress factors. In the livers of these mice, a significant induction of c-Raf-1/MAP2 kinase activity was observed (Hildt et al., manuscript in preparation). The activation of this growth-controlling signalling cascade is reflected in an increased expression level of various key enzymes of proliferation control epidermal growth factor receptor, EGF receptor; Shc; SH-PTP2ase; AP2) as compared to the wild type. By determining, the proliferating cell nuclear antigen (PCNA) content and bromodeoxyuridine (BrdU) incorporation, an increased proliferation rate of the liver was found as compared to the wild type. In accordance with this, stable cell lines producing the MHBs[t76] activator also show an increased proliferation rate (Saher et al., submitted). On the other site it has to be considered that expression of the MHBs[t] activator causes an increased sensitivity for TNF-a-dependent induction of apoptosis (E. Hildt, unpublished results). Moreover, a significantly elevated level of eps15 and eps8 was observed in the livers of the transgenic animals. Overexpression of eps15 was recently shown to cause transformation of NIH3T3 cells (Fazioli et al. 1993).

Both, in the transgenic animals and in stable cell lines producing MHBs[t76] (Saher et al., submitted), a sequestration of p53 to the ER was observed. The interaction between p53 and PreS2 was confirmed in in vitro experiments. The sequestration of p53 to the ER result in an inactivation of p53, since it prevents p53 from reaching its site of activity, the nucleus. However, the stochiometric ratio between the amount of PreS2 activators and of p53 in the human liver is unclear, and the pathogenic significance of this observation therefore needs to be carefully considered. In this context, it should be mentioned that, in the livers of MHBs[t76] transgenic mice, a significantly elevated level of mdm2 was observed. In accordance with this, activation of the mdm2 promoter by LHBs was found in a transient expression system (M. Wollersheim, personal communication). The mdm2 regulator binds to the transactivator domain of p53, thereby down-modulating p53 activity. The elevation of the mdm2 level due to the presence of PreS2 activators might represent an additional mechanism of p53 inactivation. In this system, even small amounts of PreS2 activator could result in inactivation of larger amounts of p53 by induction of mdm2 expression.

Relevance of PreS2 Activators for the Development of Human Hepatocellular Carcinoma

Based on epidemiological data in humans, it is generally accepted that HBV plays a causative role in the development of HCC.

At the molecular level, however, no classical transforming oncogene has been detected in the HBV genome. The long latency period of up to 30 years between acute infection and the development of HCC strongly suggests that a multi-step process causes the development of HCC. An analysis of integrates of tumours and tumour-derived cell lines (Yamamoto et al. 1993; Schlüter et al. 1994) demonstrated that, of 26 tumours and cell lines analyzed 80% harboured integrates coding for HBx or MHBst and 69% carried the preS/S open reading frame and could therefore code for LHBs (Schlüter et al. 1994). These epidemiological data do indeed suggest a causative role of these open reading frames in the development of HCC. Transgenic mice, which strongly overproduce LHBs in the liver, develop liver tumours. In these hepatomas, however, the synthesis of LHBs has not been observed so far. This observation permits several conclusions: (a) the expression level in the tumour is so low that it is indetectable, (b) the activator function is only essential for the initial steps of the transformation process, or (c) in later steps, the function is taken over by MHBs[t] or HBx.

Based on data on the transcriptional activator function of HBx and the PreS2 activators, we propose the following model for the role of these HBV activators in the development of an HBV-associated HCC. Both the Hbx activator (Kekulé et al. 1993) and the PreS2 activators exert their effects by activation of signalling pathways which can also be activated by chemical tumour promoters such as phorbol myristate acetate (PMA). In the case of stable cell lines producing the MHBs[t76] activator, an increased proliferation rate was indeed observed (Saher et al., submitted). According to the classical model of carcinogenesis (initiation and promotion), the PreS2 activators MHBs[t] and LHBs might act as tumour promoters through the activation of key enzymes of proliferation control (promotion). In addition, the permanent activation of NF-κB might give these cells increased apoptotic resistance. Cells harbouring critical mutations (initiation) can therefore then be positively selected by expression of the PreS2 activators (promotion). In the case of the transgenic mice overproducing the LHBs, activator, this could mean that critical mutations can be generated by the continuous inflammatory process and that, in a second step, these cells then show an increased proliferation rate due to the activator function of LHBs. The presence of a stronger activator such as TGF-α might shorten the time period up to the development of a tumour.

It has to be considered, however, that the HBV activators are only produced in very small amounts. This could explain the long latency period between infection and HCC development.

Recent data from Taiwan show that, as a result of a nationwide HBV vaccination programme in 1984, the average annual incidence of HCC among children was decreased from 0.7 per 100 000 children between 1981 and 1986 to 0.36 between 1990 and 1996 (Chang et al. 1997). The most powerful tool is thus prevention of infection by vaccination of the complete population at risk.

However, cautious estimates demonstrate that, in the year 2000, approximately 400 million people worldwide will be chronically infected with HBV. Even if vaccination programmes were to be implemented consistently, which they are not at present, chronic infection with HBV will therefore continue to be a severe health problem in the next century.

The different integration patterns and chromosomal rearrangements observed in the tumours analysed so far demonstrate that each HBV-associated HCC is an "individual tumour". However, transcriptional activation is an early critical event for the transformation process, the development of very specific inhibitors that interfere with the transcriptional activator function would be of great medical significance in reducing the risk of developing an HBV-associated HCC.

References

Beasley RP (1988) Hepatitis B virus: the major etiology of hepatocellular carcinoma. Cancer 61:1942–1956

Beasley RP, Hwang LY, Lin CC, Chien CS (1981) Hepatocellular carcinoma and hepatitis B virus. A prospective study of 22 707 men in Taiwan. Lancet 2:1129–1133

Benn J, Schneider RJ (1994) Hepatitis B virus pX protein activates Ras-GTP complex formation and establishes a Ras, Raf, MAP kinase signaling cascade. Proc Natl Acad Sci USA 91:10350–10354

Benn J, Schneider RJ (1995) Hepatitis B virus HBx protein deregulates cell cycle checkpoint controls. Proc Natl Acad Sci USA 92:11215–11219

Bruss V, Lu R, Thomssen R, Gerlich W (1994) Post translational alterations in the transmembrane topology of the hepatitis B virus large envelope protein. EMBO J 13:2273–2279

Buendia MA (1992) Mammalian hepatitis B viruses and primary liver cancer. Semin Cancer Biol 3:309–320

Caselmann WH (1996) Trans-activation of cellular genes by hepatitis B virus proteins: a possible mechanism of hepatocarcinogenesis. Adv Virus Res 47:253–302

Caselmann WH, Meyer M, Kekulé AS, Lauer U, Hofschneider PH, Koshy R (1990) A transactivator function is generated by integration of hepatitis B virus preS/S sequences in human hepatocellular carcinoma DNA. Proc Natl Acad Sci USA 87:2970–2974

Chang MH, Chen C, Lai M, Hsu H, Wu T, Kong M, Liang D, Shau W, Chen D (1997) Universal HBNV vaccination in Taiwan and the incidence of HCC in children. N Engl J Med 336 (26):1855–1859

Chisari FV (1995) Hepatitis B virus transgenic mice: insights into the virus and the disease. Hepatology 22:1316–1325

Chisari FV (1996) Hepatitis B virus transgenic mice: Models of viral immunobiology and pathogenesis. Curr Top Microbiol 186:149–173

Chisari FV, Pinkert CA, Milich DR, Filippi P, McLachlan A, Palmiter RD, Brinster RL (1985) A transgenic mouse model of the chronic hepatitis B virus surface antigen carrier state. Science 230:1157–1160

Chisari FV, Filippi P, McLachlan A, Milich D, Riggs M, Lee S, Palmiter RD, Brinster RL (1986) Expression of hepatitis B virus large envelope protein inhibits hepatitis B surface antigen secretion in transgenic mice. J Virol 60:6909–6913

Chisari FV, Klopching K, Moryiama T, Pasquinelli C, Dunsford HA, Sell S, Pinkert CA, Brinster RL, Palmiter RD (1989) Molecular pathogenesis of hepatocellular carcinoma in hepatitis B virus transgenic mice. Cell 59:1145–1156

Fazioli F, Minichiello L, Matoskova B, Wong WT, Difiore PP (1993) Eps15 a novel tyrosine kinase substrate exhibits transforming activity. Mol Cell Biol 13:5814–5828

Ganem D (1991) Assembly of hepadnaviral virions and subviral particles. Curr Top Microbiol Immunol 168:61–83

Hildt E, Urban S, Lauer U, Hofschneider PH, Kekulé AS (1993) ER-localization and functional expression of the HBV transactivator MHBs^t. Oncogene 8:3359–3367

Hildt E, Urban S, Hofschneider PH (1995) Characterization of essential domains for the functionality of the MHBs^t transcriptional activator and identification of a minimal MHBs^t activator. Oncogene 11:2055–2066

Hildt E, Urban S, Eckerskorn C, Hofschneider PH (1996a) Isolation of highly purified, functional carboxy-terminally truncated hepitatis B virus middle surface protein activators from eucaryotic expression systems. Hepatology 24:502–507

Hildt E, Saher G, Bruss V, Hofschneider PH (1996b) The hepatitis B virus large surface protein (LHBs) is a transcriptional transactivator. Virology 225:235–239

Hildt E, Hofschneider PH, Urban S (1996c) The role of hepatitis B virus in the development of hepatocellular carcinoma. Semin Virol 7:333–347

Hildt E, Saher G, Munz B, Hofschneider PH (1998) The hepatitis B virus transcriptional activator MHBs^t binds to PKC and induces PKC-dependent transcriptional activation of the Raf/MAP-kinase signal transduction pathway (submitted)

Hildt E, Reifenberg K, Hoschneider PH (1998) Activation of cRaf-1/MAP2-kinase signal transduction pathway in transgenic mice producing the preS2 activatis LHBs or MHBs^t (manuscript in preparation)

Hurtley S, Helenius A (1989) Protein oligomerization in the endoplasmic reticulum. Annu Rev Cell Biol: 5:277–307

Jakubczak JL, Chisari FV, Merlino G (1997) Synergy between TGFa and hepatitis B virus surface antigen in hepatocellular proliferation and carcinogenesis. Cancer Res 57(16): 3606–3611

Kekulé AS (1994) Hepatitis B virus transactivator proteins: the 'trans' hypothesis of liver carcinogenesis. In: Bréchot C (ed) Human primary liver cancer: etiological and progression factors. CRG Press, Boca Raton, pp 191–210

Kekulé AS, Lauer U, Meyer M, Caselmann WH, Hofschneider PH, Koshy R (1990) The preS2/S region of integrated hepatitis B virus DNA encodes a transcriptional transactivator. Nature 343:457–461

Kekule AS, Lauer U, Weiss L, Luber B, Hofschneider PH (1993) Hepatitis B virus transactivator HBx uses a tumour promoter signalling pathway. Nature 361:742–745

Lauer U, Weiss L, Hofschneider PH, Kekulé AS (1992) The hepatitis B virus preS2/St transactivator is generated by 3' truncations within a defined region of the S gene. J Virol 66:5284–5289

Lauer U, Weiss L, Lipp M, Hofschneider PH, Kekulé AS (1994) The hepatitis B virus preS2/ St transactivator utilizes AP-1 and other transcription factors for transactivation. Hepatology 19:23–31

Meyer M, Caselmann WH, Schlüter V, Schreck R, Hofschneider PH, Baeuerle PA (1992a) Hepatitis B virus transactivator MHBs^t: activation of NF-χB, selective inhibition by antioxidants and integral membrane localization. EMBO J 11:2991–3001

Meyer M, Wiedorn KH, Hofschneider PH, Koshy R, Caselmann WH (1992b) A chromosome 17:7 translocation is associated with a hepatitis B virus DNA integration in human hepatocellular carcinoma DNA. Hepatology 15:665–671

Natoli G, Avantaggiati M, Balsano C, de Marzio E, Collepadro D, Elfassi E, Levrero M (1992) Characterization of the hepatitis B virus preS/S region encoded transcriptional transactivator. Virology 187:663–670

Natoli G, Avantaggiati ML, Chirillo P, Puri PL, Lanni A, Balsano C, Levrero M (1994) Ras- and Raf dependent activation of c-jun transcriptional activity by hepatitis B virus transactivator pX. Oncogene 9:2837–2843

Ostapchuk P, Hearing P, Ganem D (1994) A dramatic shift in the transmembrane topology of a viral envelope glycoprotein accompanies hepatitis B viral morphogenesis. EMBO J 13:1048–1057

Pahl HL, Bäuerle PA (1994) Oxygen and the control of gene-expression. Bioessays 19:497–502

Parkin DM, Stjernswaerd J, Muir CS (1984) Estimates of the worldwide frequency of twelve major cancers. Bull World Health Org 62:163–182

Rogler CE, Chisari FV (1992) Cellular and molecular mechanisms of hepatocarcinogenesis. Semin Liver Dis 12:265–278

Rothmann K, Schnoelzer M, Radziwill G, Hildt E, Moelling K, Schaller H (1998) Host cell-virus cross talk: phosphorylation of a hepatitis B virus envelope protein mediates intracellular signaling. EMBO J (submitted)

Saher G, Hofschneider PH, Hildt E (1998) Increased proliferation of cells stably producing the hepatitis B virus activator MHBs^{t76}. Hepatology (submitted)

Schlüter V, Meyer M, Hofschneider PH, Koshy R, Caselmann WH (1994) Integrated hepatitis B virus X and 3' truncated preS/S sequences derived from human hepatomas encode functionally active transactivators. Oncogene 9:3335–3344

Stevenson MA, Pllock S, Coleman S, Calderwood K (1994) X-irradiation, phorbo esters and H_2O_2 stimulate mitogen activated protein kinase activity in MIH3T3 cells through the formation of reactive oxygen intermediates. Cancer Res 54:12–15

Stibbe W, Gerlich WH (1983) Structural relationship between minor and major proteins of hepatitis B surface antigen. J Virol 46:626–628

Szmuness W (1978) Hepatocellular carcinoma and the hepatitis B virus: evidence for a causal association. Progr Med Vir 24:40–69

Twu JS, Schloemer RH (1987) Transcriptional trans-activating function of hepatitis B virus. J Virol 61:3448–3453

Urban S, Hildt E, Eckerskorn C, Kekulé AS, Hofschneider PH (1996) One-step purification of hepatitis B virus X protein from a baculovirus expression system and its characterization by mass spectrometry. Heptatology 26:1045–1053

Weiss L, Hildt E, Hofschneider PH (1996) Anti HBV activity of N-acetyl-L-cysteine (NAC): new aspects of a well established drug. J Antivir Res 32:43–53

Wollersheim M, Delbelka U, Hofschneider PH (1988) A transactivating function encoded in the hepatitis B virus X gene is conserved in the integrated state. Oncogene 3:545–552

Yamamoto S, Nakatake H, Kawamoto M, Koshy R, Matsubara K (1993) Transactivation of cellular promotors by an integrated hepatitis B virus DNA. Biochem Biophys Res Commun 192:111–118

Zahm P, Hofschneider PH, Koshy R (1988) The HBV X-ORF encodes a transactivator: a potential factor in viral hepatocarcinogenesis. Oncogene 3:169–177

Antiviral Cell-Mediated Immune Responses During Hepatitis B and Hepatitis C Virus Infections

C. Ferrari[1,2], A. Penna[1], A. Bertoletti[1], A. Cavalli[1], G. Missale[1],
V. Lamonaca[1], C. Boni[1], A. Valli[1], R. Bertoni[1], S. Urbani[1],
P. Scognamiglio[1], and F. Fiaccadori[1,2]

[1] Laboratorio di Immunopatologia Virale, Azienda Ospedaliera di Parma,
  Via A. Gramsci 14, 43100 Parma, Italy
[2] Cattedra Malattie Infettive, Università di Parma, Via A. Gramsci 14,
  43100 Parma, Italy

Abstract

Cell-mediated immune responses to hepatitis B (HBV) and hepatitis C virus (HCV) antigens are vigorous and multispecific in acute, self-limited infections. Moreover, the prevalent cytokine pattern of circulating virus-specific T cells from patients who recover spontaneously from acute hepatitis is Th1-like. Longitudinal analysis of the T cell response to HCV antigens from the early stages of HCV infection in patients who recover from hepatitis and those who do not indicates that weaker responses and a prevalent Th2 pattern of cytokine production is associated with viral persistence and chronic evolution of disease. Although similar sequential studies are missing in hepatitis B, the observation that HBV-specific T cell responses are very weak or totally undetectable in the peripheral blood of patients with long-lasting chronic hepatitis B suggests that strength and quality of virus-specific T cell responses at the early stages of infection may influence the final outcome of both hepatitis B and C. While T cell hyporesponsiveness seems to be an important determinant for HBV persistence once chronic hepatitis has developed, this mechanism appears to be less critical in chronic HCV infection, because the vigor and quality of HCV-specific T cell responses seem to improve as a function of the duration of infection. This is shown by the finding that HCV-specific CD4- and CD8-mediated responses are easily detectable in the peripheral blood of patients with long-lasting chronic hepatitis C and that production of Th1 cytokines predominates within their livers. HCV therefore seems to be able to persist even in the face of an active T cell response and to acquire the capacity to survive within a host environment apparently unfavorable to its persistence. The high variability of HCV may explain its efficiency in escaping immune surveillance.

Recent Results in Cancer Research, Vol. 154
© Springer-Verlag Berlin · Heidelberg 1998

Role of the Specific Immune Response in the Defense Against Viruses

The final outcome of infections by viruses able to produce chronic diseases mostly depends upon the balance between the rate of replication of the infecting virus and the capacity of the immune system to prevent viral spread above critical threshold levels beyond which the infection cannot be efficiently controlled and becomes chronic (Doherty and Ahmed 1997). Since viruses are intracellular parasites, their recognition and neutralization once they are within a cell become a selective task of T cells. Indeed, antibodies produced by B cells are crucial for the neutralization of circulating viral particles, whereas cytotoxic T lymphocytes (CTLs) are responsible for the elimination of intracellular viruses by virtue of both their cytolytic potential, leading to destruction of infected cells, and their capacity to produce antiviral cytokines at the site of viral replication, which may be responsible for down-regulation of viral gene expression (Guidotti et al. 1994, 1996). This may represent a curative noncytolytic mechanism that is even more efficient than the killing of infected cells with respect to viral clearance. Both B cell and CTL functions are more or less tightly controlled by HLA class II-restricted T cells, which mostly express a regulatory function through the production of different sets of cytokines.

Cell-Mediated Immune Response in the Pathogenesis of Hepatitis B Virus Infection

During acute, self-limited hepatitis B, both CD4-mediated, HLA class II-restricted and CD8-mediated, HLA class I-restricted T cell responses are vigorous and efficient, whereas the same responses are much weaker in the peripheral blood of patients with chronic persistent infection (Chisari and Ferrari 1995; Ferrari et al. 1990; Jung et al. 1991; Marinos et al. 1995). The vigor of these T cell responses may increase during the reactivation phases of chronic hepatitis B (Tsai et al. 1992). Frequencies of circulating hepatitis B virus (HBV)-specific T cells in acute hepatitis may even be close to the frequencies induced by superantigens, whereas frequencies are not measurable in most chronic patients (Penna et al. 1996).

In the acute phase of hepatitis B, the T cell response is polyclonal and multispecific, as shown by analysis of the fine specificity of the CD4-mediated T cell response to HBcAg, which is the most potent immunogen for HLA class II-restricted T cells during acute HBV infection (Chisari and Ferrari 1995; Ferrari et al. 1990; Jung et al. 1991). Moreover, B cell responses to hepatitis B core antigen (HBcAg) can be either T cell dependent and independent (Milich and McLachlan 1986). Several HLA class II restricted T cell epitopes have been identified within the core molecule, and the sequence 50–69 appears to be highly immunodominant and promiscuous because it is recognized by virtually all patients with acute infection irrespective of their HLA haplotypes (Ferrari et al. 1991). The high immunogenicity and the capacity of the sequence 50–69 to associate with different HLA class II molecules makes the epitope contained within this region a good candidate for the design of a synthetic peptide-based vaccine.

While HBcAg is the most powerful immunogen for HLA class II-restricted T cells, analysis of the HLA class I-restricted CTL response to HBV indicates that this response is directed against several epitopes located within all different HBV structural and nonstructural proteins (Penna et al. 1991; Nayersina et al. 1993; Rehermann et al. 1995).

A prevalent Th1 cytokine pattern with production of high levels of interferon (IFN)-γ is associated with recovery from HBV infection, as indicated by the functional study of HBcAg-specific T cell lines and clones derived from the peripheral blood of patients with acute hepatitis B (Penna et al. 1997). This pattern may contribute not only to liver cell injury, but probably also to recovery from disease and successful control of infection.

Efficient peripheral blood T cell responses to HBV nucleocapsid proteins can be maintained for decades following clinical recovery from acute hepatitis B, without apparent reexposure to the virus. These responses are generally sustained by activated T cells, and in most subjects the frequencies of circulating HBcAg-specific T cells are similar to those observed in the acute phase of infection. Moreover, traces of virus are detectable by nested polymerase chain reaction (PCR) in approximately 50% individuals who have recovered from infection (Penna et al. 1996). These data therefore suggest that these long-lasting T cell responses may actually represent effector rather than real memory responses and that they may be crucial to keep a persisting virus under tight control. This observation raises the concept that clinical resolution does not necessarily correspond to eradication of HBV and suggests the possibility that long-lasting T cell memory following hepatitis B can be maintained by the chronic production of minute (and serologically undetectable) amounts of antigen.

Pathogenetic Role of the Cell-Mediated Immune Response in Hepatitis C Virus Infection

Although the available results suggest that a weaker T cell response to HBV antigens may represent an important determinant of viral persistence, no information is available at present about the features of the cell-mediated immune response at the early stages of acute HBV infection in patients who subsequently develop chronic hepatitis. Unfortunately, this type of analysis is very difficult in hepatitis B because clinically overt, acute HBV infections are generally self-limited and chronic evolution more commonly follows anicteric, subclinical infections. In contrast, the high rate of chronic evolution of acute hepatitis C virus (HCV) infection makes acute hepatitis C an ideal model to study the peculiar features of the T cell response which are specifically associated with recovery or chronic viral persistence and to characterize the immune events which precede and perhaps determine the final outcome of the disease.

To address this issue, the T cell response to HCV antigens has been sequentially studied from the early stages of infection in wide groups of patients with acute hepatitis C showing that the T cell reactivity to HCV is significantly more efficient in patients who succeed in normalizing alanine aminotransferase (ALT) than in those who develop a chronic infection (Diepolder et al. 1995; Missale et al. 1996). As described in hepatitis B, the CD4-mediated response is also multispecific in acute hepatitis C and immunodominant epitopes have recently been identified by the study of the fine specificity of HCV-reactive polyclonal T cell lines derived from peripheral blood mononuclear cell (PBMC) stimulated with recombinant HCV proteins. Of particular interest with respect to the design of preventive or immunotherapeutic vaccines is the NS3 sequence 1248–1261, which is highly promiscuous and is located within a highly conserved HCV region (Diepolder et al. 1997; C. Ferrari et al., unpublished observations).

Not only the strength but also the quality of the T cell response is different between patients who recover and those who develop a chronic HCV infection, because recovery is associated with a prevalent Th1 profile of peripheral blood HCV-specific T cells, whereas Th2 and Th0 patterns are prevalent among circulating HCV-specific T cells of patients with chronic evolution (Tsai et al. 1997).

The HLA class II-restricted T cell response at the early stages of infection is therefore vigorous, polyclonal, and multispecific in patients who spontaneously recover from acute HCV infection, but the same response is weak or totally undetectable in the peripheral blood of patients who subsequently develop a chronic infection. Similarly to what has been described for hepatitis B, this response remains vigorous for several years following resolution of hepatitis C (Ferrari et al. 1994). Moreover, the HLA class II-restricted T cell responses appear to be stronger in patients with a long-lasting chronic HCV infection than in the acute stage of infection in patients who subsequently develop chronic hepatitis (Bottarelli et al. 1993; Ferrari et al. 1994). In patients who develop a chronic infection, the peripheral blood response therefore seems to progressively increase as a function of the duration of infection, because it is very weak at the very early stages of infection but stronger in long-lasting chronic HCV infections.

In patients with chronic HCV infection, HCV-specific helper cells and CTLs able to recognize structural and nonstructural HCV proteins have also been detected within the liver (Koziel et al. 1992, 1993; Minutello et al. 1993). All these results suggest that the virus can persist, at least in some patients, even in the presence of an active T cell response.

The same conclusion seems to be suggested by the study of the cytokine pattern within the liver of patients chronically infected by HCV. While most intrahepatic T cells are Th1-like and secrete large amounts of IFN-γ, in chronic hepatitis B the majority of liver-infiltrating T lymphocytes are Th0 cells able to produce both Th2 cytokines and lower levels of IFN-γ (Bertoletti et al. 1997; Napoli et al. 1996). The liver environment in chronic hepatitis C therefore appears to be dominated by antiviral Th1 cytokines and should be favorable to viral clearance. Instead, HCV persists in the infected host highly efficiently. In contrast, the liver cytokine environment in chronic hepatitis B is more strongly influenced by Th2 cytokines which may contribute to viral persistence.

Conclusion

In conclusion, it is tempting to speculate that, once a chronic infection has been established, a critical factor that may influence the mechanisms of viral persistence in HCV and HBV infections is the relative antigen load, which is very high in HBV infection and lower in hepatitis C. While a high viral and antigen load may be responsible for T cell hyporesponsiveness in HBV infection as a possible result of T cell exhaustion and preferential expansion of T cells able to produce suppressive Th2 cytokines, this pathway probably does not apply to chronic hepatitis C, in which viral persistence may occur even in the face of an apparently efficient antiviral T cell response.

In HCV infection, escape from antibody and CTL responses or interference with other host immune functions may play a more important role in view of the extremely high mutation rate of this virus, which seems to have acquired the capacity to adapt itself in order to survive in an apparently adverse environment.

Although the high mutation rate of HCV (Simmonds 1995) suggests that escape from CTL surveillance through mutations within immunodominant epitopes may theoretically represent an efficient strategy for the virus to persist and to adapt itself in order to survive, no definitive data are available at present to confirm that this mechanism is actually operative in human HCV infection. Instead, the possibility of viral escape from CTL surveillance has been suggested by recent studies in patients with chronic HBV infection (Bertoletti et al. 1994). Even if these results establish the principle that escape is a possible event when the CTL response is narrowly focused on a single or a few immunodominant epitopes, they also suggest that this mechanism is probably uncommon during acute HBV infection as a primary cause of persistence, because the multispecificity of the CTL response at this stage of infection likely reduces the chances that CTL escape mutants can emerge. The requirements for viral escape to occur seem to be met in a limited subgroup of patients with chronic HBV infection who show a weak and oligospecific CTL response focused on a few dominant epitopes (Bertoletti et al. 1994a,b). In this situation, variant viruses carrying mutations within critical epitopes would be protected from CTL lysis, whereas "wild-type" viruses would be cleared by the immune system, leading to selection of the mutant strains. Escape from CTL responses may occur in these patients not only by mutational inactivation of CTL epitopes, but also by inhibition of the CTL response by T cell receptor antagonism, causing active suppression of wild-type virus recognition by specific CTL (Bertoletti et al. 1994b). This effect could be important immediately after the generation of a mutant DNA, when a single cell is infected by a mixed population of mutated and nonmutated viruses. In this setting, the simultaneous presentation of mutated and nonmutated epitopes on the surface of infected hepatocytes might inhibit the specific CTL response and protect the cell from lysis, facilitating the selection of the variant virus (Meier et al. 1995). Since these results do not demonstrate that selection of HBV variants by the CTL response represents a primary cause of viral persistence, additional studies are needed to better define the relevance of this mechanism in HBV and HCV pathogenesis.

References

Bertoletti A, Costanzo A, Chisari FV, Levrero M, Artini M, Sette A, Penna A, Giuberti T, Fiaccadori F, Ferrari C (1994a) Cytotoxic T lymphocyte response to a wild type hepatitis B virus epitope in patients chronically infected by variant viruses carrying substitutions within the epitope. J Exp Med 180:933–943

Bertoletti A, Sette A, Chisari FV, Penna A, Levrero M, De Carli M, Fiaccadori F, Ferrari C (1994b) Natural variants of cytotoxic epitopes are T cell receptor antagonists for anti-viral cytotoxic T cells. Nature 369:407–410

Bertoletti A, D'Elios M, Boni C, De Carli M, Zignego AL, Durazzo M, Missale M, Penna A, Fiaccadori F, Del Prete G, Ferrari C (1997) Different cytokine profiles of intrahepatic T-cells in chronic hepatitis B and hepatitis C virus infections. Gastroenterology 112:193–199

Bottarelli P, Brunetto MR, Minutello MA, Calvo P, Unutmaz D, Weiner AJ, Choo QL, Shuster JR, Kuo G, Bonino F, Houghton M, Abrignani S (1993) T-lymphocyte response to hepatitis C virus in different clinical courses of infection. Gastroenterology 104:580–587

Chisari FV, Ferrari C (1995) Hepatitis B virus immunopathogenesis. Annu Rev Immunol 13:29–60

Diepolder HM, Zachoval R, Hoffmann RM, Wierenga EA, Santantonio T, Jung MC, Eichenlaub D, Pape GR (1995) Possible mechanism involving T-lymphocyte response to non-structural protein 3 in viral clearance in acute hepatitis C Virus infection. Lancet 346:1006–1007

Diepolder HM, Gerlach JT, Zachoval R, Hoffmann RM, Jung MC, Wierenga EA, Scholz S, Santantonio T, Houghton M, Southwood S, Sette A, Pape GR (1997) Immunodominant CD4+ T-cell epitope within nonstructural protein 3 in acute hepatitis C virus infection. J Virol 71:6011–6019

Doherty PC, Ahmed R (1997) Immune response to viral infection. In: Nathanson N (ed) Viral pathogenesis. Lippincott-Raven, Philadelphia, pp 143–161

Ferrari C, Penna A, Bertoletti A, Valli A, Degli Antoni A, Giuberti T, Cavalli A, Petit M, Fiaccadori F (1990) Cellular immune response to hepatitis B virus (HBV) encoded antigens in acute and chronic HBV infection. J Immunol 145:3442–3449

Ferrari C, Bertoletti A, Penna A, Cavalli A, Valli A, Missale G, Fiaccadori F (1991) Identification of immunodominant T cell epitopes of the hepatitis B virus nucleocapsid antigen. J Clin Invest 88:214–222

Ferrari C, Valli A, Galati L, Penna A, Scaccaglia P, Giuberti T, Schianchi C, Missale G, Marin MG, Fiaccadori F (1994) T-cell response to structural and nonstructural hepatitis C virus antigens in persistent and self-limited hepatitis C virus infections. Hepatology 19:286–295

Guidotti LG, Ando K, Hobbs MV, Ishikava T, Runkel L, Schreiber RD, Chisari FV (1994) Cytotoxic T lymphocytes inhibit hepatitis B virus gene expression by a non cytolitic mechanism in transgenic mice. Proc Natl Acad Sci USA 91:3764–3768

Guidotti LG, Ishikava T, Hobbs MV, Matzke B, Schreiber RD, Chisari FV (1996) Intracellular inactivation of the hepatitis B virus by cytotoxic T lymphocytes. Immunity 4:25–36

Jung C, Spengler U, Schraut W, Hoffmann R, Zachoval R, Eisenburg J, Eichenlaub D et al (1991) Hepatitis B virus antigen-specific T-cell activation in patients with acute and chronic hepatitis B. J Hepatol 13:310–317

Koziel MJ, Dudley D, Wong J, Dienstag J, Houghton M, Ralston R, Walker BD (1992) Intrahepatic cytotoxic T lymphocytes specific for hepatitis C virus in persons with chronic hepatitis. J Immunol 149:3339–3344

Koziel MJ, Dudley D, Afdhal N, Choo QL, Houghton M, Ralston R, Walker BD (1993) Hepatitis C virus (HCV)-specific cytotoxic T lymphocytes recognize epitopes in the core and envelope proteins of HCV. J Virol 67:7522–7532

Marinos G, Torre F, Chokshi S, Hussain M, Clarke BE, Rowlands DJ, Eddleston AL, Naumov NV, Williams R (1995) Induction of T helper cell response to hepatitis B core antigen in chronic hepatitis B: a major factor in activation of the host immune response to the hepatitis B virus. Hepatology 22: 1040–1049

Meier UC, Klenerman P, Griffin T, James W, Koppe B, Larder B, McMichael A, Phillips R (1995) Cytotoxic T lymphocytes lysis inhibited by viable HIV mutants. Science 270: 1360–1362

Milich DR, McLachlan A (1986) The nucleocapsid of the hepatitis B virus is both a T cell-independent and T cell-dependent antigen. Science 234:1398–1401

Minutello MA, Pileri P, Unutmaz D, Censini S, Kuo G, Houghton M, Brunetto MR, Bonino F, Abrignani S (1993) Compartmentalization of T-lymphocytes to the site of the disease: intrahepatic CD4+ T-cells specific for the protein NS4 of hepatitis C virus in patients with chronic hepatitis C. J Exp Med 178:17–26

Missale G, Lamonaca V, Bertoni R, Valli A, Massari M, Mori C, Rumi MG, Fiaccadori F, Ferrari C (1996) Different clinical behaviours of acute hepatitis C virus infection are associated with different vigor of the anti-viral cell-mediated immune response. J Clin Invest 98:706–714

Napoli J, Bishop GA, McGuinness PH, Painter DM, McCaughan GW (1996) Progressive liver injury in chronic hepatitis C infection correlates with increased intrahepatic expression of Th1-associated cytokines. Hepatology 24:759–765

Nayersina R, Fowler P, Guilhot S, Missale G, Cherny A, Schlicht HJ, Vitiello A, Chesnut R, Person JL, Redeker AG (1993) HLA-A2-restricted cytotoxic T lymphocyte responses to multiple hepatitis B surface antigen epitopes during hepatitis B virus infection. J Immunol 150:4659–4671

Penna A, Chisari FV, Bertoletti A, Missale G, Fowler P, Giuberti T, Fiaccadori F (1991) Cytotoxic T lymphocytes recognize an HLA-A2-restricted epitope within the hepatitis B virus nucleocapsid antigen. J Exp Med 174:1565–1570

Penna A, Artini M, Cavalli A, Levrero M, Bertoletti A, Pilli M, Chisari FV, Rehermann B, Del Prete G, Fiaccadori F, Ferrari C (1996) Long lasting memory T-cell responses following self-limited acute hepatitis B. J Clin Invest 98:1185–1194

Penna A, Del Prete G, Cavalli A, Bertoletti A, D'Elios M, Sorrentino R, D'Amato M, Boni C, Pilli M, Fiaccadori F, Ferrari C (1997) Predominant T-helper 1 cytokine profile of hepatitis B virus nucleocapsid-specific T cells in acute self-limited hepatitis B. Hepatology 25:1022–1027

Rehermann B, Fowler P, Sidney J, Person J, Redeker A, Brown M, Moss B, Sette A, Chisari FV (1995) The cytotoxic T lymphocyte response to multiple hepatitis B polymerase epitopes during and after acute viral infection. J Exp Med 181:1047–1058

Simmonds P (1995) Variability of hepatitis C virus. Hepatology 21:570–581

Tsai SL, Chen MY, Yang PM (1992) Acute exacerbations of chronic type B hepatitis are accompanied by increased T cell responses to hepatitis B core and e antigens. Implications for hepatitis B e antigen seroconversion. J Clin Invest 89:87–96

Tsai SL, Liaw YF, Chen MH, Huang CY, Kuo GC (1997) Detection of type 2-like T-helper cells in hepatitis C virus infection: implications for hepatitis C virus chronicity. Hepatology 25:449–458

The Role of Hepatitis C Virus in Hepatocellular Carcinoma

M. Colombo

"Angela Maria e Antonio Migliavacca" Center for Liver Disease
and the FIRC University Unit for Liver Cancer, IRCCS Maggiore Hospital,
University of Milan, Italy

Abstract

The sequential development of cirrhosis and hepatocellular carcinoma (HCC) in patients with post-transfusion hepatitis was a clue that led to the identification of hepatitis C virus (HCV) as a risk factor for HCC. The average time lag between transfusion-associated infection and cancer development was 30 years, with a range of 15–45 years. Using the polymerase chain reaction (PCR) technique, HCV-RNA has been almost invariably detected in serum and tumor tissue of anti-HCV-seropositive patients with HCC In many patients, HCV-RNA was found to belong to the more pathogenic type 1b. However, it is unlikely that HCV plays a direct role in liver tumorigenesis, since no reverse transcriptase activity has been found in infected livers. One current opinion is that HCV may promote cancer through cirrhosis, which is per se an important risk factor for this tumor: almost all patients with HCC have cirrhosis and up to 30% of them have coexisting serological evidence of hepatitis B virus (HBV) or alcohol abuse, further supporting the idea that both HCC and cirrhosis might result from the interplay of several risk factors. However, there are also data suggesting that HCV may interact with cellular genes regulating cell growth and differentiation independently of the onset of cirrhosis.

Introduction

Hepatocellular carcinoma (HCC) is a multistage disease whose occurrence is linked to environmental and life-style factors. The great variations in levels of carcinogenic factors in the environment account for the different incidences of the tumor (Bosch and Munoz 1991). Recent advances made in molecular biology and genetics have initiated a whole new field, i.e., molecular epidemiology of HCC. The identification of risk factors for HCC has provided insights into the etiology and natural history of this tumor and has made it possible to implement screening campaigns aimed at early detection of the tumor. Worldwide, chronic infection with HCV is a leading cause of

Recent Results in Cancer Research, Vol. 154
© Springer-Verlag Berlin · Heidelberg 1998

morbidity and mortality, and a link seems to exist between HCV and HCC (Okuda 1997). However, the mechanisms by which HCV is oncogenic to the liver have not yet been determined.

Epidemiological Studies

In many parts of the world, including most European countries, the role of HBV in human HCC is steadily declining. Between 1961 and 1982, the absolute numbers of fatal liver cancers in Osaka (Japan) dramatically increased (Okuda 1997). During the same period, HBV-independent HCC increased by 50%. In a study of 54 119 autopsies in Venice, HCC incidence rose from 0.6% in the years 1906–1929 up to 1.6% in the years between 1947 and 1988 (Martelli et al. 1991). While the proportion of HCC cases developing in normal livers did not change over time (0.3%), the proportion of HCC cases related to cirrhosis rose from 0.3% to 1.6%, indicating that the observed increase in HCC incidence was due to increased numbers of patients with cirrhosis. Many data suggest that most cases of cirrhosis associated with HCC were caused by infection with HBV and HCV. In Italy and Japan, the iatrogenic spread of HCV with infected needles and blood transfusions also increased the background incidence of HCV infection in the older population (Guadagnino et al. 1997; Okuda 1997).

Case Reports

Early evidence connecting HCC with HCV was the sequential development of chronic liver disease and liver cancer that has been observed in many patients with either community-acquired or transfusion-related hepatitis C (Table 1) (Ayoola et al. 1982; Resnick et al. 1983; Gilliam et al. 1984; Kiyosawa et al. 1984; Cohen et al. 1987; Tremolada et al. 1990). The time lag between exposure to HCV and development of HCC varied greatly from patient to patient, and in all cases HCC was a long-term sequela of HCV-related

Table 1. Reports of progression from non-A, non-B hepatitis to hepatocellular carcinoma (HCC)

Author	Modality of infection	Histologic follow-up	Time lag between infection and HCC (Years)
Ayoola et al. (1982)	Sporadic	CAH → HCC	3
Resnick et al. (1983)	Transfusion	HCC	17
Gilliam et al. (1984)	Transfusion	CAH → CIRRH → HCC	9
Kiyosawa et al. (1984)	Transfusion	CPH → CAH → CIRRH → HCC	13
Cohen et al. (1987)	Sporadic	CAH → CIRRH → HCC	8
Tremolada et al. (1990)	Transfusion	CAH → CIRRH → HCC	12

CAH, chronic active hepatitis; CPH, chronic persistent hepatitis; CIRRH, cirrhosis.

chronic liver disease, with cirrhosis almost invariably preceding the development of cancer. In a study of Japanese patients with transfusion-associated HCV infection (Kiyosawa et al. 1990), HCC developed with an average incubation period of 19 years. The time lag between exposure to HCV and HCC development was similar in hemophilic patients among whom HCC patients were identified by a questionnaire-based multicenter international survey (Colombo et al. 1991). Further studies provided additional evidence of the existence of a close association between HCV, cirrhosis, and HCC (Tradati et al. 1998).

Serologic Studies

With the advent of a serum assay for antibody to HCV (anti-HCV), it became possible to measure the magnitude of the role of HCV in HCC. Many patients with HCC throughout the world had anti-HCV, a serum marker of past or ongoing infection with HCV, with a wide range (6%–75%) of seropositive rates (Table 2) (Bruix et al. 1989; Colombo et al. 1989; Bottelli et al. 1991; Chen et al. 1991; Chiaramonte et al. 1990; Dazza et al. 1990; Ducreux et al. 1990; Hasan et al. 1990; Kaklamani et al. 1991; Kew et al. 1990; Levrero et al. 1991; Nalpas et al. 1991, Nishioka et al. 1991; Poynard et al. 1991; Saito et al. 1990; Santantonio et al. 1990; Sbolli et al. 1990; Simonetti et al. 1989; Srivantanakul et al. 1991; Vargas et al. 1990; Velosa et al. 1990; Watanabe et al. 1991; Yu et al. 1990). Studies of HCV RNA in serum and liver using different probes demonstrated that many HCC patients were actually harboring HCV at the time of sampling, with preference for the genotype 1b (Ohkashi et al. 1990; Ruiz et al. 1991; Shibata et al. 1991; Zala et al. 1991; Gerber et al. 1992; Tang et al. 1995). Early serological studies with anti-HCV provided some important preliminary information about the distinctive features of HCV -related and non-HCV-related liver cancer. Patients with HCV-related tumors were likely to be 10 years older than patients with HBV-related tumors and almost invariably had associated liver cirrhosis (97%). Not surpris-

Table 2. Prevalence of anti-HCV in 2293 patients with hepatocellular carcinoma and in blood donors (23 studies)

	Anti-HCV (%)
Europe	28–75
USA	29–41
Far East	6–55
Africa	29–58
Blood donors	0.5–2.2

Authors: Bottelli et al. 1991; Bruix et al. 1989; Chen et al. 1991; Chiaramonte et al. 1990; Colombo et al. 1989; Dazza et al. 1990, Ducreux et al. 1990; Hasan et al. 1990; Kaklamani et al. 1991; Kew et al. 1990; Levrero et al. 1991; Nelpas et al. 1991; Nishioka et al. 1991; Poynard et al. 1991; Saito et al. 1990; Santantonio et al. 1990; Sbolli et al. 1990; Simonetti et al. 1989; Srivantanakul et al. 1991; Vargas et al. 1990; Velosa et al. 1990; Watanabe et al. 1991; Yu et al. 1990.

ingly, many anti-HCV-seropositive patients had additional risk factors for HCC, particularly alcohol abuse, suggesting that more than one factor may have operated to cause HCC in the patients. In Spanish and French alcoholics with chronic liver disease, infection with HCV was shown to a aggravate the risk of HCC development (Bruix et al. 1989; Vargas et al. 1990; Zarski et al. 1991). The same is true for patients with chronic hepatitis B who became infected with HCV. In these patients the severity of the disease correlated positively with the prevalence of serum anti-HCV, and the highest rates of HCV infection were indeed found in patients with HCC (Chen et al. 1991). In one study, patients infected simultaneously with HCV and HBV had a relative risk of developing HCC of 40, compared to 14 for patients infected with HBV only (Chuang et al. 1992). There are, however, exceptions. In Japan, anti-HCV was detected only rarely in hepatitis B surface antigen (HBsAg)-positive patients with HCC, as were the HBV markers in the anti-HCV-positive patients with liver cancer (Okuda 1997). This indicates that, in some areas, there are distinct populations of cancer patients, probably reflecting different epidemiologies and infection modalities. In Japan, chronic HBsAg carriers often originated from transmission of HBV within families, while HCV was likely to be transmitted later in life by iatrogenic modalities. In South Africa, HBV-related tumors were more common than HCV-related tumors among young men living in the countryside (Kew et al. 1990). HCV-dependent tumors were more often detected in elderly women living in urban communities.

Prospective Studies

The molecular epidemiology analysis of a cohort of patients with well-compensated cirrhosis who were enrolled in 1986 in a surveillance programme for HCC offered us the opportunity to prospectively investigate the relationships between HCV and HCC. A total of 417 HCC-free patients were studied for 10 years to assess the risk of de-novo appearance of HCC, with annual measurements of serum α-fetoprotein (AFP) and abdominal ultrasound. A total of 280 patients were retrospectively found to be anti-HCV seropositive with a third-generation enzyme-linked immunosorbent assay (ELISA). Serum HCV-RNA was detected in 246 patients by PCR and typed with a hybridization assay based on PCR. Of these patients, 138 (52%) had genotype 1b, 67 (25%) had 2a/c, 20 (8%) had 1a, and 39 (15%) had other genotypes. During a 10-year follow-up period, 56 patients with HCV-related cirrhosis developed HCC, with an annual incidence of 2.2%. Stratifying the prevalence of each genotype according to the outcome of follow-up, the 1b to 2a/c genotype ratio of 2:1 observed in the cohort at enrollment remained unchanged during follow-up in the patients who developed HCC or not, who were alive or dead, and who subsequently were lost to follow-up. On multivariate analysis, age over 55 years, male sex, and high baseline AFP were the only variables independently correlated with the risk of developing HCC. To study the risk of HCC in patients with serologic markers of chronic infection and elevated alanine aminotransferase (ALT) levels, we followed up 385 hemophiliacs with these characteristics who had undergone multiple transfusions for a period of 4 years annual HCC incidence was lower than that observed in nonhemophilic patients with HCV-related cirrhosis (0.4% vs. 2.2%) (Tradati et al. 1998). The HCC risk in hemophiliacs was found to correlate with clinical signs of cirrhosis, baseline levels of AFP greater than 11 ng, and age over 45 years, but not with HCV genotype. Interestingly, HCC developed in patients who became infected late during life more often than in those infected earlier. Thus, in two studies, we found no evidence that HCV genotypes correlated with the risk of HCC in patients with chronic hepatitis C. Our data contrast with the results of a prospective study of 163 Italian patients with HCV-related cirrhosis (Bruno et al. 1997), which demonstrated a strict association between HCC and HCV type 1b. After a 68-month follow-up period, HCC developed in 22 of the patients, mostly infected by HCV type 1b, and multivariate analysis showed that HCV type 1b was the most important risk factor for HCC (odds ratio, 6.14). Older age of patients and male sex were less important independent risk factors for HCC. Thus whether severity of HCV-related hepatitis is influenced by selected virus strains is uncertain. A study in France and Italy (Nousbaum et al. 1995) showed reduced incidence of genotype 1b in young patients and in more recently infected individuals with cirrhosis, suggesting that the prevalence of this HCV strain is declining among the general population. Since the pattern of molecular epidemiology of HCV in Italy is changing as a consequence of increasing infection with genotype 1a and 3a due to needle-sharing among young drug users (Silini et al. 1995), more cases of cirrhosis and HCC can be expected in the near future with the increasing contribution of genotypes other than 1b.

HCV RNA Studies

Cross-sectional and prospective studies in patients with chronic hepatitis C indicate that cirrhosis per se might be the relevant pathogenic factor for HCC during chronic HCV infection. However, experimental studies also suggest that HCV might be more directly implicated in liver cell cancer. HCV might activate cellular genes via nuclear localization of core proteins or nonstructural regions of its genome. The nucleotide sequences of the core region of HCV extracted from a HCC revealed deletions and mutuations resulting in truncated core proteins. Interestingly, mutated HCV sequences were not found in the peritumoral liver and serum (Ruster et al. 1996). The putative core proteins of HCV may have an important role in regulating cell growth, i.e., by inhibiting apoptotic cell death, transforming primary rat embrio fibroblast cells with a cooperative oncogene, and promoting cell growth by repressing p53 transcription (Ray et al. 1997). Finally, the HCV genome segment encoding NS3 was shown to transform NIH 3T3 mouse cells, forming tumors in nude mice (Takegami et al. 1995).

Conclusions

Worldwide epidemiological and clinical investigations have clearly demonstrated a link between HCV and HCC. HCV, alone or in conjunction with other environmental risk factors such as alcohol or hepatitis B, is the most important pathogenic factor in the development of HCC in many countries. The proportion of HCC attributable to HCV alone is 25% in Italy. HCV-related tumors arise in older patients, are almost invariably associated with cirrhosis, and often have a less aggressive course than HCC related to other risk factors. HCV is unlikely to be directly responsible for hepatic carcinogenesis, since there is no reverse transcriptase activity in the infected livers. However, the constant finding of viral RNA in the tumor tissue suggests that viral persistence is important in hepatic carcinogenesis. It is unclear whether HCC develops as a consequence of persistent liver cell mytoses during hepatitis C or due to virus-mediated dysregulation of cell genes controlling liver cell growth.

References

Ayoola EA, Odelola HA, Johnson AOK (1982) Primary liver cancer (PLC) after non-A, non-B hepatitis (NANBH) Hepatology 2:154

Bosch FX, Munoz N (1991) Hepatocellular carcinoma in the world: epidemiologic questions. In: Tabor E, Di Bisceglie AM, Purcell RH (eds) Etiology, pathology and treatment of hepatocellular carcinoma in North America. Gulf, Houston, pp 35–54

Bottelli R, Mondazzi L, Asti L, Rezakovic I, Bellati G, Marotta F, Ideo G (1991) Confronting different methods in determination of anti-HCV antibodies in chronic liver disease. 3rd International Symposium on HCV, Strasbourg, Sept 16–17, abstr. E32

Bruix J, Barrera JM, Calvet X, Costa J, Ventura M, Bruguera M, Castillo R, Ercilla G, Sanchez-Tapias JM, Vall M, Bru C, Rodes J (1989) Prevalence of antibodies to hepatitis C virus in Spanish patients with hepatocellular carcinoma and hepatic cirrhosis. Lancet 2:1004–1006

Bruno S, Silini E, Crosignani A, Bonino F, Leandro G, Bono F, Asti M, Rossi S, Larghi A, Cerino A, Podda M, Mondelli MU (1997) Hepatitis C virus genotypes and risk of hepatocellular carcinoma in cirrhosis: a prospective study. Hepatology 25:754–758

Chen DS, Kuo GC, Sung JL, Lai MY, Sheu HC, Chen PJ, Yang PM, Hsu HM, Chang MH, Chen CJ, Hahn LC, Choo QL, Wang TH, Houghton M (1991) Hepatitis C virus infection in an area hyperedemic for hepatitis B and chronic liver disease: the Taiwan experience. J Infect Dis 162:817–822

Chiaramonte M, Farinati F, Fagiuoli S, Ongaro S, Aneloni V, De Maria N, Naccarato R (1990) Antibody to hepatitis C virus in hepatocellular carcinoma. Lancet 1:300–302

Chuang WL, Chang WY, Lu SN, Su WP, Lin ZY, Chen SC, Hsieh MY, Wang LY, You SL, Chen SJ (1992) The role of hepatitis B and C in hepatocellular carcinoma in a hepatitis B endemic area. Cancer 69:2052–2054

Cohen EB, Gang DL, Zeldis JB (1987) Primary hepatocellular carcinoma following non specific non-B hepatitis with tumor DNA negative for HBV-DNA. Dig Dis Sci 32:1428–1430

Colombo M, Kuo G, Choo QL, Donato MF, Del Ninno E, Tommasini MA, Dioguardi N, Houghton M (1989) Prevalence of antibodies to hepatitis C virus in Italian patients with hepatocellular carcinoma. Lancet 2:1006–1008

Colombo M, Mannucci PM, Brettler DB, Girolami A, Lian ECY, Rodeghiero F, Scharrer I, Smith PS, White GC II (1991) Hepatocellular carcinoma in hemophilia. Am J Hematol 37:243–246

Dazza MC, Meneses LV, Girard PM, Villaroel C, Brechot C, Larouze B (1990) Hepatitis C antibody and hepatocellular carcinoma. Lancet 1:1216

Ducreux M, Buffet C, Dussaix EA, Pelletier G, Briantais MJ, Yvart Y, Jaques L, Etienne JP (1990) Antibody to hepatitis C virus in hepatocellular carcinoma. Lancet 1:301

Gerber MA, Shieh YS, Shim KS, Thung SN, Demetris AJ, Schwartz M, Akyol G, Dash S (1992) Detection of replicative hepatitis C virus sequences in hepatocellular carcinoma. Am J Pathol 144:1271–1277

Gilliam JH, Geisinger KR, Richter JE (1984) Primary hepatocellular carcinoma after choronic non-A, non-B post-transfusion hepatitis. Ann Intern Med 101:794–795

Guadagnino V, Stroffolini T, Rapicetta M, Costantino A, Kondili LA, Menniti-Ippolito F, Caroleo B, Costa C, Griffo G, Loiacono L, Pisani V, Focà A, Piazza M (1997) Prevalence, risk factors, and genotype distribution of hepatitis C virus infection in the general population: a community-based survey in Southern Italy. Hepatology 26:1006–1011

Hasan F, Jeffers LJ, De Medina M, Rajender Reddy K, Parker T, Schiff ER, Houghton M, Choo QL, Kuo G (1990) Hepatitis C-associated hepatocellular carcinoma. Hepatology 12: 589–591

Kaklamani E, Trichopoulos D, Tzonou A, Zavitsanos X, Koumantaki Y, Hatzakis A, Hsieh CC, Hadziyannis S (1991) Hepatitis B and C viruses and their interaction in the origin of hepatocellular carcinoma. Jama 265:1974–1976

Kew MC, Houghton M, Choo QL, Kuo GA (1990) Hepatitis C virus antibodies in Southern African blacks with hepatocellular carcinoma. Lancet 1:873–874

Kiyosawa K, Akahana Y, Nagata A, Furuta S (1984) Hepatocellular carcinoma after non-A, non-B post-transfusion hepatitis. Am J Gastroenterol 79:777–781

Kiyosawa K, Sodeyama T, Tanaka E, Gibo Y, Yoshizawa K, Nakano Y, Furuta S, Akahane Y, Nishioka K, Purcell RH, Alter HJ (1990) Interrelationship of blood transfusion, non-A, non-B hepatitis and hepatocellular carcinoma: analysis by detection of antibody to hepatitis C virus. Hepatology 12:671–675

Levrero M, Tagger A, Balsano C, De Marzio E, Avantaggiati ML, Natoli G, Diop D, Villa E, Diodati G, Alberti A (1991) Antibodies to hepatitis C virus in patients with hepatocellular carcinoma. J Hepatol 12:60–63

Martelli C, Massaro C, Zulian M, Blandamura S (1991) Sulla frequenza del carcinoma epatico primitivo nel settorato di Venezia dal 1906 al 1988. Pathologica 83:249–258

Nalpas B, Driss F, Pol S, Hamelin B, Housset C, Brechot C, Berthelot P (1991) Association between HCV and HBV infection in hepatocellular carcinoma and alcoholic liver disease. J Hepatol 1:70–74

Nishioka K, Watanabe J, Furuta S, Tanaka E, Iino S, Suzuki H, Tsuji T, Yano M, Kuo G, Choo QL, Houghton M, Oda T (1991) A high prevalence of antibody to the hepatitis C virus in patients with hepatocellular carcinoma in Japan. Cancer 67:429–433

Nousbaum JB, Pol S, Nalpas B, Landais P, Berthelot P, Brechot C, the Collaborative Study Group (1995) Hepatitis C virus type 1b (II) infection in France and Italy. Ann Intern Med 122:161–168

Ohkoshi S, Kato N, Kinoshita T, Hijikata M, Ohtsuyama Y, Okazaki N, Ohkura H, Hiroashi S, Honma A, Ozaki T, Yoshikawa A, Kajama H, Asakura H, Shimotohno K (1990) Detection of hepatitis C virus RNA in sera and liver tissues of non-A, non-B hepatitis patients using the polymerase chain reaction. Jpn J Cancer Res 81:862–865

Okuda K (1997) Hepatitis C virus and hepatocellular carcinoma. In: Okuda K (ed) Liver cancer. Churchill Livingstone, New York, pp 39–49

Poynard T, Aubert A, Lazizi Y, Bedossa P, Hamelin B, Terris B, Naveau S, Dubreuil P, Pillot J, Chaput JC (1991) Independent risk factors for hepatocellular carcinoma in French drinkers. Hepatology 13:896–901

Ray RB, Steele R, Meyer K, Ray R (1997) Transcriptional repression of p53 promoter by hepatitis C virus core protein. J Biol Chem 272:10983–10986

Resnick RH, Stone K, Antonioli D (1983) Primary hepatocellular carcinoma following non-A, non-B post-transfusion hepatitis. Dig Dis Sci 28:908–911

Ruiz J, Cuende JI, Sangro B, Herrero JI, Beloqui O, Prieto J (1991) Hepatitis C virus (HCV) viremia in patients with hepatocellular carcinoma (HCC) detected by nested PCR. J Hepatol 413:S165

Ruster B, Zeuzem S, Roth WK (1996) Hepatitis C virus sequences encoding truncated core proteins detected in a hepatocellular carcinoma. Biochem Biophys Res Commun 219: 911–915

Saito I, Miyamura T, Ohbayashi A, Harada H, Katayama T, Kikuchi S, Watanabe Y, Koi S, Onji M, Ohta Y, Choo QL, Houghton M, Kuo G (1990) Hepatitis C virus infection is associated with the development of hepatocellular carcinoma. Proc Natl Acad Sci USA 87:6547–6549

Santantanio T, Monno L, Milella M, Fico C, Pastore G (1990) HCV infection in liver cirrhosis and hepatocarcinoma in South Italy. International Symposium on Viral Hepatitis and Liver Disease, Contemporary Issues and Future Prospects, April 4–8, Houston, Texas, abstr 634

Sbolli G, Zanetti AR, Tanzi E, Cavanna L, Civardi G, Fornari F, Di Stasi M, Buscarini L (1990) Serum antibodies to hepatitis C virus in Italian patients with hepatocellular carcinoma. J Med Virol 30:230–232

Shibata M, Takeda S, Kudo T, Kimura H, Kuzushita K, Moroshima T, Nagai Y (1991) Minus strand RNA of hepatitis C virus in liver tissues. J Hepatol 13:379–380

Silini E, Bono F, Cividini A, Cerino A, Maccabruni A, Tinelli C, Bruno S, Bellobuono A, Mondelli MU (1995) Molecular epidemiology of hepatitis C virus infection among intravenous drug users. J Hepatol 22:691–695

Simonetti RG, Cottone M, Craxì A, Pagliaro L, Rapicetta M, Chionne P, Costantino A (1989) Prevalence of antibodies to hepatitis C virus in hepatocellular carcinoma. Lancet 2:1338

Srivantanakul P, Parkin DM, Khlat M, Chenvidhya D, Chotiwan P, Insiripong S, L'Abbe KA, Wild CP (1991) Liver cancer in Thailand. II. A case control study of hepatocellular carcinoma. Int J Cancer 48:329–332

Takegami T, Sakamuro D, Peng XX, Hasumura Y, Furukawa T (1995) Hepatitis C virus genome segment encoding NS3 transforms NIH 3T3 mouse cells. 5th International Symposium on Hepatitis C Virus and Related Viruses. 24 Aug – 3 Sept, Brisbane, abstr C43

Tang L, Tanaka Y, Enomoto N, Marumo F, Sato C (1995) Detection of hepatitis C virus RNA in hepatocellular carcinoma by in situ hybridization. Cancer 76:2211–2216

Tradati F, Colombo M, Mannucci PM, Rumi MG, De Fazio C, Gamba C, Ciavarella N, Rocino A, Morfini M, Scaraggi A, Taioli E, The Study Group of the Association of Italian Hemophilia Centers (1998) A prospective multicenter study of hepatocellular carcinoma in Italian hemophiliacs with chronic hepatitis C. Blood 91:1173–1177

Tremolada F, Benvegnu L, Casarin C, Pontisso P, Tagger A, Alberti A (1990) Antibody to hepatitis C virus in hepatocellular carcinoma. Lancet 1:300–301

Vargas V, Castells L, Esteban JI (1990) High frequency of antibodies to hepatitis C virus among patients with hepatocellular carcinoma. Ann Intern Med 112:232–233

Velosa M, Marinho R, Sariva A, Ramalho F, Carneiro de Moura M (1990) Prevalence of anti HCV antibodies in patients with chronic hepatitis and hepatocellular carcinoma. International Symposium on Viral Hepatitis and Liver Disease, Contemporary Issue and Future Aspects, April 4–8, Houston, Texas

Watanabe Y, Harada S, Saito I, Miyamura T (1991) Prevalence of antibody against the core protein of hepatitis C virus in patients with hepatocellular carcinoma. Int J Cancer 48:340–343

Yu MC, Tong MJ, Coursaget P, Ross RK, Govindarajan S, Henderson BE (1990) Prevalence of hepatitis B and C viral markers in black and white patients with hepatocellular carcinoma in the United States. J Natl Cancer Inst 82:1038–1041

Zala G, Mevelka J, Joller-Jemelka HJ, Garson JA, Risti B, Meier B, Schmid M, Buhler H (1991) Hepatitis C virus (HCV) and hepatocellular carcinoma (HCC) J Hepatol 13:S183

Zarski JP, Lunel P, Dardelet D, Thelu MA, Baccard M, Perrin M, Huraux JM, Seigneurin JM (1991) Hepatitis C virus and hepatocellular carcinoma in France: detection of antibodies using two second generation assays. J Hepatol 13:376–377

Overview of Viruses, Cancer,
and Vaccines in Concept and in Reality

M. R. Hilleman

Merck Institute for Therapeutic Research, Merck Research Laboratories,
West Point, PA 19486, USA

Abstract

Cancer is a consequence of malfunction of the replicative cell cycle caused
by acquisition of independence from proliferative and restrictive controls in
the process. Such alteration may be driven by unrepaired mutations in proto-
oncogenes and anti-oncogenes or by genetic insults of environmental, infectious, or spontaneous origin. The consequence of mutations may be reflected
at any of a number of locations in the transductive pathways from receptor
to nucleus which upset normal homeostatic balance between the opposing
forces for promotion or restraint of cell proliferation.

About 15% of human cancers are caused primarily by viruses that bring
about aberrations in gene structure and function or that express proteins
that bind to cell regulatory proteins. The means for achieving immunoprophylaxis of viral cancers, such as hepatitis B or Marek's disease, are based on
prior specific perturbation of the immune system, causing it to respond rapidly and effectively in preventing infection on subsequent contact with the
corresponding agent. Existing cancers of viral origin and those of nonviral
causation come together in attempted immunotherapy. Cure is far more difficult to achieve than prevention and relies on the principle that tumor cells
can display abnormal markers on the cell surface that are capable of being
detected and engaged by an effective immune response.

Efforts to prevent and cure cancer of viral, spontaneous, or environmental
origin are a worthy pursuit and must take account of the most advanced
information relating to the chemistry of the cell cycle and to the function of
the immune system.

Cell Cycle and Cancer

In the simple sense, cancer (Clurman and Roberts 1995; Draetta and Pagano
1996; Hartwell and Kastan 1994; Hunter 1997; Jacks and Weinberg 1996;
Pines 1994; Sherbet and Lakshmi 1997a) is malignant cell growth generated
by malfunction of the replicative cell cycle (Fig. 1). Malignancy arises

Recent Results in Cancer Research, Vol. 154
© Springer-Verlag Berlin · Heidelberg 1998

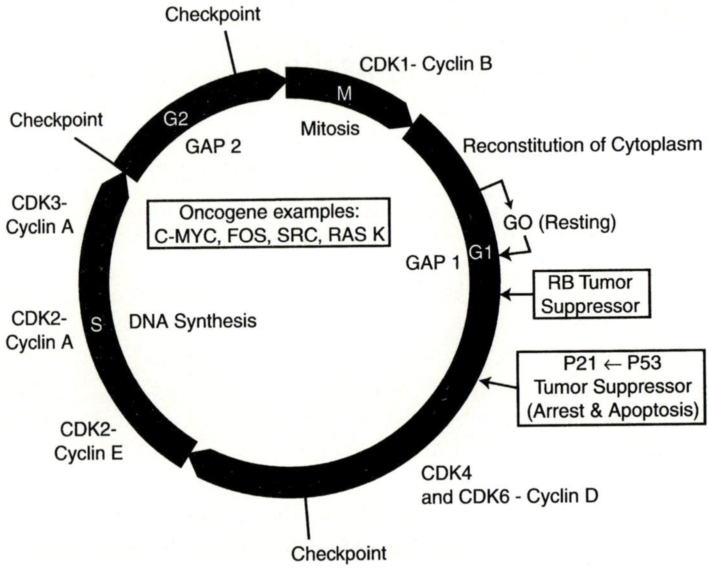

Fig. 1. Mammalian cell cycle. *CDK*, Cholecystokinin

through acquisition of independence from proliferative and restrictive
controls that normally guide the orderly procession through the four phases
(G_1, S, G_2, and M) involved in cell replication.

In most instances, cell mitosis is initiated by binding of extracellular proliferative signaling ligands to complementary tyrosine kinase receptors on
the cell surface. The receptors act as signal transducers which initiate a cascade of cell cycle events driven by sequential phosphorylation of cyclin-dependent kinases. The kinases may be restricted by cyclin-dependent kinase
inhibitors (Clurman and Roberts 1995).

There are at least 60 different cell proliferative proteins (such as *myc*, *ras*, *fos*,
src) that are encoded by cell proto-oncogenes and may be present at any of a
number of locations in the transductive pathway from receptor to nucleus. Proto-oncogenes that have been altered by mutation or other mechanisms to encode abnormally active proteins at any point along the signal cascade are
called oncogenes (Sherbet and Lakshmi 1997a, b) and may induce cancer by
causing cells to proliferate in the absence of external signals for proliferation.

The Gap 1, or G_1 phase of the cell cycle is one of restoration of cell size
following mitosis and may also be one of resting, referred to as Gap 0. Differentiation may take the cell out of the replicative cycle completely. The G_1
phase is followed by DNA synthesis (S phase), preparation for mitosis (G_2
phase), and finally by cell division itself in the M phase. The entire cell cycle
is closely monitored, and there are periods of great activity during which
there is arrest and repair of newly formed but miscoded DNA, especially as
detected at critical checkpoint sites. The regulatory rb (Herwig and Strauss

1997; Wang et al. 1994) and p53 (Guinn and Mills 1997; Levine 1997; Sherbet and Lakshmi 1997c) tumor-suppressive anti-oncogenes are the best known of a large number of defined and as yet undefined proteins that are gatekeepers for the cell cycle. They detect and arrest the cycle in cells bearing miscoded DNA and other errors. There is ample time for DNA repair (Hanawalt 1995; Culotta and Koshland 1994) but irreparable errors may trigger cell destruction by apoptosis. The recently described (Haines 1997; Piette et al. 1997) mdm2 proto-oncogene may become oncogenic by overexpression with resultant binding to the p53 and rb tumor-suppressive proteins.

Most somatic cell alterations responsible for the induction of cancer include mutations that activate oncogenes or, equally importantly mutations that bring about loss or inactivation of tumor-suppressing anti-oncogenes. These mutations may arise from errors in DNA replication of spontaneous origin, from inherited genetic predispositions, or from factors encountered in the environment such as irradiation or carcinogens in foods or cigarette smoke. Physical factors include exposure to ionizing or ultraviolet radiation. Chemical substances may cause mutations involving alteration or deletion of genetic information, chromosomal breaks, or frameshift changes in cell DNA. Neoplasia of hormone-responsive tissues may arise from facilitation of mutation, enhanced fixation, or defects in DNA that arise during mitosis. Another complication may occur when cells that have exceeded their normal replicative life span undergo oncogenic transformation that is associated with the activation of telomerase. RNA telomeres are present on the two strands of DNA at the ends of chromosomes and are needed to prevent unraveling of these strands (Wynford-Thomas 1996; Holt et al. 1996). Progressive shortening of the telomeres on cell replication leads to cell senescence and ultimately provides a signal for cell death. Inappropriate activation of telomerase lengthens the telomeres and is associated with rescue and induction of immortality in senescent cells that may become malignant. With regard to human cancer, the telomere hypothesis, has not yet been proved. At least 15% of all cancers are primarily of viral cause. Another suspected possibility is rare bacterial carcinogenesis, such as that associated with *Helicobacter* infection (O'Connor et al. 1996; Genta et al. 1997); however, this has also not yet been proved.

Homeostasis in cell function clearly depends on the appropriate balance between a myriad of mostly undefined opposing forces such as those of oncogenes and anti-oncogenes that promote or restrain mitosis, much as in a tug-of-war. Genetic mutation results in altered protein folding, which changes the three-dimensional fit and charge patterns of the proteins involved so that they are no longer complementary to each other.

Selected Examples of Viruses in Human and Animal Cancer

Examples of viruses (Darcel 1994; Hilleman 1993; Hoppe-Seyler and Butz 1995; Vousden and Farrell 1994; zur Hausen 1991, 1996a) known to cause or to be associated with carcinogenesis are listed in Table 1 and will not be dis-

Table 1. Selected examples of viruses that may cause cancer

Family	Nucleic acid	Group	Agent	Species of origin	Comments Highlights
Retroviridae			RNA		
	Oncovirus	HTLV-1 and -2		Human	Adult T cell and possibly hairy cell leukemias in humans
		Leukemia-sarcoma Viruses		Animals	Leukemias and sarcomas, many species
	Lentivirus				
		HIV (AIDS)		Human	Multiple neoplasia in humans associated with immunodeficiency
		SIV (SAIDS)		Monkey	Neoplasia in monkeys
Flaviviridae			RNA		
	Hepatitis C			Human	Cirrhosis and hepatocellular carcinoma in humans
Hepadnaviridae			DNA		
	Hepatitis B			Human	Liver cirrhosis and hepatocarcinoma in humans
	Woodchuck			Animal	Hepatocarcinoma
Papovaviridae			DNA		
	Papillomavirus			Human	Anogenital cancer, especially cervical carcinoma, and skin cancer
	Polyomavirus				
		JC, BK		Human	Tumorogenic in animals; possible rare neoplasia in humans
		SV_{40}		Monkey	Diverse tumors in rodents
		Polyoma (mouse)		Mouse	Tumors in rodents
Herpesviridae			DNA		
	Epstein-Barr virus			Human	Burkitt and other lymphomas, nasopharyngeal carcinoma in humans
	Herpes simplex			Human	Possibly associated with papillomavirus cervical cancer in humans
	Human herpes-virus-8			Human	Sarcoma associated with HIV in humans
	Marek's disease			Chicken	Neural and generalized lymphomatosis in chickens
Adenoviridae			DNA		Human	Tumors in rodents by certain types; none in humans
				Animal	Tumors in rodents by certain types

HTLV, human T cell leukemia virus; HIV, human immmunodeficiency virus; AIDS, acquired immunodeficiency; SIV, simian immunodeficiency; SAIDS, simian AIDS.

cussed individually in this brief overview. These viruses belong to six different phylogenetic groups, the first two of which are RNA viruses and the remaining four of which are DNA agents. The organisms disrupt the normal cell cycle. The oncovirus subgroup of the retroviruses cause T cell leukemias in humans (Gallo 1995; Kaplan 1993). The lentivirus subgroup, or "slow viruses", exemplified by the human immunodeficiency virus (HIV), may be oncogenic in some instances, but the associated neoplasia probably usuallly arises through association with another agent or through loss of immunologic control of neoplasia caused by severe immunodeficiency. Hepatitis C (Kew 1994) flavivirus commonly causes cancer, but there is no defined direct role. In most cases, hepatocarcinoma may result from the increased likelihood of mutational errors occuring during extensive hepatocyte replacement. Hepatitis B hepadnavirus hepatocarcinoma (Hildt et al. 1996) occurs as a sequel to a long-term viral carrier state and may be promoted by aflatoxin.

Certain papillomavirus (Laimins 1996; Zur Hausen 1996b) serotypes of the Papoviridae cause squamous carcinoma and cancers of the anogenital region, especially cervical carcinoma. Human polyomaviruses, e.g., JC and KB (Carallini et al. 1987; Arthur et al. 1994), may cause fatal degenerative disease of the central nervous system in the face of immunodeficiency. Possible oncogenicity is infrequent and is not firmly established (Carallini et al. 1987; Arthur et al. 1994). Simian and mouse polyomaviruses (Girardi et al. 1962; Levine 1994) are oncogenic for rodents. At least three viruses of the Herpesviridae may cause or be associated with cancer in humans. These include the Epstein-Barr (E-B) virus (EBV) (Raab-Traub 1996) which causes both carcinomas and lymphomas in humans. The recently discovered human herpesvirus-8 has an apparent causal role in most Kaposi's sarcomas, especially in HIV-infected individuals (Kempf and Adams 1996; Ambroziak et al. 1995). Herpes simplex viruses, which are commonly found in association with cervical carcinomas, are an unlikely primary cause for cancer, but might play a secondary role in cervical carcinoma caused by papillomavirus (Jones 1995). All human adenoviruses transform rodent cells in culture, but only a few induce tumors in rodents. These include types 12 and 18 (Shenk 1996), which are highly oncogenic, and types 3 and 7 (Girardi et al. 1964), which are weakly oncogenic. None has been found to cause cancer in humans, and evidence for oncogenicity in humans is lacking.

Mechanisms of Viral Oncogenesis

The mechanisms whereby individual viruses of each of the six different families initiate cancer (Table 2) are complex, diverse, and poorly or incompletely understood. As with nonviral cancers, most virus-caused cancers require cumulative secondary cell mutations and cofactors that deliver spurious signals and misdirect normal cell function as a necessary prerequisite for progression to full neoplasia. Demonstration of tumorigenesis in animals by infection with human viruses may not be predictive for humans.

Table 2. Diverse, defined or obscure mechanisms in selected examples of viral oncogenesis

Virus	Probable or proven mechanisms
Retroviridae	
Oncovirus HTLV-1	Genomic integration, insertional mutation, *cis-* and *trans*-activation
Lentivirus HIV	Rarely oncogenic, possible herpesvirus promotion, host immune collapse
Flaviviridae	
Hepatitis C	Nononcogenic; high risk for mutation on hepatocyte replacement
Hepadnaviridae	High risk for mutation on hepatocyte turnover; integration, with possible *cis-*
Hepatitis B	and *trans*-activation, X regulatory protein promotion, and possible binding to p53
Papovaviridae	Best defined are HPV types 16 and 18, causing cervical neoplasia
Papillomavirus	Viral E6 oncoprotein binds to and degrades p53 regulatory protein (anti-oncogene) and activates cell promoters and telomerase
	Viral E7 oncoprotein binds to rb regulatory and other proteins, releasing genes for cell cycle progression
	Both E6 and E7 oncoproteins plus added mutations and cofactors are needed for neoplasia
Polyomavirus	Large T antigen oncoprotein shares a sequence with HPV E7 oncoprotein
SV$_{40}$	Binding to p53 and rb regulatory proteins is essential in rodent neoplasia
Herpesviridae	Complex virus-induced B lymphocyte proliferation leads to lymphoproliferative
Epstein-Barr virus	disease with predisposition to *c-myc* oncogene translocation and emergence of malignant clones; enhanced by immunosuppression, malaria cofactor
HHV-8	Recently discovered HHV-8 infection appears to be central to spindle cell formation in Kaposi's sarcoma; HIV-infected cells may release cell cytokines and tat protein, enormously promoting spindle cell formation
Adenoviridae	E1A and E1B oncoproteins of oncogenic adenovirus types, like those for papillomaviruses and polyomaviruses, bind to rb and p53 cellular regulatory proteins, respectively, and are essential for induction of neoplasia in animals

HTLV, human T cell leukemia virus; HIV, human immunodeficiency virus; HHV, human herpesvirus-8; HPV, human papillomavirus.

Rather than reviewing the details for each virus or virus family, it may be instructive (Ambroziak et al. 1995; Arthur et al. 1994; Carallini et al. 1987; Darcel 1994; Gallo 1995; Girardi et al. 1962, 1964; Hall 1996; Hildt e al. 1996; Hilleman 1993; Hoppe-Seyler and Butz 1995; Jansen-Dürr 1996; Jones 1995; Kaplan 1993; Kempf and Adams 1996; Kew 1994; Laimins 1996; Levine 1994; Raab-Traub 1996; Shenk 1996; Vousden 1994; Zur Hausen 1991, 1996a, b) to define the general mechanisms whereby viruses may be involved in the neoplastic process. Several such mechanisms are highlighted in Table 3. These mechanisms are essentially the following:

a) Viral genetic material that is integrated into the cell genome in whole or in part may bring about insertional mutations and *cis-* or *trans*-activation of host mitogenic genes.

b) Nononcogenic viruses associated with tumor may bring about a need for host cell replacement and an increased likelihood of mutations, with random and spontaneous tumor cell appearance.

c) Viruses encoding oncoproteins that bind to or destroy the regulatory anti-oncogene products such as rb or p53 may be prominently oncogenic and may enhance the likelihood of nonrestricted cell replication.

Table 3. Collective summary of mechanisms in viral neoplasia

Genomic integration with insertional mutation and cell mitogenic activation
Enhanced spontaneous neoplasia from errors arising in increased cell replication
Binding of cell regulatory antioncogene proteins by viral oncoproteins
Chromosomal breaks and translocations leading to abnormal cell signaling
Viral-encoded mitogenic promoters together with cellular cytokines
Loss of immunosuppression of tumor by depression of host immunity
Collectively, mechanisms are highly complex: increasing recognition of a central role for disruption of p53, rb antioncogenes, and similar substances in most viral oncogenesis

d) Certain viruses may bring about host chromosomal breaks and translocations leading to abnormal cell replication.

e) Virally encoded mitogenic promoters, together with cell released cytokines, may play a substantive role in certain neoplastic processes.

f) Viruses that bring about a state of immunodeficiency may facilitate the appearance of clinical neoplasia that might otherwise be detected and repressed by the host immune system.

It is clear that the mechanisms for viral carcinogenesis are highly complex and poorly understood, though their role in overriding control mechanisms in the cell cycle is well established. In addition, the importance of disruption of p53 and rb tumor suppressor proteins by oncoproteins of viruses that may now include certain of the herpesviruses is increasingly being recognized.

Vaccinology and Immunology

The science of vaccinology involves microbiology, virology, molecular biology, and immunology in an attempt to prevent disease in practice by immunoprophylaxis. Modern vaccinology is largely a branch of applied immunology on which it has come to rely for enlightenment and guidance in understanding mechanisms and development of approaches to immunoprophylaxis and immunotherapy. Prophylactic vaccines against viruses that cause acute infectious diseases or a chronic disease state or that are the primary initiators of neoplasia have been notably effective. In contrast, immunotherapeutic vaccines against chronic infections and neoplasia have brought little more than an unrealized promise.

The science of immunology has grown over the past two decades from black box empiricism to become the heart of all endeavors seeking to achieve active intervention through immunization. The mechanisms of the immune response are highly complex, and understanding them is critical to the successful pursuit of vaccines.

In the simplest sense, the immune system recognizes what is not self and also those parts of self that are usually covert or poorly expressed and are not usually seen by the mature immune system. The mechanisms for engagement of the adoptive immune processes are shown in Fig. 2. The effectors of

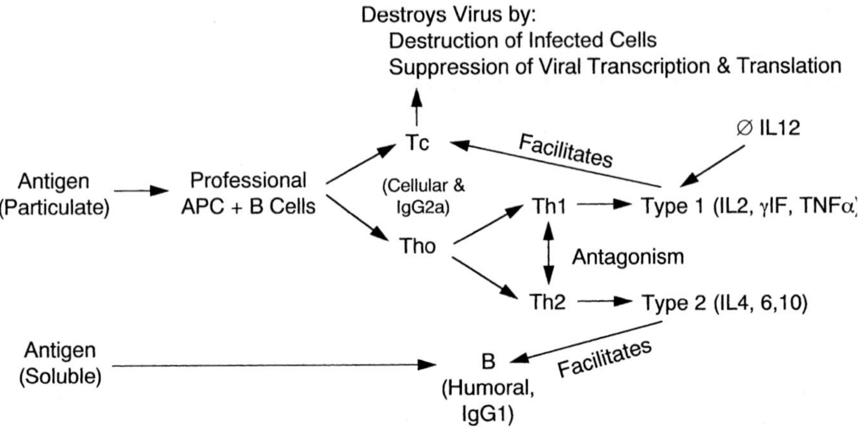

Fig. 2. Immune response (simplified, conjectural); *APC*, antigen-presenting cells; *IL*, interleukin; *IF*, interferon; *TNF*, tumor necrosis factor

humoral responses are B cells that produce antibodies. T cell effectors are of two kinds, each having different functions: cytotoxic T cells detect and destroy abnormal cells and form the basis of cell-mediated immunity, while activated T helper cells aid and assist in the differentiation and expansion of specific B cells and cytotoxic T cells. The Th1 subset of T helper cells elaborates cytokines that favor a cytotoxic T cell response, while the Th2 subset favors antibody responses. The cytokines elaborated in the type 1 and 2 responses are antagonistic to and suppressive of each other, respectively. Immune recognition of nonself proteins by T cells is aided through antigen presentation by professional antigen-presenting cells (dendritic cells, macrophages, B cell). In this process, immunologic determinants that are present in short linear fragments of proteins are displayed on the cell surface bound to class I or II major histocompatibility complex (MHC) receptors in a context in which they are seen and recognized. Understanding immune mechanisms permits the development of rational approaches to vaccine design and to elicitation of chosen and appropriate responses.

Prevention Versus Cure

Vaccinology and immunology (Table 4) have progressed over a period of two centuries following the first scientific investigations by Edward Jenner into immunization of humans against smallpox by prior inoculation of the attenuated but antigenically related cowpox virus. Immunoprophylaxis against viral and other infective agents is relatively simple in that these entities present novel antigenic determinants, against which specific adaptive immune responses can be directed that are destructive to the invaders. Many prophylactic vaccines are highly effective and are routinely used, and infective

Table 4. Prevention versus cure

Vaccinology and immunology began with Edward Jenner in 1796
Prophylaxis of infections by vaccine is relatively simple, since it erects a barrier prior to exposure to
  the infectious agent
Therapy of persistent infections and of cancer by vaccine is difficult and needs to achieve detection
  and elimination of already infected or otherwise altered cells; this may be complicated by existent
  damage to the immune system
In immunotherapy, persistent viral infections and chronic proliferative and degenerative
  diseases find a common pursuit

agents such as poliovirus and measles virus are targeted for worldwide eradication by the same mass immunization strategy as that used against smallpox virus. Vaccines that attempt immunologic recognition and immunotherapeutic intervention in already existing conditions, such as cancer or chronic and persistent viral infections, are immensely difficult to develop and suffer from a lack of knowledge in this area. However, it is important, conceptually, to note that transformed neoplastic cells and cells which are persistently infected with viruses come together in the common pursuit of immunotherapy. They both pose the difficult problems of specific immune recognition and the stimulation of effectors that will bring about selective identification and removal of abnormal cells without destroying normal cells. The problems may be magnified by existing damage to the immune system, e.g., by anergy, by evasion and escape from immune recognition, by the overwhelming presence of abnormal cells, and by reduction of immune responses as a result of a decrease in the number and function of relevant effector cells. It is here that infections and chronic proliferative and degenerative diseases have a common cause.

Prophylactic Vaccines Against Oncolytic Viruses

Numerous and highly effective live and killed viral and bacterial vaccines against infectious diseases, most of which were developed in the last 50 years, are now being used routinely. Viral infections, whether they cause acute illness or cancer, are alike in that prevention of infection prevents both kinds of outcome.

My own career in basic and applied research has included pioneering discoveries of viruses that cause cancer and in the development of vaccines that prevent cancer (Table 5). I can use these to illustrate the principles for prevention of virus-caused cancer. Discovery of the adenoviruses (Hilleman and Werner 1954; Rowe et al. 1953), some of which cause cancer (Shenk 1996; Girardi et al. 1964), led to highly effective vaccines (Hillemann et al. 1953). Our discoveries of the simian SV_{40} polyomavirus (Sweet and Hilleman 1960a,b) in 1960 and of its oncogenicity (Girardi et al. 1962) in 1962 were followed by studies showing abortive prevention of viral cancer by irradiated

Table 5. Pioneering events in cancer virus and vaccine discovery

Virus	Source	Highlights	
		Year	Event
Adenovirus	Human	1953	Codiscoveries by Hilleman and Werner (1954) and by Rowe et al. (1953)
		1956	Highly effective killed vaccine
			Oncogenicity for rodents of type 7 virus demonstrated
SV_{40}	Macaque	1960	Discovery of virus
		1962	Discovery of oncogenicity
		1964	Irradiated whole tumor cell vaccine prevents cancer in adult hamsters infected with virus when newborn
		1967	Passive maternal antibody prevents tumor in animals challenged neonatally
Marek's herpesvirus	Chickens	1971	Licensure; first live whole cell vaccine against Marek's disease (Hilleman 1974a, b)
		1974	First live cell-free dried vaccine against Marek's disease (Witter 1971)
			These vaccines for use in chickens were the first licensed vaccines against any viral cancer in any species
Hepatitis B	Human	1968	Basic vaccine initiative began
		1975	Proof of safety and efficacy in chimpanzees; proof of safety and immunogenicity for humans
		1981	Licensure of the first killed subunit vaccine against viral infection
		1986	Licensure of the first recombinant vaccine; hepatitis B vaccine was the first vaccine against human cancer, the first subunit virus vaccine, and the first recombinant-expressed vaccine

SV_{40} and adenovirus discoveries were seminal to:
carcinogenesis by DNA viruses and the basic model for virus in cancer; prevention of oncogenesis by vaccines; discovery of p53 anti-oncogene (Levine 1994); and evolvement of modern viral genetics and molecular biology.

whole cell vaccine (Goldner et al. 1964; Coggin et al. 1967) and by demonstrating the prevention of viral infection by maternal antibodies (Larson et al. 1967). The SV_{40} and adenovirus discoveries provided seminal data relative to carcinogenesis and tumor vaccine immunogenesis, and, in addition, were of critical significance to the evolution of modern viral genetics and molecular biology, including the discovery of the p53 anti-oncogene (Levine 1994).

Whole cell (Hilleman 1972, 1974a) and killed dried (Hilleman 1974b) vaccines against neural lymphomatosis in chickens, employing the Witter-Burmester turkey herpesvirus (Witter 1971), were the first licensed vaccines of any kind against any viral cancer. Their effectiveness on application revolutionized the economics of the poultry industry. The plasma-derived vaccine against hepatitis B (Buynak et al. 1976; Hilleman et al. 1978, 1982; Hilleman 1984, 1992a, 1996a, b), which was introduced in 1981 after 13 years of research, was the first licensed subunit viral vaccine and the first licensed vaccine against a human cancer. The new yeast recombinant hepatitis B vaccine

(Hilleman 1996a, b; McAleer et la. 1984a) was developed and licensed by 1986. This was the first and is still the only licensed recombinant vaccine. A vaccine that employed purified hepatitis B surface antigen secreted from carrier Alexander hepatocarcinoma cells (McAleer 1984b) in culture was developed in our laboratories. It was not pursued to licensure, however, because of the success with the yeast recombinant program. Present worldwide selective and universal immunization against hepatitis B will eliminate hepatitis B regionally and may eventually lead to worldwide eradication within a few generations (Hilleman 1996a, b). The significance of preventing hepatitis B infection is illustrated by the present world census of 350 million viral carriers and the inevitable death by necroinflammatory disease, cirrhosis, and hepatocarcinoma of about 75 million of these carriers (Hilleman 1996a, b).

The known universe of oncogenic viruses is small, as is the number of target vaccines worthy of pursuit. It is notable, however, that research to develop vaccines against papillomaviruses (Hines et al. 1995; Schiller and Lowy 1996; Tindle 1996), including DNA vaccine (Donnelly et al. 1996) and against (EBV (Gu et al. 1993; Morgan 1992; Rickinson et al. 1996), is currently being actively pursued. Early findings in human trials in China of EBV gp350 recombinant vaccine by Wolfe have shown protection against natural infection in a majority of vaccinees in a small study (Rickinson et al. 1996). Vaccines against hepatitis C will be very difficult to develop because of the multiple subtypes, antigenic hypervariability, and non-neutralizability (Prince 1994) of the agent. Vaccines against leukemia of cats (retrovirus) have been licensed in the United States for commercial distribution since 1985. Findings have been presented which indicate that certain vaccines may afford protection in some cats against natural challenge, as evidenced by a reduction in viremia, latency, transmissibility, and clinical disease (Legendre et al. 1991).

Therapeutic Vaccines Against Cancer and Against Persistent Viral Infections

Although immunotherapy of cancer has been pursued for more than a century (Table 6), and promise has been shown in experimental animal models, no vaccines have been developed that have been significantly beneficial clinically in humans. All this might change as a result of the application of the latest concepts and technologies in molecular biology and specific immune responses. Present information relating to cancer vaccines and to clinical trials is overwhelming in volume and complexity, reflecting the ingenuity and energy of those who are pursuing them (Baltz 1995; Boon and van der Bruggen 1996; Celis et al. 1995; Disis and Cheever 1996; Durrant and Spendlove 1996; Hilleman 1992b, 1993; Irvine and Restifo 1995; Kabrin and Kwak 1994; Lewis and Houghton 1995; Linehan et al. 1996; Ragupathi 1996; Schlag et al. 1994; Slingluff 1996; Tuttle 1996).

It is important that specific tumor-associated antigens exist in individual patients and sometimes between patients, as exemplified by antigens in mela-

Table 6. Therapeutic vaccines against cancer and persistent viral infections

No licensed therapeutic vaccine in spite of decades of research
The venture is worthy of pursuit since:
Specific tumor cell antigens do exist (e.g., melanoma)
  Specific viral antigens are present in virus-induced tumors (e.g., hepatitis B)
Success in developing therapeutic cancer vaccines relies mainly on:
  Identification of truly unique antigens
  Presentation of antigen fragments by professional antigen-presenting cells
  Induction of a cell-mediated immune response (cytotoxic T cells)

noma (Dalgleish 1996; Kuhn and Hanke 1997; Robins and Kawakami 1996). Tumor target antigens may be mutant proteins, over-expressed normal antigens, antigens ordinarily expressed only in embryonic or neonatal life, or antigens in virus-induced cancer. The key to success for therapeutic vaccines is first, to identify those antigens that are truly unique and second, to present them to the immune system in a way in which they can be recognized and will elicit an effective cell-mediated immune response. Antigens carry immunologic determinants called epitopes, and it is hoped that simplified antigens bearing them can be made highly immunogenic or can be incorporated into recombinant vectors that will gain ready access to the cytoplasm of professional antigen-presenting cells.

Central to the elicitation of relevant cell-mediated immune responses is the presentation of appropriate antigen fragments in MHC receptors on the cell surface of professional antigen-presenting cells. The MHC receptors themselves are highly variable and conformationally selective for any of perhaps 100 different alleles. The HLA-A2 receptor is the most common of all the shared MHC alleles, and it is important, when possible, to engage this receptor to achieve broadest generic clinical application. The complex and convoluted processes for immunologic recognition and response are presented in simplified form in Figs. 3–5.

Somatic cells of the body, including cancer cells, conduct continuous sampling, fragmentation, and display of their internal substances in MHC class I receptors on the cell surface (Fig. 3). This presentation provides a signal for recognition and destruction, by complementary cytotoxic T lymphocytes, of cells that are seen as immunologically abnormal. Importantly, such somatic cell presentation does not activate naive T cells, because the former cells do not present the second signal needed for T cell activation. In fact, occupancy by antigen alone may suffice to render naive T cells of complementary immunologic specificity anergic.

Immune activation of T cells is achieved (Fig. 4) when professional antigen-presenting cells, such as bone marrow-derived mononuclear and dendritic cells, fragment exogenous and endogenous proteins and present them on their cell surface in MHC class I or II receptors. Most importantly, these professional cells also provide a necessary second or costimulatory signal ligand, such as B7-1 or B7-2, that engages the CD28 receptor on T cells needed to ac-

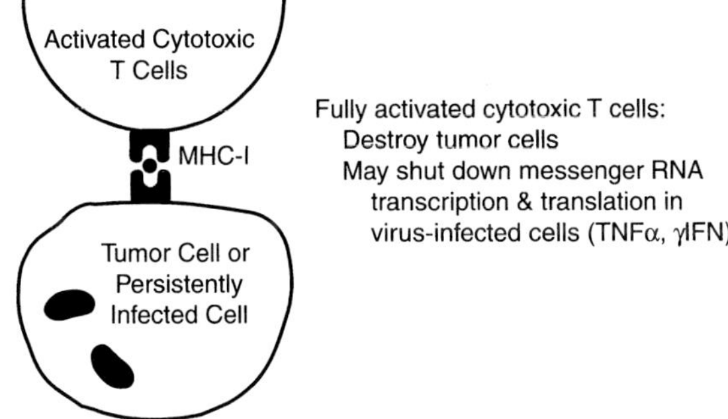

Fig. 3. Antigen presentation without costimulation

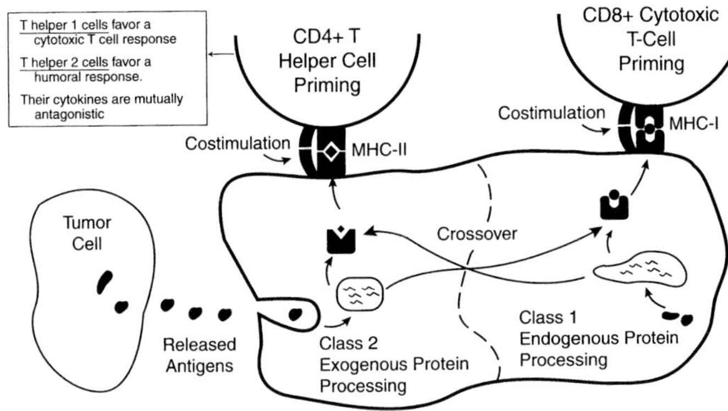

Fig. 4. Activation of CD^{4+} and CD^{8+} T cells by professional bone marrow-derived antigen-presenting cells. *MHC*, major histocompatibility complex

tivate them. Professional antigen-presenting cells present by two pathways: class I presentation activates $CD8^+$ cytotoxic T cells, while class II presentation activates $CD4^+$ T helper cells of subset 1 or 2, which in turn secrete cytokines that favor and facilitate either a type 1 cytotoxic T cell or a type 2 humoral antibody response. The respective collections of cytokines responsible for the two kinds of responses are antagonistic to each other.

Naive cytotoxic T cells are specifically activated by combined antigen and coreceptor presentations. Further differentiation and clonal expansion is aided by the elaboration of cytokines from the T helper cells of subgroup 1. Appropriately activated cytotoxic T lymphocytes (Fig. 5) seek out and destroy tumor cells and other cells displaying complementary abnormal antigens. They do this by means of cytolytic or apoptotic processes. Viral suppression in persistent viral infection can also be achieved by noncytolytic mechanisms. Chisari (1996, 1997) demonstrated that gamma interferon and tumor necrosis factor alpha may prevent transcription and translation of viral messenger and may even be curative in transgenic mice bearing the hepatitis B virus genome.

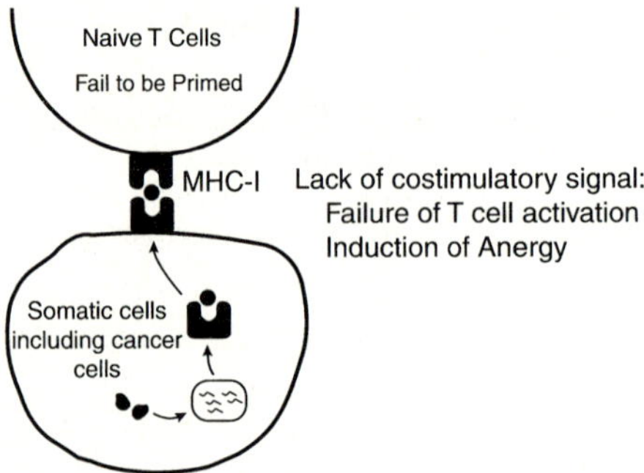

Fig. 5. Destructive damage of abnormal target cells by activated cytotoxic T cells. *MHC*, major histocompatibility; *TNF*, tumor necrosis factor; *IFN*, interferon

Table 7. Priming and facilitation of specific cancer immunotherapy. Priming: Identification and acquisition of tumor specific antigens. Autogenous vaccine – perhaps by cell culture. Sequenced common antigens that are recombinant expressed

Formulation/Facilitation	Examples
Adjuvants and immune potentiators	
Aluminum compounds (for antibody)	Aluminum hydroxide, phosphate
Water-oil emulsions	MF59, SAF-1, oil with nonionic block copolymers
Phospholipid/cholesterol/water complexes	Liposomes, cationic liposomes, cochleates
Saponin	QS21
Immunostimulants	Muramyl peptides, detoxified lipid A
Presentation systems	
ISCOMS	Quil A with antigen and cholesterol
Particulates	Virus-like particles, virosomes
Protein conjugation	With haptens or polysaccharides
Multiple antigen peptides	Organic scaffolds for peptides, virosomes
Targeted delivery and release	
Microencapsulation	Polylactide/glycolide polymers, glucans
Mucosal immunization	Cationic liposomes, cochleates, microencapsulation
Ligand-linked antigens	Cholera toxin B subunit, Fc receptor: antigen linked
Cytokines	
Types 1 and 2	IFN-γ, TNF-α, IL-2, -4, -5, -6, -10, -12
MHC combined with antigens	Dendritic cells pulsed with antigen fragments
Recombinant vectors	
Nonreplicating viruses	Canarypox; prime and boost
DNA vaccines	Mixtures of diversely encoded plasmid vectors

MHC, major histocompatibility complex; IL, interleukin; IFN, interferon; TNF, tumor necrosis factor.

As stated above, the requirements for specific immunotherapy of cancer (Table 7) by vaccination consist in the identification, acquisition, and presentation of appropriate tumor antigens. Such antigens may be formulated to stimulate recognition and to evoke an appropriate cytotoxic T cell response. Numerous technologies for facilitating immune responses already exist and consist of adjuvants and immune potentiators, presentation systems, targeted delivery and timed release mechanisms, cytokines, or pulsed or recombinant dendritic cells. Most promising are the recombinant viral vectors that express foreign proteins when delivered to the cytosol of target cells and, in particular, the recombinant DNA plasmid vaccines that may actively express reporter proteins for sustained periods of time. DNA vaccines do not need an envelope, which might be immunogenic, and may thus be repeatedly reused and may be given in diverse mixtures of plasmids that express antigens, receptors, coreceptors, cytokines, ligands, and the like. It is important that recombinant vector vaccines reside in a universe of potential diversity through selective mixing and can be made to transfect antigen-presenting cells, thereby gaining direct access to both the MHC I and MHC II pathways essential to cytotoxic T cell and T helper activation. Responses raised by vectors may be increased by boosting with the corresponding expressed proteins following vector priming.

Conclusion

In conclusion, efforts to prevent and cure spontaneously, environmentally, and virally-induced cancers are a worthy pursuit. In this endeavor, the two most important disciplines to follow are those that relate to the chemistry of the cell cycle and to basic immunology. Vaccinology is an applied discipline in immunology and will be guided by the latest concepts in immunology as they evolve.

References

Ambroziak JA, Blackburn DJ, Hernadier BG, Glogan RG, Gullett JH, McDonald AR, Lennette ET, Levy JA (1995) Herpes-like sequences in HIV-infected and uninfected Kaposi's sarcoma patients. Science 268:582–583

Arthur RR, Grossman SA, Ronnett BM, Bigner SH, Vogelstein B (1994) Lack of association of human polyomaviruses with human brain tumors. J Neurooncol 20:55–58

Baltz JK (1995) Vaccines in the treatment of cancer. Am J Health Syst Pharm 52:2574–2585

Boon T, van der Bruggen P (1996) Human tumor antigens recognized by T lymphocytes. J Exp Med 183:725–729

Buynak EB, Roehm RR, Tytell AA, Bertland AU, Lampson GP, Hilleman MR (1976) Vaccine against human hepatitis B. JAMA 235:2832–2834

Carallini A, Pagnani M, Viadana P, Silini E, Mottes M, Milanesi G, Gerna G, Vettor R, Trapella G, Silvani V, Gaist G, Barbanti-Brodano G (1987) Association of BK virus with human brain tumors and tumors of pancreatic islets. Int J Cancer 39:60–67

Celis E, Sette A, Grey HM (1995) Epitope selection and development of peptide based vaccines to treat cancer. Semin Cancer Biol 6:329–336

Chisari FV (1996) Hepatitis B virus transgenic mice: models of viral immunobiology and pathogenesis. Curr Top Microbiol Immunol 206:149–173

Chisari FV (1997) Cytotoxic T cells and viral hepatitis. J Clin Invest 99:1472–1477

Clurman BE, Roberts JM (1995) Cell cycle and cancer. J Natl Cancer Inst 87:1499–1501

Coggin JH, Larson VM, Hilleman MR (1967) Prevention of SV$_{40}$ virus tumorigenesis by irradiated, disrupted and iododeoxyuridine treated tumor cell antigens. Proc Soc Exp Biol Med 124:774–784

Culotta E, Koshland, DE Jr (1994) DNA repair works its way to the top. Science 266:1926–1929

Dalgleish A (1996) The case for therapeutic vaccines. Melanoma Res 6:5–10

Darcel C (1994) Reflections on viruses and cancer. Vet Res Communications 18:43–61

Disis ML, Cheever MA (1996) Oncogenic proteins as tumor antigens. Curr Opin Immunol 8:637–642

Donnelly JJ, Martinez D, Jansen KV, Ellis RW, Montgomery DL, Liu M (1996) Protection against papillomavirus with a polynucleotide vaccine. J Infect Dis 713:314–320

Draetta G, Pagano M (1996) Cell cycle control and cancer. Annu Rep Med Chem 31:241–248

Durrant LG, Spendlove I (1996) Cancer vaccines. Q J Med 89:645–651

Gallo RC (1995) Human retroviruses in the second decade: a personal perspective. Nature [Medicine] 1:753–759

Genta RM, Anti M, Gasbarrini G (1997) Summary report: malignancies. Eur J Gastroenterol Hepatol 9:621–623

Girardi AJ, Sweet BH, Slotnick BV, Hilleman MR (1962) Development of tumors in hamsters inoculated in the neonatal period with vacuolating virus, SV_{40}. Proc Soc Exp Biol Med 109:649–660

Girardi AJ, Hilleman MR, Zwickey RE (1964) Tests in hamsters for oncogenic quality of ordinary viruses including adenovirus type 7. Proc Soc Exp Biol Med 115:1141–1150

Goldner H, Girardi AJ, Larson VM, Hilleman MR (1964) Interruption of SV_{40} virus tumorigenesis using irradiated homologous tumor antigen. Proc Soc Exp Biol Med 117:851–857

Gu S-Y, Huang T-M, Ruan L, Miao Y-H, Lu H, Chu C-M, Motz M, Wolf H (1993) On the first EBV vaccine trial in humans using recombinant vaccinia virus expressing the major membrane antigen. In: Tursz T, Pagano JS, Ablashi DV, de Thé G, Lenoir G, Pearson GR (eds) The Epstein Barr virus and associated diseases. Libby, London, pp 579–584 (Colloque INSERM, vol 225)

Guinn B-A, Mills KI (1997) p53 mutations, methylation and genomic instability in the progression of chronic myeloid leukaemia. Leuk Lymphoma 26:211–226

Haines DS (1997) The mdm2 proto-oncogene. Leuk Lymphoma 26:227–238

Hall PA (1996) p53 – integrating the complexity. J Pathol 180:1–5

Hanawalt PD (1995) DNA repair comes of age. Mut Res 336:101–113

Hartwell LH, Kastan MB (1994) Cell cycle control and cancer. Science 266:1821–1828

Herwig S, Strauss M (1997) The retinoblastoma protein: a master regulator of cell cycle, differentiation and apoptosis. Eur J Biochem 246:581–601

Hildt E, Hofschneider PH, Urban S (1996) The role of hepatitis B virus (HBV) in the development of hepatocellular carcinoma. Semin Virol 7:333–347

Hilleman MR (1972) Marek's disease vaccine. Its implication in biology and medicine. Avian Dis 16:191–199

Hilleman MR (1974a) Prospects for vaccines against cancer. In: Kurstak E, Maramorosch K (eds) Viruses, evolution, and cancer. Academic, New York, pp 549–560

Hilleman MR (1974b) Human cancer virus vaccines and the pursuit of the practical. Cancer 34:1439–1445

Hilleman MR (1984) Immunologic prevention of human hepatitis. Perspect Biol Med 27:543–557

Hilleman MR (1992a) Plasma-derived hepatitis B vaccine: a breakthrough in preventive medicine. In: Ellis RW (ed) Hepatitis B vaccines in clinical practice. Dekker, New York, pp 17–39

Hilleman MR (1992b) Historical and contemporary perspectives in vaccine developments: from the vantage of cancer. Prog Med Virol 39:1–18

Hilleman MR (1993) The promise and the reality of viral vaccines against cancer. Ann N Y Acad Sci 690:6–18

Hilleman MR (1996a) Three decades of hepatitis vaccinology in historic perspective. A paradigm of successful pursuits. In: Plotkin S, Bantini B (eds) Vaccinia, vaccination and vaccinology: Jenner, Pasteur and their successors. Elsevier, Paris, pp 199–209

Hilleman MR (1996b) Immunology, vaccinology, and pathogenesis of hepatitis B. In: Koprowski H, Olstone, MBS (eds) Microbe hunters: then and now. Medi-Ed Bloomington, IL, pp 221–233

Hilleman MR, Werner JH (1954) Recovery of new agent from patients with acute respiratory illness. Proc Soc Exp Biol Med 85:183–188

Hilleman MR, Stallones RA, Gauld RL, Warfield MS, Anderson SA (1956) Prevention of acute respiratory illness in recruits by adenovirus (RI-APC-ARD) vaccine. Proc Soc Exp Biol Med 92:377–383

Hilleman MR, Bertland AU, Buynak EB, Lampson GP, McAleer WJ, McLean AA, Roehm RR, Tytell AA (1978) Clinical and laboratory studies of HBsAg vaccine. In: Vyas GN, Cohen SN, Schmid R (eds) Viral hepatitis. Franklin Institute, Philadelphia, pp 525–537

Hilleman MR, Buynak EB, McAleer WJ, McLean AA, Provost PJ, Tytell AA (1982) Hepatitis A and hepatitis B vaccines. In: Szmuness W, Alter H, Maynard J (eds) Viral hepatitis. 1981 International Symposium. Franklin Institute, Philadelphia, pp 385–397

Hines JF, Ghim S-J, Schlegel R, Jenson AB (1995) Prospects for a vaccine against human papillomavirus. Obstet Gynecol 85:860–866

Holt SE, Shay JW, Wright WE (1996) Refining the telomere-telomerase hypothesis of aging and cancer. Nature [Biotechnol] 14:836–839

Hoppe-Seyler F, Butz K (1995) Molecular mechanisms of virus-induced carcinogenesis: the interaction of viral factors with cellular tumor suppressor proteins. J Mol Med 73:529–538

Hunter T (1997) Oncoprotein networks. Cell 88:333–346

Irvine KR, Restifo NP (1995) The next wave of recombinant and synthetic anticancer vaccines. Semin Cancer Biol 6:337–347

Jacks T, Weinberg RA (1996) Cell-cycle control and its watchman. Nature 381:643–644

Jansen-Dürr P (1996) Viral oncogenesis and cell cycle control. Virus Res 42:187–191

Jones C (1995) Cervical cancer: is herpes simplex virus type II a cofactor? Clin Microbiol Rev 8:549–556

Kaplan MH (1993) Human retroviruses and neoplastic disease. Clin Infect Dis 17:S400–S406

Kempf W, Adams V (1996) Viruses in the pathogenesis of Kaposi's sarcoma – a review. Biochem Mol Med 58:1–12

Kew MC (1994) Hepatitis C virus and hepatocellular carcinoma. FEMS Microbiol Rev 14:211–220

Kobrin CB, Kwak LW (1994) The current status of human cancer vaccines. Exp Opin Invest Drugs 3:1241–1253

Kuhn CA, Hanke CW (1997) Current status of melanoma vaccines. Dermatol Surg 23:649–655

Laimins LA (1996) Human papillomaviruses target differentiating epithelia for virion production and malignant conversion. Semin Virol 7:305–313

Larson VM, Raupp WG, Hilleman MR (1967) Prevention of SV_{40} tumorigenesis in newborn hamsters by maternal immunization. Proc Soc Exp Biol Med 126:674–677

Legendre AM, Hawks DM, Sebring R, Rohrbach B, Chavez L, Chu H-J, Acree WM (1991) Comparison of the efficacy of three commercial feline leukemia virus vaccines in a natural challenge exposure. J Am Vet Med Assoc 199:1456–1462

Levine AJ (1994) The origins of the small DNA tumor viruses. Adv Cancer Res 65:141–168

Levine AJ (1997) p53, the cellular gatekeeper for growth and division. Cell 88:323–331

Lewis JJ, Houghton AN (1995) Definition of tumor antigens suitable for vaccine construction. Semin Cancer Biol 6:321–327

Linehan DC, Goedegebuure PS, Eberlein TJ (1996) Vaccine therapy for cancer. Ann Surg Oncol 3:219–228

McAleer WJ, Buynak EB, Maigetter RZ, Wampler DE, Miller WJ, Hilleman MR (1984a) Human hepatitis B vaccine from recombinant yeast. Nature 307:178–180

McAleer WJ, Markus HZ, Wampler DE, Buynak EB, Miller WJ, Welbel RE, McLean AA, Hilleman MR (1984b) Vaccine against human hepatitis B virus prepared from antigen derived from human hepatoma cells in culture. Proc Soc Exp Biol Med 175:314–319

Morgan AJ (1992) Epstein-Barr virus vaccines. Vaccine 10:563–570

O'Connor F, Buckley M, O'Morain C (1996) Helicobacter pylori: the cancer link. J R Soc Med 89:674–678

Piette J, Neel H, Maréchal V (1997) Mdm2: keeping p53 under control. Oncogene 15:1001–1010

Pines J (1994) The cell cycle kinases. Semin Cancer Biol 5:305–313

Prince AM (1994) Challenges for development of hepatitis C virus vaccines. FEMS Microbiol Rev 14:273–278

Raab-Traub N (1996) Pathogenesis of Epstein-Barr virus and its associated malignancies. Semin Virol 7:315–323

Ragupathi G (1996) Carbohydrate antigens as targets for active specific immunotherapy. Canc Immunol Immunother 43:152–157

Rickinson AB, Kieff E (1996) Epstein-Barr virus. In: Fields BN, Knipe DM, Howley PM et al (eds) Fields virology, 3 edn. Lippincott-Raven, Philadelphia, pp 2397–2446

Robbins PF, Kawakami Y (1996) Human tumor antigens recognized by T cells. Curr Opin Immunol 8:628–636

Rowe WP, Huebner RJ, Gilmore LK, Parrott RH, Ward TG (1953) Isolation of a cytopathogenic agent from human adenoids undergoing spontaneous degeneration in tissue culture. Proc Soc Exp Biol Med 84:570–573

Schiller JT, Lowy DR (1996) Papillomavirus-like particles and HPV vaccine development. Semin Cancer Biol 7:373–382

Schlag PM, Milleck J, Liebrich W (1994) Progress with tumour vaccines. Clin Immunother 2:23–31

Shenk T (1996) Adenoviridae: the viruses and their replication. In: Fields BN, Knipe DM, Howley PM et al (eds) Fields virology. 3 edn. Lippincott-Raven, Philadelphia, pp 2111–2148

Sherbet GV, Lakshmi MS (eds) (1997a) The genetics of cancer. Genes associated with cancer invasion, metastasis and cell proliferation. Academic, San Diego, pp 27–75

Sherbet GV, Lakshmi MS (eds) (1997b) The genetics of cancer. Genes associated with cancer invasion, metastasis and cell proliferation. Academic, San Diego, pp 144–154

Sherbet GV, Lakshmi MS (eds) (1997c) The genetics of cancer. Genes associated with cancer invasion, metastasis and cell proliferation. Academic, San Diego, pp 171–182

Slingluff CL Jr (1996) Tumor antigens and tumor vaccines: peptides as immunogens. Semin Surg Oncol 12:446–453

Sweet BH, Hilleman MR (1960a) Detection of a "non-detectable" simian virus (vacuolating agent) present in rhesus and cynomolgus monkey-kidney cell culture material. A preliminary report. 2nd International Conference on Live Poliovirus Vaccines, Pan American Health Organization and the World Health Organization, June 6–7, Washington, DC, pp 79–85

Sweet BH, Hilleman MR (1960b) The vacuolating virus. S.V. 40. Proc Soc Exp Biol Med 105:420–427

Tindle RW (1996) Human papillomavirus vaccines for cervical cancer. Curr Opin Immunol 8:643–650

Tuttle TM (1996) Oncogene products represent potential targets of tumor vaccines. Cancer Immunol Immunother 43:135–141

Vousden KH, Farrell PJ (1994) Viruses and human cancer. Br Med Bull 50:560–581

Wang JYJ, Knudsen ES, Welch PJ (1994) The retinoblastoma tumor suppressor protein. Adv Cancer Res 64:25–85

Witter RL (1971) Marek's disease research – history and perspectives. Poultry Sci 50:333–342

Wynford-Thomas D (1996) Telomeres, p53 and cellular senescence. Oncology Res 8:387–398

Zur Hausen H (1991) Viruses in human cancers. Science 254:1167–1173

Zur Hausen H (1996a) Foundations in cancer research. Viruses in human tumors – reminiscences and perspectives. Adv Cancer Res 68:1–22

Zur Hausen H (1996b) Roots and perspectives of contemporary papillomavirus research. J Cancer Res Clin Oncol 122:3–13

Recent Results in Cancer Research
Volumes published since Vol. 146

Printing and binding: Druckerei Triltsch, Würzburg